T0229057

MRI of Cartilage

Guest Editor

RICHARD KIJOWSKI, MD

MAGNETIC RESONANCE IMAGING CLINICS OF NORTH AMERICA

www.mri.theclinics.com

Consulting Editors
VIVIAN S. LEE, MD, PhD, MBA
LYNNE STEINBACH, MD
SURESH MUKHERJI, MD

May 2011 • Volume 19 • Number 2

SAUNDERS an imprint of ELSEVIER, Inc.

W.B. SAUNDERS COMPANY
A Division of Elsevier Inc.

1600 John F. Kennedy Boulevard • Suite 1800 • Philadelphia, Pennsylvania 19103-2899

http://www.theclinics.com

MRI CLINICS OF NORTH AMERICA Volume 19, Number 2
May 2011 ISSN 1064-9689, ISBN 13: 978-1-4557-0742-3

Editor: Barton Dudlick
Developmental Editor: Donald Mumford

© 2011 Elsevier Inc. All rights reserved.

This journal and the individual contributions contained in it are protected under copyright by Elsevier, and the following terms and conditions apply to their use:

Photocopying
Single photocopies of single articles may be made for personal use as allowed by national copyright laws. Permission of the Publisher and payment of a fee is required for all other photocopying, including multiple or systematic copying, copying for advertising or promotional purposes, resale, and all forms of document delivery. Special rates are available for educational institutions that wish to make photocopies for non-profit educational classroom use. For information on how to seek permission visit www.elsevier.com/permissions or call: (+44) 1865 843830 (UK)/ (+1) 215 239 3804 (USA).

Derivative Works
Subscribers may reproduce tables of contents or prepare lists of articles including abstracts for internal circulation within their institutions. Permission of the Publisher is required for resale or distribution outside the institution. Permission of the Publisher is required for all other derivative works, including compilations and translations (please consult www.elsevier.com/permissions).

Electronic Storage or Usage
Permission of the Publisher is required to store or use electronically any material contained in this journal, including any article or part of an article (please consult www.elsevier.com/permissions). Except as outlined above, no part of this publication may be reproduced, stored in a retrieval system or transmitted in any form or by any means, electronic, mechanical, photocopying, recording or otherwise, without prior written permission of the Publisher.

Notice
No responsibility is assumed by the Publisher for any injury and/or damage to persons or property as a matter of products liability, negligence or otherwise, or from any use or operation of any methods, products, instructions or ideas contained in the material herein. Because of rapid advances in the medical sciences, in particular, independent verification of diagnoses and drug dosages should be made.

Although all advertising material is expected to conform to ethical (medical) standards, inclusion in this publication does not constitute a guarantee or endorsement of the quality or value of such product or of the claims made of it by its manufacturer.

Magnetic Resonance Imaging Clinics of North America (ISSN 1064-9689) is published quarterly by Elsevier Inc., 360 Park Avenue South, New York, NY 10010-1710. Months of issue are February, May, August, and November. Business and Editorial Offices: 1600 John F. Kennedy Blvd., Ste. 1800, Philadelphia, PA 19103-2899. Customer Service Office: 3251 Riverport Lane, Maryland Heights, MO 63043. Periodicals postage paid at New York, NY and additional mailing offices. Subscription prices are $309.00 per year (domestic individuals), $501.00 per year (domestic institutions), $158.00 per year (domestic students/residents), $345.00 per year (Canadian individuals), $628.00 per year (Canadian institutions), $448.00 per year (international individuals), $628.00 per year (international institutions), and $228.00 per year (international and Canadian students/residents). International air speed delivery is included in all *Clinics* subscription prices. All prices are subject to change without notice. **POSTMASTER:** Send address changes to *Magnetic Resonance Imaging Clinics*, Elsevier Health Sciences Division, Subscription Customer Service, 3251 Riverport Lane, Maryland Heights, MO 63043. Customer Service (orders, claims, online, change of address): Elsevier Health Sciences Division, Subscription Customer Service, 3251 Riverport Lane, Maryland Heights, MO 63043. Tel:1-800-654-2452 (U.S. and Canada); 314-447-8871 (outside U.S. and Canada). Fax: 314-447-8029. E-mail: journalscustomerservice-usa@elsevier.com (for print support); journalsonlinesupport-usa@elsevier.com (for online support).

Reprints. For copies of 100 or more of articles in this publication, please contact the Commercial Reprints Department, Elsevier Inc., 360 Park Avenue South, New York, NY 10010-1710. Tel.: 212-633-3812; Fax: 212-462-1935; E-mail: reprints@elsevier.com.

Magnetic Resonance Imaging Clinics of North America is covered in the *RSNA Index of Imaging Literature, MEDLINE/PubMed (Index Medicus),* and *EMBASE/Excerpta Medica.*

Printed and bound by CPI Group (UK) Ltd, Croydon, CR0 4YY

Transferred to Digital Print 2011

GOAL STATEMENT

The goal of *Magnetic Resonance Imaging Clinics of North America* is to keep practicing physicians up to date with current clinical practice by providing timely articles reviewing the state of the art in patient care.

ACCREDITATION

The *Magnetic Resonance Imaging Clinics of North America* is planned and implemented in accordance with the Essential Areas and Policies of the Accreditation Council for Continuing Medical Education (ACCME) through the joint sponsorship of the University of Virginia School of Medicine and Elsevier. The University of Virginia School of Medicine is accredited by the ACCME to provide continuing medical education for physicians.

The University of Virginia School of Medicine designates this educational activity for a maximum of 15 *AMA PRA Category 1 Credits*™ for each issue, 60 credits per year. Physicians should only claim credit commensurate with the extent of their participation in the activity.

The American Medical Association has determined that physicians not licensed in the US who participate in this CME activity are eligible for a maximum of 15 *AMA PRA Category 1 Credits*™ for each issue, 60 credits per year.

Credit can be earned by reading the text material, taking the CME examination online at http://www.theclinics.com/home/cme, and completing the evaluation. After taking the test, you will be required to review any and all incorrect answers. Following completion of the test and evaluation, your credit will be awarded and you may print your certificate.

FACULTY DISCLOSURE/CONFLICT OF INTEREST

The University of Virginia School of Medicine, as an ACCME accredited provider, endorses and strives to comply with the Accreditation Council for Continuing Medical Education (ACCME) Standards of Commercial Support, Commonwealth of Virginia statutes, University of Virginia policies and procedures, and associated federal and private regulations and guidelines on the need for disclosure and monitoring of proprietary and financial interests that may affect the scientific integrity and balance of content delivered in continuing medical education activities under our auspices.

The University of Virginia School of Medicine requires that all CME activities accredited through this institution be developed independently and be scientifically rigorous, balanced and objective in the presentation/discussion of its content, theories and practices.

All authors/editors participating in an accredited CME activity are expected to disclose to the readers relevant financial relationships with commercial entities occurring within the past 12 months (such as grants or research support, employee, consultant, stock holder, member of speakers bureau, etc.). The University of Virginia School of Medicine will employ appropriate mechanisms to resolve potential conflicts of interest to maintain the standards of fair and balanced education to the reader. Questions about specific strategies can be directed to the Office of Continuing Medical Education, University of Virginia School of Medicine, Charlottesville, Virginia.

The faculty and staff of the University of Virginia Office of Continuing Medical Education have no financial affiliations to disclose.

The authors/editors listed below have identified no professional or financial affiliations for themselves or their spouse/partner:
Donna G. Blankenbaker, MD; Gregory Chang, MD; Jung-Ah Choi, MD, PhD; Derik Davis, MD; Eduard de Lange, MD (Test Author); Jennifer L. Demertzis, MD; Barton Dudlick, (Acquisitions Editor); Michael Forney, MD; Douglas W. Goodwin, MD; Vivian S. Lee, MD, PhD, MBA (Consulting Editor); Guillaume Madelin, PhD; Michael Recht, MD; Ravinder Regatte, PhD; Humberto G. Rosas, MD; David A. Rubin, MD; Colin D. Strickland, MD; Naveen Subhas, MD; Michael J. Tuite, MD; Eric A. Walker, MD; and Carl S. Winalski, MD.

The authors/editors listed below identified the following professional or financial affiliations for themselves or their spouse/partner:
Michel D. Crema, MD is a shareholder with Boston Imaging Core Lab (BICL).
Brian Donley, MD is a consultant, stockholder, and a patent holder with Extremity Medical, is a consultant for Tenstegrity.
Garry E. Gold, MD is an industry funded research/investigator for GE Healthcare, and is a consultant for Arthrocare, Zimmer, and ICON Medica.
Ali Guermazi, MD owns stock in Synarc and BICL; is an industry funded research/investigator for GE Healthcare; and is a consultant for Novartis, Genzyme, Stryker, Merck, and Serono.
Richard Kijowski, MD (Guest Editor) is a consultant for Flex Biomedical, Inc.
Timothy J. Mosher, MD owns stock in Johnson and Johnson, and is a consultant for Kensey Nash Corporation.
Suresh K. Mukheri, MD (Consulting Editor) is a consultant for Philips.
Frank W. Roemer, MD owns stock in Boston Imaging Core Lab (BICL) LLC.
Orrin Sherman, MD is a consultant for Knee Creations.
Lynne Steinbach, MD (Consulting Editor) is a consultant for Synarc and Pfizer, Inc.

Disclosure of Discussion of non-FDA approved uses for pharmaceutical products and/or medical devices:
The University of Virginia School of Medicine, as an ACCME provider, requires that all faculty presenters identify and disclose any "off label" uses for pharmaceutical and medical device products. The University of Virginia School of Medicine recommends that each physician fully review all the available data on new products or procedures prior to instituting them with patients.

TO ENROLL

To enroll in the Magnetic Resonance Imaging Clinics of North America Continuing Medical Education program, call customer service at 1-800-654-2452 or visit us online at www.theclinics.com/home/cme. The CME program is available to subscribers for an additional fee of $196.00.

Contributors

CONSULTING EDITORS

VIVIAN S. LEE, MD, PhD, MBA
Professor of Radiology, Physiology, and
Neurosciences; Vice-Dean for Science; and
Senior Vice-President and Chief Scientific
Officer at New York University Langone
Medical Center, New York, New York

LYNNE STEINBACH, MD
Professor of Clinical Radiology and
Orthopaedic Surgery at the University of
California San Francisco, San Francisco,
California

SURESH MUKHERJI, MD
Professor and Chief of Neuroradiology and
Head and Neck Radiology; Professor of
Radiology, Otolaryngology Head Neck
Surgery, Radiation Oncology, Periodontics and
Oral Medicine, University of Michigan Health
System, Ann Arbor, Michigan

GUEST EDITOR

RICHARD KIJOWSKI, MD
Associate Professor, Department of Radiology,
University of Wisconsin School of Medicine
and Public Health, Madison, Wisconsin

AUTHORS

DONNA G. BLANKENBAKER, MD
Associate Professor of Radiology, Department of
Radiology, University of Wisconsin School of
Medicine and Public Health, Madison, Wisconsin

GREGORY CHANG, MD
Quantitative Multinuclear Musculoskeletal
Imaging Group (QMMIG), Center for
Biomedical Imaging, Department of Radiology,
New York University Langone Medical Center,
New York, New York

JUNG-AH CHOI, MD, PhD
Department of Radiology, Stanford University,
Stanford, California; Department of Radiology,
Seoul National University Bundang Hospital,
Seoul National University College of Medicine,
Bundang-gu, Seongnam, Gyeongido, Seoul,
South Korea

MICHEL D. CREMA, MD
Adjunct Assistant Professor of Radiology,
Department of Radiology, Quantitative
Imaging Center, Boston University School
of Medicine; Boston Imaging Core Lab (BICL),
Boston, Massachusetts; Institute of
Diagnostic Imaging (IDI); Division of
Radiology, Department of Internal
Medicine, Ribeirão Preto School of
Medicine, University of São Paulo (USP),
Ribeirão Preto, São Paulo, Brazil

DERIK DAVIS, MD
Assistant Professor of Radiology,
Department Diagnostic Radiology and Nuclear
Medicine, University of Maryland Medical
Center, Baltimore, Maryland

JENNIFER L. DEMERTZIS, MD
Assistant Professor of Radiology, Division of Musculoskeletal Radiology, Mallinckrodt Institute of Radiology, St Louis, Missouri

BRIAN DONLEY, MD
Director, Center of Foot and Ankle Surgery, Orthopaedic and Rheumatologic Institute, Cleveland Clinic, Cleveland, Ohio

MICHAEL FORNEY, MD
Imaging Institute, Cleveland Clinic, Cleveland, Ohio

GARRY E. GOLD, MD
Assistant Professor, Departments of Radiology, Bioengineering, and Orthopedic Surgery, Stanford University, Stanford, California

DOUGLAS W. GOODWIN, MD
Associate Professor of Radiology and Orthopaedic Surgery; Director of Musculoskeletal Imaging, Department of Radiology, Dartmouth-Hitchcock Medical Center, Dartmouth Medical School, Lebanon, New Hampshire

ALI GUERMAZI, MD
Professor of Radiology, Department of Radiology, Quantitative Imaging Center, Boston University School of Medicine; Boston Imaging Core Lab (BICL), Boston, Massachusetts

RICHARD KIJOWSKI, MD
Associate Professor, Department of Radiology, University of Wisconsin School of Medicine and Public Health, Madison, Wisconsin

GUILLAUME MADELIN, PhD
Quantitative Multinuclear Musculoskeletal Imaging Group (QMMIG), Center for Biomedical Imaging, Department of Radiology, New York University Langone Medical Center, New York, New York

TIMOTHY J. MOSHER, MD
Professor of Radiology and Orthopaedic Surgery, Department of Radiology, Penn State University College of Medicine, Penn State Milton S. Hershey Medical Center, Hershey, Pennsylvania

MICHAEL RECHT, MD
Quantitative Multinuclear Musculoskeletal Imaging Group (QMMIG), Center for Biomedical Imaging, Department of Radiology, New York University Langone Medical Center, New York, New York

RAVINDER REGATTE, PhD
Quantitative Multinuclear Musculoskeletal Imaging Group (QMMIG), Center for Biomedical Imaging, Department of Radiology, New York University Langone Medical Center, New York, New York

FRANK W. ROEMER, MD
Adjunct Associate Professor of Radiology, Department of Radiology, Quantitative Imaging Center, Boston University School of Medicine; Boston Imaging Core Lab (BICL), Boston, Massachusetts; Department of Radiology, Klinikum Augsburg, Augsburg, Germany

HUMBERTO G. ROSAS, MD
Assistant Professor of Radiology, Musculoskeletal Imaging, University of Wisconsin School of Medicine and Public Health, University of Wisconsin Hospital and Clinics, Madison, Wisconsin

DAVID A. RUBIN, MD
Professor of Radiology; Section Chief of the Division of Musculoskeletal Radiology, Mallinckrodt Institute of Radiology, St Louis, Missouri

ORRIN SHERMAN, MD
Associate Professor, Department of Orthopedic Surgery, New York University Langone Medical Center, New York, New York

COLIN D. STRICKLAND, MD
Assistant Professor, Department of Radiology, University of Colorado Denver, Aurora, Colorado

NAVEEN SUBHAS, MD
Staff Radiologist, Imaging Institute, Cleveland Clinic, Cleveland, Ohio

MICHAEL J. TUITE, MD
Professor of Radiology, Department of
Radiology; Section Chief, Musculoskeletal
Radiology, University of Wisconsin School of
Medicine and Public Health, Madison,
Wisconsin

ERIC A. WALKER, MD
Assistant Professor of Radiology, Department
of Radiology, Penn State University College of

Medicine, Penn State Milton S. Hershey
Medical Center, Hershey, Pennsylvania;
Departments of Radiology and Nuclear
Medicine, Uniformed Services University
of the Health Sciences, Bethesda, Maryland

CARL S. WINALSKI, MD
Imaging Institute, Cleveland Clinic,
Cleveland, Ohio

Contents

Preface: MRI of Cartilage xiii

Richard Kijowski

MRI Appearance of Normal Articular Cartilage 215

Douglas W. Goodwin

At each joint, the extracellular matrix of cartilage is arranged in a complex and characteristic organization that is specific for that joint. This structure exerts a strong influence on the appearance of magnetic resonance (MR) images through orientation-related alterations in T2 decay. As a result, the MR appearance of cartilage at each joint is predictable and specific for that joint. The diagnostic utility of MR imaging for evaluating cartilage is enhanced when the acquisition and review of the images is informed by an understanding of this relationship between normal structure and the MR appearance of cartilage.

Morphologic Imaging of Articular Cartilage 229

Colin D. Strickland and Richard Kijowski

Magnetic resonance (MR) imaging plays an integral role in the assessment of articular cartilage. This article discusses the role of MR imaging in the evaluation of articular cartilage, the appearance of cartilage lesions on MR imaging, and the currently available MR imaging techniques for evaluating cartilage morphology. A limitation of currently available sequences is their inability to consistently detect superficial degenerative and posttraumatic cartilage lesions that may progress to more advanced osteoarthritis. In the future, improved image quality may allow for better evaluation of articular cartilage and earlier detection of cartilage lesions.

MR Imaging of Articular Cartilage Physiology 249

Jung-Ah Choi and Garry E.Gold

The newer magnetic resonance (MR) imaging methods can give insights into the initiation, progression, and eventual treatment of osteoarthritis. Sodium imaging is specific for changes in proteoglycan (PG) content without the need for an exogenous contrast agent. T1ρ imaging is sensitive to early PG depletion. Delayed gadolinium-enhanced MR imaging has high resolution and sensitivity. T2 mapping is straightforward and is sensitive to changes in collagen and water content. Ultrashort echo time MR imaging examines the osteochondral junction. Magnetization transfer provides improved contrast between cartilage and fluid. Diffusion-weighted imaging may be a valuable tool in postoperative imaging.

Rapidly Progressive Osteoarthritis: Biomechanical Considerations 283

Eric A. Walker, Derik Davis, and Timothy J. Mosher

An underlying hypothesis for rapid cartilage loss in patients with osteoarthritis (OA) is that perturbation from normal joint mechanics produces locally high biomechanical strains that exceed the material properties of the tissue, leading to rapid destruction. Several imaging findings are associated with focally high biomechanical forces and thus are potential candidates for predictive biomarkers of rapid OA progression. This article focuses on 3 aspects of knee biomechanics that have potential magnetic resonance imaging correlates, and which may serve as prognostic biomarkers: knee malalignment, meniscal dysfunction, and injury of the osteochondral unit.

Magnetic Resonance Imaging in Knee Osteoarthritis Research: Semiquantitative and Compositional Assessment   **295**

Michel D. Crema, Frank W. Roemer, and Ali Guermazi

Semiquantitative assessment of the knee by expert magnetic resonance imaging readers is a powerful research tool for understanding the natural history of osteoarthritis (OA). Several reliable semiquantitative scoring systems have been applied to large observational cross-sectional and longitudinal epidemiologic studies and interventional clinical trials. Such evaluations have enabled understanding of the relevance of disease in structures within the knee joint to explain pain and progression of OA. Compositional imaging of cartilage has added to our ability to detect early degeneration before morphologic changes are present, which may help to prevent the permanent morphologic changes commonly seen in knee OA.

MR Imaging Assessment of Articular Cartilage Repair Procedures   **323**

Gregory Chang, Orrin Sherman, Guillaume Madelin, Michael Recht, and Ravinder Regatte

Because articular cartilage is avascular and has no intrinsic capacity to heal itself, physical damage to cartilage poses a serious clinical problem for orthopedic surgeons and rheumatologists. No medication exists to treat or reconstitute physical defects in articular cartilage, and pharmacotherapy is limited to pain control. Developments in the field of articular cartilage repair include microfracture, osteochondral autografting, osteochondral allografting, repair with synthetic resorbable plugs, and autologous chondrocyte implantation. MR imaging techniques have the potential to allow in vivo monitoring of the collagen and proteoglycan content of cartilage repair tissue and may provide useful additional metrics of cartilage repair tissue quality.

MR Imaging Assessment of Inflammatory, Crystalline-Induced, and Infectious Arthritides   **339**

Jennifer L. Demertzis and David A. Rubin

The role of magnetic resonance imaging in evaluating patients with inflammatory arthritides has evolved with the recent introduction of drugs capable of modifying disease activity and natural history. In conditions like rheumatoid arthritis, active synovitis and bone marrow inflammation precede and predict bone and cartilage erosion. These imaging findings identify patients who can be treated early and aggressively to prevent future morbidity. Similarly, in gout and other crystalline disorders, specific diagnosis aided by imaging may lead to earlier medical and surgical management. Infected joints need the most rapid identification to institute immediate therapy and prevent irreversible cartilage destruction.

MR Imaging of Early Hip Joint Degeneration   **365**

Donna G. Blankenbaker and Michael J. Tuite

MR imaging is one of the most commonly used imaging techniques to evaluate patients with hip pain. Intra-articular abnormalities of the hip joint are better assessed with recent advances in MR imaging technology, such as high-field strength scanners, improved coils, and more signal-to-noise ratio-efficient sequences. This article discusses the causes of early hip joint degeneration and the current use of morphologic and physiologic MR imaging techniques for evaluating the articular cartilage of the hip joint. The article also discusses the role of MR arthrography in clinical cartilage imaging.

MR Imaging of the Articular Cartilage of the Knee and Ankle   379

Michael Forney, Naveen Subhas, Brian Donley, and Carl S. Winalski

Cartilage abnormalities in the knee and ankle are a common source of pain and are often difficult to diagnose clinically or radiographically. MR imaging is a valuable tool for diagnosing and characterizing cartilage lesions of both the knee and ankle. An understanding of the appearance of cartilage, and an understanding of how and when to report cartilage injury in the knee and ankle based on current grading systems allows the radiologist to provide the most helpful reports to referring clinicians. This article presents the range of cartilage pathologies in the knee and ankle and provides clinically relevant guidelines.

The Current State of Imaging the Articular Cartilage of the Upper Extremity   407

Humberto G. Rosas and Michael J. Tuite

MR imaging has increasingly been used to image joints since its inception. Historically, there has been more emphasis on the evaluation of internal derangement rather than cartilaginous disease. This article reviews cartilaginous diseases of the upper extremity emphasizing those that can be assessed using current clinical MR imaging protocols and addresses the limitations of current imaging techniques in evaluating the articular cartilage of smaller joints. It also provides a brief overview of novel techniques that may be instituted in the future to improve the diagnostic performance of MR imaging in the evaluation of the articular cartilage of the upper extremity.

Index   425

Magnetic Resonance Imaging Clinics of North America

FORTHCOMING ISSUES

Normal MR Anatomy
Peter Liu, MD,
Guest Editor

MRI of the Newborn
Claudia Hillenbrand, PhD and
Thierry Huisman, MD,
Guest Editors

RECENT ISSUES

February 2011

Diffusion Imaging: From Head to Toe
L. Celso Hygino Cruz Jr, MD,
Guest Editor

November 2010

**Normal Variants and Pitfalls in
Musculoskeletal MRI**
William B. Morrison, MD and
Adam C. Zoga, MD,
Guest Editors

August 2010

MRI of the Liver
Alisha Qayyum, MD,
Guest Editor

RELATED INTEREST

Emergency Neuroradiology
Alexander J. Nemeth, MD, and Matthew T. Walker, MD, *Guest Editors*
Radiologic Clinics of North America, January 2011

THE CLINICS ARE NOW AVAILABLE ONLINE!

Access your subscription at:
www.theclinics.com

Preface
MRI of Cartilage

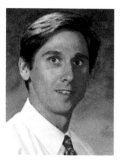

Richard Kijowski, MD
Guest Editor

Evaluation of articular cartilage plays an integral role in the assessment of the musculoskeletal system. Osteoarthritis is a highly prevalent chronic disease affecting millions of Americans and is one of the most common causes of disability in the United States. Many individuals in our country and worldwide also suffer from the debilitating effects of inflammatory, crystalline-induced, and infectious arthritis. New medical and surgical treatment options are now available to treat these individuals. However, noninvasive methods are needed to identify patients who can be treated early and aggressively to prevent future morbidity and to monitor the response to medical and surgical interventions.

Due to its high spatial resolution, multiplanar capability, and excellent tissue contrast, MRI is the noninvasive modality of choice for evaluating articular cartilage in both the clinical and the research setting. Cartilage imaging in the past has focused primarily on large joints such as the knee and hip. However, with recent development of high field strength scanners, three-dimensional cartilage-sensitive sequences, and multichannel coils, images of joints with higher spatial resolution, thinner slices, and greater tissue contrast can be obtained in clinically feasible scan times. With this new technology, MRI is now being used to evaluate the articular cartilage of the shoulder, elbow, ankle, and small joints of the upper and lower extremity.

This edition of *Magnetic Resonance Imaging Clinics of North America* gives a broad overview of the role of MRI in the evaluation of articular cartilage. Articles in this issue describe the role of histological structure on the MRI appearance of normal articular cartilage and discuss currently used MRI techniques to evaluate both cartilage morphology and cartilage physiology. Factors related to rapid progression of osteoarthritis and the use of MRI in evaluating patients in osteoarthritis research studies and following cartilage repair procedures are also revewed. Articles discussing the role of MRI in the evaluation of patients with inflammatory, crystalline-induced, and infectious arthritis and patients with various articular disorders of the hip, knee and ankle, and upper extremity are included.

I express my utmost appreciation to the authors who have spent much time and effort writing these articles. I was fortunate to receive the participation of many excellent musculoskeletal radiologists who are international experts in the area of cartilage imaging. I have enjoyed reading these articles and have learned a great deal about cartilage imaging in my role as guest editor. I have no doubt that the readers will do so as well.

Richard Kijowski, MD
Department of Radiology
University of Wisconsin School of Medicine
and Public Health
600 Highland Avenue
Madison, WI 53792, USA

E-mail address:
rkijowski@uwhealth.org

Magn Reson Imaging Clin N Am 19 (2011) xiii
doi:10.1016/j.mric.2011.03.001
1064-9689/11/$ – see front matter
© 2011 Elsevier Inc. All rights reserved.

MRI Appearance of Normal Articular Cartilage

Douglas W. Goodwin, MD

KEYWORDS

• Cartilage • Collagen • T2 • Matrix • Layers • MRI

The ability of magnetic resonance (MR) imaging to identify injuries of articular cartilage continues to improve because of the development of new sequences and advances in coil and magnet technology. As demonstrated in studies of knee MR imaging, the technique can be highly reliable if the images are of adequate quality and optimized for the visualization of the joint surface in question.[1–4] The interpretation must also be performed by a motivated and knowledgeable observer who is familiar with the appearance of normal articular cartilage on MR images.

CARTILAGE HISTOLOGY

Understanding the MR appearance of normal articular cartilage requires some appreciation of the underlying histology. Articular cartilage contains a relatively small number of chondrocytes.[5,6] The bulk of this tissue consists of an extracellular matrix composed of water, collagen, and proteoglycans. Large proteoglycans are trapped in a compressed configuration within a collagen network.[7] The negatively charged carboxyl and sulfate groups attached to the glycosaminoglycan side chains of proteoglycans create an osmotic gradient across the surface of cartilage that draws water into the tissue. Collagen provides the tensile resistance to the swelling pressure created by the trapped proteoglycans.[5] Collagen fibers also anchor cartilage to the underling bone.

This description of cartilage histology is a useful model for understanding how the stiffness of cartilage is created and maintained. It is, however, an obviously simplistic model. With any connective tissue there is relationship between the structure and physical qualities, and the extraordinary physical properties of articular cartilage suggest that the structure of cartilage is likely equally remarkable. In the normal state, cartilage is capable of resisting substantial deforming forces over the course of a lifetime while also providing a nearly frictionless articular surface. One would therefore reasonably predict that the structure of the cartilage extracellular matrix is arranged in a fashion that is optimal for providing the required biomechanical properties. Moreover, the considerable variation in the typical deforming forces experienced at different joint surfaces and different regions of a given joint surface suggests that the typical structure of cartilage is likely to be different depending on which joint or even what part of the joint surface is considered.

The results of biomechanical studies of articular cartilage are consistent with this premise that a complex and variable organization of the extracellular matrix must be present. The stresses experienced at different joint surfaces vary considerably from one to another. This variation between joint surfaces is matched by corresponding variations in the measured stiffness of articular cartilage.[8] As would be expected, the biomechanical properties of joint surfaces vary in accordance with variations in the physical demands placed on each joint. Moreover, variations in the stress experienced at different regions of a particular joint surface parallel regional variations in stiffness.[8,9] These biomechanical properties of cartilage

Department of Radiology, Dartmouth-Hitchcock Medical Center, Dartmouth Medical School, One Medical Center Drive, Lebanon, NH 03756, USA
E-mail address: douglas.goodwin@hitchcock.org

Magn Reson Imaging Clin N Am 19 (2011) 215–227
doi:10.1016/j.mric.2011.02.007
1064-9689/11/$ – see front matter © 2011 Elsevier Inc. All rights reserved.

indicate that the structure of cartilage must be joint specific and organized such that specific areas of cartilage are ideally organized to resist the deforming forces routinely experienced at a particular location. For example, one would predict that the structure of the cartilage of the tibial plateau should be different from the structure of cartilage at the radial head. Moreover, the periphery of the tibial plateau should have a structure that is different from that of the central region of the joint surface.

Despite the smooth featureless appearance on gross inspection, cartilage is not uniform. Water concentration, chondrocyte size, orientation, density, proteoglycan concentration, and collagen size all vary with depth across the thickness of cartilage.[5] These depth-dependent variations seen on histology studies are a further indication that the matrix of cartilage is structured. Unfortunately, traditional histology uses tissue sectioning, which cuts through the matrix. This approach compromises attempts to understand the 3-dimensional tissue organization of cartilage.

If instead of cutting through the extracellular matrix of cartilage, the tissue is studied by breaking it, causing it to cleave along planes of internal structure, an internal organization becomes more apparent. The earliest example of such a technique is the use of surface split lines. Hultkrantz, in 1896, punctured the surfaces of human articular cartilage with a round awl, creating linear defects in the surface of cartilage.[10] Using this method, the fibrous surface structure of the cartilage is in effect fractured or teased apart. As shown in **Fig. 1**, these split-line studies revealed characteristic patterns that were distinct and reproducible at each of the different joint surfaces he investigated. His study demonstrated that cartilage, at least at the surface, is organized in a joint-specific manner. Hultkrantz[10] speculated that this structure was ideally suited to meet the biomechanical demands typically faced by a given joint.

More recently, fracture sectioning of cartilage has proven to be a useful technique for directly visualizing internal matrix structure. This fracturing of cartilage is usually done after tissue freezing and in preparation for scanning electron microscopy. Low-magnification images of the fractured cartilage reveal a fibrous structure that radiates from the subchondral bone and curves through an arc of 90°, eventually curving into the plane of the joint surface. Higher-magnification images reveal that small collagen fibrils are organized into the much larger curving structure described by Jeffery and colleagues as parallel leaves of collagen and are also referred to as "fibers" by other investigators.[11–14] This macroscopic structure revealed in the curved fracture plane is even apparent on gross inspection of osteochondral fractures, as shown in **Fig. 2**. Jeffery and colleagues[14] also found that the plane of matrix curvature is perpendicular to the orientation of surface split lines. This link between the surface organization described by Hultkrantz[10] and the structure of cartilage at deeper levels strongly suggests that the organization or architecture of the extracellular matrix of cartilage is joint specific.

Further evidence that articular surfaces are joint specific and organized in a purposeful manner is apparent in the regional variation of cartilage structure.[13,15] The structure of tibial plateau, as described through the use of scanning electron microscopy by Clark and illustrated in **Fig. 3**, is an instructive example.[13] At the central region of the tibial plateau, matrix is organized into prominent columns that radiate in parallel arrays from the subchondral bone and curve to become parallel with the joint surface only at very superficial levels. In the periphery or submeniscal region, however, a more complex and oblique curvature is present. This regional and joint-specific variation in structure is consistent with the presence of a typical extracellular matrix architecture at each joint surface. It is reasonable to assume that the matrix architecture of a given joint surface is characteristic in much the same way that trabecular bone is organized in distinctive and predictable patterns. For example, one would predict that the structure of the cartilage of the femoral head is just as characteristic as the trabecular bone organization of the femoral neck.

MR Imaging of Cartilage

On most spin-echo and fast spin-echo images, the signal intensity of cartilage is not uniform. Typically, when a joint surface is imaged with the surface perpendicular to the main magnetic field (B_0), 3 different layers are apparent. As seen in **Fig. 4**, a low signal intensity deep or radial layer, a transitional layer of higher signal intensity, and a thin surface layer of lower signal intensity are present. These layers reflect the presence of depth-dependent variations in the T2 of cartilage.[16–18] These variations in T2 are displayed in **Fig. 5**. The boundaries between layers are not discreet or well defined and reflect gradual variation in T2. As a result, the relative thickness of each layer will change as the T2 weighting of the image is altered.

The second characteristic feature of MR images of cartilage is T2 anisotropy. Changes in tissue orientation relative to B_0 alter the appearance of

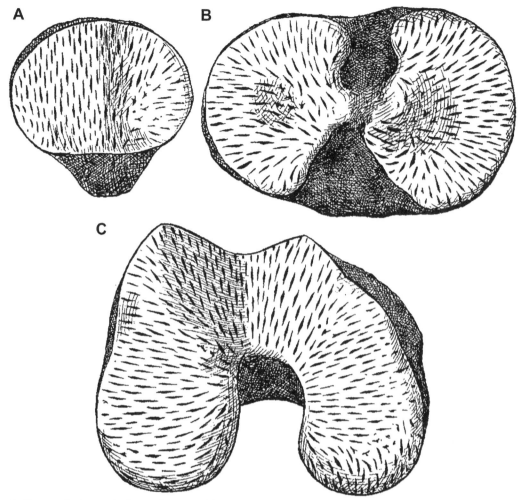

Fig. 1. By puncturing articular surfaces, Hultkrantz identified characteristic split-line patterns at each of the different joints he studied. The typical patterns of the patella (*A*), tibial plateau (*B*), and femoral condyles (*C*) are displayed. (*Adapted from* Hultkrantz W. Ueber die Spaltrichtungen der Gelenkknorpel. Verh Anat Ges 1898;12:248–56.)

the layers described previously. As demonstrated in **Figs. 4** and **5**, the appearance of layers and T2 measurements will change depending on tissue orientation.[16–19]

Both of the characteristic features of MR images of cartilage T2 decay—depth dependence and anisotropy—can be explained by the influence of the magic angle effect. Highly organized collagenous structures, such as articular cartilage, promote rapid T2 decay and low signal intensity. However, as the orientation of these fibrous structures is tilted away from the direction of B_0, prolongation of the T2 occurs. Maximal T2 prolongation is observed at approximately 55°, the so-called magic angle. It is important to remember that this T2 prolongation is continuous and any tilt away from parallel will influence the T2. Although the effect is maximal at the magic angle, the effect is

not limited to that one orientation. As a tissue curves, the T2 will lengthen and then shorten as it curves up to and past the 55° orientation.[20–22] The bell-shaped curve of the T2 profile displayed on high-resolution T2 maps of cartilage is precisely what one would predict given this arc-shaped internal structure.[18]

An interrelationship between cartilage structure and T2 has been shown on studies that correlate changes in signal intensity and T2 with the curvature of matrix structure as revealed by fracture sectioning, as displayed in **Fig. 5**.[15,23] This anisotropy of cartilage is apparent at all levels: there is no random or isotropic layer. It is frequently difficult to demonstrate T2 anisotropy within the transitional layer, as doing so requires aligning a curved structure with the magnetic field and avoiding the averaging of multiple orientations within a single voxel.

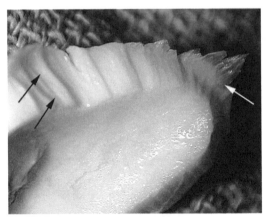

Fig. 2. Acute osteochondral fracture of the patella. The curved fracture plane (*white arrow*) and the internal columnar structure (*black arrows*) of cartilage are apparent on this acute fracture.

Because the spatial resolution of MR imaging is limited, especially in the slice-thickness direction, it is extremely difficult to avoid this volume averaging at any orientation, especially on images and maps with high in-plane resolution. The result is that the T2 usually remains relatively long in the transitional layer. This difficulty in demonstrating anisotropy, however, should not be considered proof that this region is isotropic, as orientation effects can be documented across the entire depth of cartilage.[15,23]

In addition to the well-described layers, there is an additional level of heterogeneity of cartilage signal intensity. On close inspection of the deepest layer of cartilage, vertically oriented striations caused by variations in cartilage T2 within the layer can be seen.[15,24] Using freeze-fracture sectioning and scanning electron microscopy of the rabbit

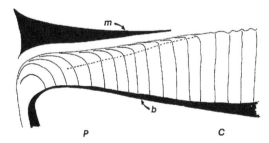

Fig. 3. A diagram of the structure of the tibial plateau as displayed after fracture sectioning. In the peripheral region of the joint surface deep to the meniscus (m), the cartilage matrix varies considerably in structure compared with the central region of the joint surface. (*From* Clark JM. Variation of collagen fiber alignment in a joint surface: a scanning electron microscope study of the tibial plateau in dog, rabbit, and man. J Orthop Res 1991;9:246–57; with permission.)

tibial plateau, ap Gwynn and colleagues[11] described a tubular organization of the extracellular matrix. This tubular structure within the matrix may explain this additional degree of T2 heterogeneity. A columnlike organization within the deepest layer of cartilage in the tibial plateau is apparent on both the MR image and the fractured gross specimen, as displayed in **Fig. 6**.

The normal appearance of cartilage on MR images is therefore a reflection of the characteristic matrix structure of the particular joint surface under consideration. The structure of cartilage determines the pattern of signal through the interrelationship between orientation to B_0 and alterations in T2 decay owing to the magic angle effect. As shown in **Fig. 7**, the "layered" pattern of cartilage signal intensity is predictable but not constant, as any change in orientation will alter the appearance of the tissue.

Clinical Imaging of Cartilage

There is no one "cartilage sequence" that will satisfy all needs in the evaluation of cartilage. A variety of different imaging sequences have been shown to be accurate. Many advocate the use of fast spin-echo imaging, whereas others have promoted imaging with volumetric sequences.[1,3,4,25] Regardless of the specific choices one makes regarding sequence selection, the images need to be optimized for the visualization of cartilage and cartilage injury. Normal variation in the appearance of cartilage must be recognized and artifacts should be limited. Finally, correlating the MR images with findings at surgery can improve the performance of the interpreter and help to optimize imaging at a given center. This requires that MR imaging and surgical findings are reported in a manner that is precise enough in the localization of lesions that correlation is possible.

Because T2-weighted images are directly influenced by the internal structure of cartilage and also produce a high-contrast interface between cartilage and adjacent synovial fluid, it is not surprising that T2-weighted images have proven useful in the clinical evaluation of cartilage. This has been especially true following the introduction of fast spin-echo techniques that allow for the acquisition of images with greater signal-to-noise ratio (SNR) and decreased imaging time. A number of studies have documented the accuracy of fast spin-echo imaging, and this approach to imaging can be successful using a variety of different imaging parameters.[1,3] One of the great benefits of using fast spin-echo imaging is that these sequences are typically used in the routine evaluation of joints and a thorough evaluation of

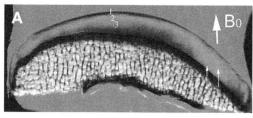
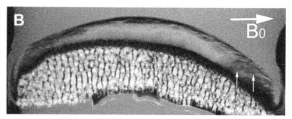

Fig. 4. Images of an osteochondral fragment of the femoral condyle with normal cartilage acquired with a 7T scanner. (A) With the surface perpendicular to B_0, 3 layers, a low-signal surface layer (1), a high-signal transitional layer (2), and a lower signal intensity deep layer (3), are apparent. (B) When the same sample is imaged with identical imaging parameters and the surface is parallel to B_0, the layers change. Note that the anisotropy can occur at all depths of cartilage (*small white arrows*). (*From* Goodwin DW, Zhu H, Dunn JF. In vivo MR imaging of hyaline cartilage: correlation with scanning electron microscopy. AJR Am J Roentgenol 2000;174:405–9; with permission.)

cartilage can be accomplished without the need to add sequences to the examination.

The distinction between proton density–weighted and T2-weighted images is somewhat arbitrary, as even on so-called proton density images acquired with a short effective echo time (TE), the contrast is because of variations in T2. An effective T2 weighting for visualization of cartilage should produce images that distinguish cartilage from synovial fluid and also allow for visualization of the internal structure of cartilage as revealed in the presence of layers. By pairing shorter effective TE "proton density"–weighted images with more heavily T2-weighted images, the observer can take advantage of the differences in contrast on the two sequences to provide a more complete evaluation of the joint surface.

When reviewing a fast spin-echo image of cartilage, one must account for normal variations in signal intensity related to the structure of cartilage at that particular joint. Care should be taken to not confuse normal variations in signal intensity with cartilage injury. Particularly when considering a frequently studied joint like the knee, these normal variations are familiar to most experienced observers. Less commonly studied joints, however, may be more challenging. As a general rule, the normal variations in signal intensity related to variations in cartilage structure and orientation appear as gradual changes in signal intensity. An abrupt change in signal intensity, as displayed in **Fig. 8**, should raise concern for cartilage injury. Because of the influence of T2 anisotropy, the normal appearance of cartilage will also be altered by changes in orientation. This is especially important to consider when imaging patients with a vertically oriented magnet, because the appearance of a normal joint will likely be very different from the appearance on a more commonly used horizontal bore scanner.

Magnetization transfer, an additional source of tissue contrast on fast spin-echo images, occurs because of the influence of less mobile protons bound to macromolecules on mobile or "liquid" protons.[26,27] The use of multiple echoes produces a greater number of resonance radiofrequency pulses during each repetition time (TR), thereby enhancing the magnetization transfer effect. The result is a decrease in signal intensity within cartilage and an increase in image contrast between cartilage and synovial fluid. This may be an advantage for the identification of chondral lesions because of the improved contrast between cartilage and fluid. Whether or not more subtle lesions may occasionally be obscured by the loss of signal within cartilage is unclear.

The persistence of high fat signal within bone marrow on T2-weighted images is a characteristic feature of fast spin-echo imaging. Suppression of this signal, typically through the use of frequency-selective fat saturation or selective excitation of water, produces images of cartilage with an enhanced dynamic range. Fat suppression also produces more accurate images of subchondral bone by eliminating chemical shift artifact. In addition, cartilage injury is often associated with the presence of fluid signal intensity within marrow, a finding obscured by high fat signal on images without suppression.[28]

Signal intensity and contrast resolution are also influenced by the receive bandwidth—the range of frequencies accepted by the receiver to sample the MR signal. The bandwidth is adjustable and, as is the case with most MR imaging parameters, choosing an optimal bandwidth requires balancing the advantages and disadvantages of a particular frequency. The signal to noise of an image can be increased by using a shorter bandwidth, but this advantage is realized at the cost of increased chemical shift artifact. These trade-offs are illustrated in **Fig. 9**. Cartilage is typically a thin tissue, and chondral injuries and regions of degeneration often require relatively high spatial resolution for visualization. For these reasons, the advantages

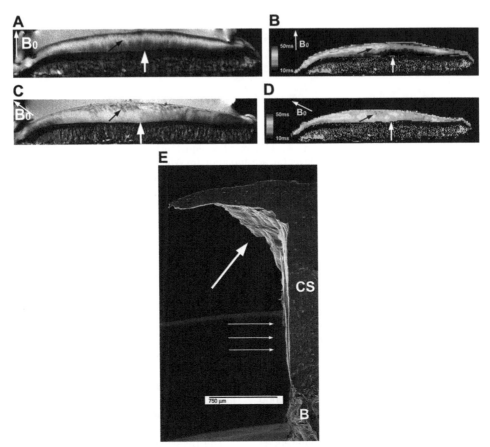

Fig. 5. The influence of structure and orientation on T2 and signal intensity is apparent on these sagittal images and T2 maps of the tibial plateau and the corresponding electron micrograph. (*A*) On this spin-echo image, the typical layered appearance of articular cartilage is present. A higher signal intensity transitional layer (*black arrow*) is bordered by lower signal intensity at more superficial and deeper layers. (*B*) On the corresponding T2 map, the variations in signal intensity present in (*A*) correlate with variations in the T2 of cartilage. (*C*) When the same sample is tilted 55° to B₀ and reimaged in the same plane, the signal intensity changes. This effect is present at the transitional layer (*black arrow*). (*D*) On the corresponding T2 map at 55° to B₀, the changes in signal intensity again correspond to changes in the T2 decay. (*E*) The sample was cut parallel to the plane of MR imaging and then fractured perpendicular to the fracture plane in the midportion of the sample (*thick white arrows* on images A–D). The fracture plane reflects a straight orientation of the matrix at deeper levels (*arrows*) that curves into the plane of the surface at the level of the transitional layer seen on the spin-echo images and T2 maps (*large arrow*). (*From* Goodwin DW, Wadghiri YZ, Zhu H, et al. Macroscopic structure of articular cartilage of the tibial plateau: influence of a characteristic matrix architecture on MRI appearance. AJR Am J Roentgenol 2004;182:311–8; with permission.)

of improved spatial resolution when using higher bandwidth for imaging cartilage usually outweigh the potential advantages of higher signal intensity when using shorter bandwidth.

The use of smoothing filters may also compromise the ability of MR images to identify subtle chondral injuries. Used to decrease image noise, these filters may obscure cartilage lesions by diminishing spatial resolution, thereby "improving" the appearance of an image at the expense of diagnostic quality. Unfortunately, choices regarding how images are filtered are likely based on a desire to optimize the visualization of structures other than articular cartilage, such as tendons, menisci, and ligaments. Frequently embedded within the proprietary software of scanners, the filters may not be available for manipulation. The cost of removing noise from the image may be the obscuration of subtle chondral lesions, as shown in **Fig. 10**.

One of the great challenges of cartilage imaging is the need to achieve a spatial resolution adequate for the identification cartilage injury. Chondral lesions are often small, particularly in relation to the slice thickness of most MR images.[29] The more complex the articular surface

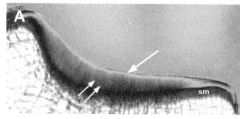
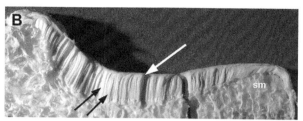

Fig. 6. Variations in the signal intensity seen on the T2-weighted spin-echo image (A) of the tibial plateau parallel changes in the orientation the matrix as displayed on the gross specimen (B), which has fractured in the plane of MR imaging. In the central region of the plateau, note the columnar organization (double arrows) and the superficial curve of tissue into the plane of the joint surface (single arrow) and the associated signal intensity changes on the MR image (B). In the submeniscal region of the plateau (sm), the more complex organization of the matrix produces a different signal intensity pattern. (From Goodwin DW, Wadghiri YZ, Zhu H, et al. Macroscopic structure of articular cartilage of the tibial plateau: influence of a characteristic matrix architecture on MRI appearance. AJR Am J Roentgenol 2004;182:311–8; with permission.)

and the thinner the cartilage, the greater the challenge becomes. Routine 2-dimensional images may miss small cartilage lesions if the abnormality is obscured by partial volume averaging with normal tissue in a thick slice. Injuries to the surface of the joint will be difficult to see if the articular surface is poorly defined as a consequence of partial volume averaging of cartilage with adjacent synovial fluid. Small high signal intensity structures adjacent to curved surfaces, such as a blood

vessel, may also be mistaken for focal abnormalities, owing to partial volume averaging, as illustrated in Fig. 11.

Limited spatial resolution is addressed, in part, by acquiring images in more than one plane. A lesion may be poorly visualized in one plane but obvious in another. More directed imaging can also be used by defining specific imaging planes other than the standard axial, coronal, and sagittal planes, which will optimize the imaging of

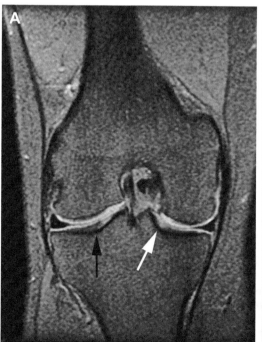
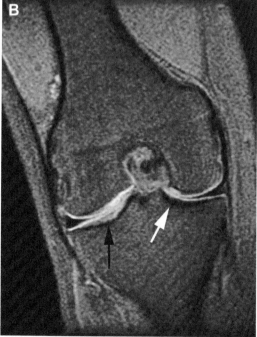

Fig. 7. Coronal fat-suppressed T2-weighted fast spin-echo images in 2 orientations reveal the influence of orientation on the normal appearance for cartilage. Signal intensity changes are apparent in the cartilage of the medial tibial plateau (white arrows) and the lateral plateau (black arrows) when the orientation is changed from straight (A) to angled relative to B_0 (B).

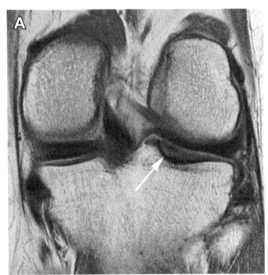
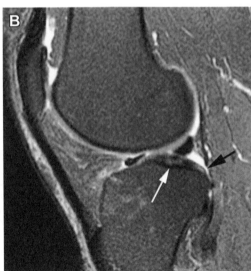

Fig. 8. (*A*) The presence of a focal abrupt change in signal intensity (*white arrow*) within the lateral tibial plateau cartilage on this proton density–weighted coronal image of the knee is consistent with a focus of cartilage injury or degeneration. (*B*) A more heavily T2-weighted fast spin-echo image acquired with fat-suppression confirms the presence of this cartilage injury by displaying it in the sagittal plane (*white arrow*). Subtle foci of increased signal intensity such as this must be distinguished from regions such as the periphery of the tibial plateau (*black arrow*), where similar signal intensity is a result of the normal structure of the articular cartilage.

a particular region of the joint. This approach is particularly helpful when investigating known osteochondral injuries and sites of cartilage repair.

Many of the limitations of spatial resolution associated with cartilage imaging can be addressed by taking advantage of the improved SNR available when imaging on a 3-Tesla (3T) scanner. As shown in **Fig. 12**, the higher SNR can be used to acquire thinner images of cartilage. Sequences that were too long to be practical in a clinical setting can now be performed routinely using a 3T scanner. When imaging at 3T, however, there are some limitations and trade-offs that must be considered. The increased chemical shift often

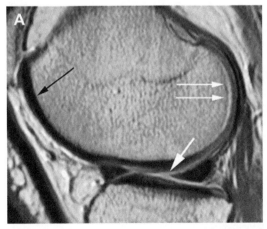
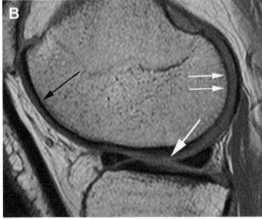

Fig. 9. The effect of bandwidth on signal intensity and spatial resolution. These 2 sagittal proton density–weighted fast spin-echo images of the knee were acquired using identical parameters, with the single exception of the receiver bandwidth, and filmed at the same window and level. On image (*A*), acquired with a receive bandwidth of 20 Hz, fat signal is shifted over the cartilage of the posterior femoral condyle (*double white arrows*) and away from the subchondral of the anterior femoral condyle, which appears abnormally thickened (*black arrow*). Because of the significantly higher SNR at lower bandwidth, the signal intensity is higher and the contrast between synovial fluid and cartilage is enhanced (*single white arrow*). On image (*B*), acquired with a receiver bandwidth of 63 Hz, the chemical shift is significantly less (*black arrow* and *double white arrows*) at the cost of diminished SNR and decreased contrast between cartilage and synovial fluid (*single white arrow*).

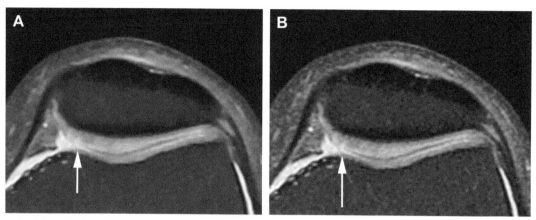

Fig. 10. The effect of filtering on spatial resolution. The same axial fat-suppressed T2-weighted fast spin-echo image filmed at identical window and level settings. (*A*) A smoothing filter has been applied and the margins of a small medial facet cartilage fissure (*white arrow*) are less sharp. (*B*) The image appears noisier without the filter, but the margins of the cartilage fissure (*white arrow*) are sharper and the lesion is more conspicuous.

requires the use of fat-suppression techniques and a longer receiver bandwidth. The frequency dependence of relaxation times also requires an adjustment of scanning parameters. Finally, increased artifact caused by metal may be limiting in postoperative patients, including those who have undergone a cartilage repair procedure.

The widespread availability of 3T scanners also makes possible the more frequent use of 3-dimensional cartilage-imaging sequences in routine clinical examinations. Sequences such as fat-saturated spoiled gradient recalled echo (SPGR) have already been shown to be accurate in identifying cartilage lesions even when used on 1.5T scanners.[2,4] Acquisition of images with thinner contiguous slices minimizes the partial volume averaging that compromises thicker images. As a result, these sequences are particularly useful in visualizing cartilage surfaces of small and irregularly shaped joint surfaces where partial volume averaging is a challenge. Using the 3-dimensional dataset, images can be reformatted

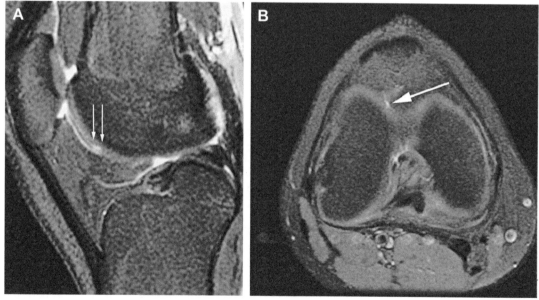

Fig. 11. The effect of partial volume averaging. (*A*) A focus of high signal within the articular cartilage of the femoral trochlea on this sagittal fat-suppressed T2-weighted fast spin-echo image of the knee is consistent with a focal cartilage erosion (*arrows*). (*B*) An axial fat-suppressed T2-weighted fast spin-echo image reveals that the signal is instead the result of the presence of a blood vessel (*arrow*). The high signal from the vessel is averaged within the volume of the 4-mm-thick sagittal plane image.

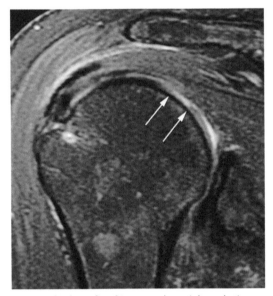

Fig. 12. The benefit of improved spatial resolution on 3T images. Because of the spherical shape and associated volume averaging, focal defects within the articular cartilage of the humeral head are often difficult to identify. As seen on this sagittal fat-suppressed T2-weighted fast spin-echo image acquired on a 3T scanner, the SNR is high enough to obtain high-quality 2-mm-thick images, which facilitate identification of the focal cartilage defect (*arrows*).

in any plane, making possible the acquisition of an image in a single plane and subsequent reconstruction images in orthogonal planes, as shown in **Fig. 13**. Rather than prospectively defining image planes, this technique allows one to acquire an image and then reformat the data in a plane that optimally displays the region of interest. Cartilage volume measurements can also be made using 3-dimensional sequences.

The routine use of 3-dimensional cartilage-imaging sequences in clinical practice, however, has not been widespread. Most volumetric sequences have limited value beyond imaging cartilage and provide little useful information regarding the status of other tissues such as ligaments and menisci. Considering that the time required for volumetric imaging at 1.5T is substantial, it is therefore not surprising that these sequences are not included in the routine MR examination. Compared with fast spin-echo imaging, these sequences are also more severely degraded by susceptibility artifact. Many of the most commonly available volumetric sequences display cartilage as a high signal intensity tissue and fluid appears dark. This results in relatively little contrast between cartilage and synovial fluid. In this setting, superficial cartilage lesions are often difficult to identify. The absence of T2 contrast within the tissue also limits evaluation of the internal structure of the tissue reflected in the normal variations of T2 so well displayed on fast spin-echo images.

Many of these limitations to the routine application of 3-dimensional cartilage-imaging sequences can be addressed through the use of 3T scanners and the development of new volumetric sequences. The increased SNR at 3T can be exploited to decrease imaging time, and the development of newer sequences have improved T2 contrast. On these bright-fluid sequences, the high signal intensity of synovial fluid relative to cartilage creates an arthrogram effect that more clearly delineates lesions on the articular surface. With the added SNR available at 3T, 3-dimensional fast spin-echo imaging is now possible. As a result, the potential to accomplish a complete study of a joint with 1 or 2 acquisitions now exists.

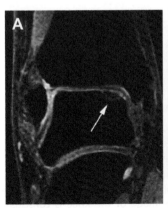
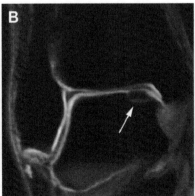
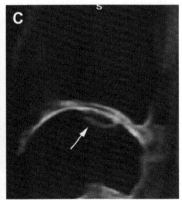

Fig. 13. By acquiring volumetric images as seen on this 3-dimensional SPGR sequence, the osteochondral lesion (*arrow*) can be imaged directly on the coronal acquisition (*A*) and can be reformatted into oblique coronal (*B*) and sagittal images (*C*), allowing for a better characterization of the lesion's size and imaging characteristics.

Although the increased use of 3T scanners and the development of new sequences will enhance the evaluation of cartilage, reliable cartilage assessment can already be performed using routinely available equipment. Cartilage imaging, however, requires a focused understanding of common artifacts and patterns of cartilage injury and a thorough review of the MR images.

As previously mentioned, the presence of chemical shift artifact may obscure cartilage because of the misregistration of fat signal from adjacent bone marrow—an artifact that is particularly prominent when imaging at 3T. The artifact can be reduced or eliminated by increasing the receive bandwidth or through the use of fat-suppression techniques. Although inversion-recovery techniques can be used, their relatively long imaging time limits their use for evaluating cartilage in clinical practice. Frequency-selective fat suppression is typically used in cartilage imaging and increasingly the suppression of fat signal through selective excitation of water provides an alternative technique.[30,31]

Truncation artifact may also compromise the evaluation of cartilage. Bright or dark lines may be found at interfaces characterized by severe differences in signal intensity, such as the articular surface. This "ringing" artifact is caused by the incomplete digitization of an echo at a sharp signal intensity interface.[32-34] Most apparent on smaller matrix images, the effect can be minimized by increasing matrix dimensions. Unlike chemical shift, the artifact occurs in both the frequency-encoding and phase-encoding directions and will parallel curved surfaces, such as the subchondral bone. This artifact, which can be seen frequently on fat-suppressed SPGR images, was in the past mistaken for true variations in signal intensity and was incorrectly presumed to correlate with the zonal organization of cartilage.[33] Although the artifact is not a frequent cause of confusion, it can in the setting of a fluid-filled joint imitate the appearance of the cartilage surface when the articular is completely lost, as seen in **Fig. 14**.

Flowing blood will cause misregistration in the phase-encoding direction. Although this artifact is well known and usually recognized without difficulty, it may still compromise the evaluation of cartilage. Misplaced signal within the articular cartilage may mimic chondral injury. Even if one is aware that flow artifact is extending through the area of interest, the reader may not be able to distinguish true pathology from artifact, as shown in **Fig. 15**.

Regardless of what equipment and imaging sequences are available, the reliable use of MR imaging to identify chondral lesions requires

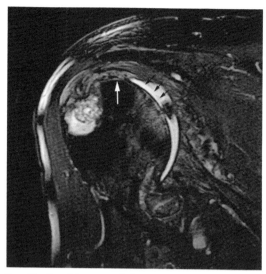

Fig. 14. On this coronal fat-suppressed T2-weighted fast spin-echo image of the shoulder with extensive loss of articular cartilage, a small area of residual cartilage is present at the superior aspect of the humeral head (*white arrow*). Truncation artifact has produced a thin low signal intensity line parallel to the subchondral bone (*black arrows*), which mimics the appearance of an articular surface and gives the false impression that a thick layer of cartilage is present.

a dedicated, thorough review of the images. This begins with the use of appropriate windowing and leveling of the image to enhance the visualization of cartilage. Window and level settings typically useful for the evaluation of ligaments, tendons, and bone are frequently not optimal for visualization of cartilage. Just as it would be impossible to review a CT scan of the chest without varying the window and level settings, evaluation of cartilage requires constant adjustment of the image display. At appropriate window and level settings, small surface lesions otherwise obscured by high signal intensity fluid at suboptimal settings can be adequately displayed. Adjustments in the window and level settings can help to distinguish focal alterations in structure caused by chondral degeneration and injury from normal variations in cartilage signal intensity.

Optimal review of the MR image is also facilitated by an understanding of where chondral injuries tend to occur and what MR findings are associated with those injuries. At any joint, the identification of a chondral lesion at one articular surface should prompt a thorough evaluation of the opposing surface. Moreover, typical patterns of malalignment are associated with predictable injury patterns. For example, varus deformity of the knee because of cartilage loss in the medial compartment will also cause abnormal alignment

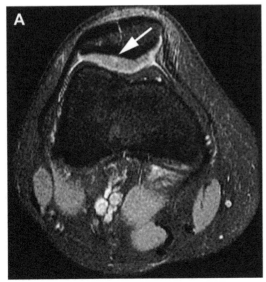 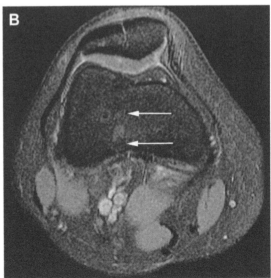

Fig. 15. (*A*) The presence of a focus of high signal intensity (*white arrow*) within the cartilage of the patella on an axial fat-suppressed T2-weighted fast spin-echo image is consistent with a small focus of cartilage injury. (*B*) When the imaged is filmed at a different window and level, however, it is apparent that pulsation artifact extends through the area of interest (*white arrows*), raising the question of whether this small abnormality is simply artifact.

of the lateral compartment. As a consequence, chondral injuries will frequently be found high along the surface of the tibial eminence, owing to the abnormal articulation of the tibial eminence with the lateral femoral condyle.

Any joint injury increases the likelihood that chondral pathology is also present. Cartilage injury, whether chronic and degenerative or caused by acute trauma, is frequently associated with bone injury and related alterations in the adjacent bone marrow signal. The presence of this edema-like signal should direct the reviewer's attention to the overlying cartilage. Similarly, injuries of the knee meniscus are frequently associated with adjacent chondral degeneration and fissuring.

In large commonly imaged joints, such as the knee, MR imaging can be highly reliable in the identification of chondral injury provided that both signal intensity and spatial resolution are adequate. When considering smaller joints with thin cartilage and irregular surfaces, cartilage imaging is more difficult largely because of the insufficient spatial resolution. Although imaging of chondral surfaces in these joints will likely remain challenging, the increased availability of 3T scanners and improvements in coil design, as well as continued advances in the development of new sequences, will likely lead to improved diagnostic performance. Regardless of what equipment is available, accurate cartilage assessment requires high-quality images with optimized tissue contrast and spatial resolution. When

reviewing a study of satisfactory quality, an understanding of the influence of cartilage structure on the normal appearance of cartilage can help distinguish cartilage pathology from normal variations in cartilage signal intensity.

REFERENCES

1. Bredella MA, Tirman PF, Peterfy CG, et al. Accuracy of T2-weighted fast spin-echo MR imaging with fat saturation in detecting cartilage defects in the knee: comparison with arthroscopy in 130 patients. AJR Am J Roentgenol 1999;172:1073–80.
2. Disler DG, McCauley TR, Kelman CG, et al. Fat-suppressed three-dimensional spoiled gradient-echo MR imaging of hyaline cartilage defects in the knee: comparison with standard MR imaging and arthroscopy. AJR Am J Roentgenol 1996;167(1):127–32.
3. Potter HG, Linklater JM, Allen AA, et al. Magnetic resonance imaging of articular cartilage in the knee. An evaluation with use of fast-spin-echo imaging. J Bone Joint Surg Am 1998;80(9):1276–84.
4. Recht MP, Piraino DW, Paletta GA, et al. Accuracy of fat-suppressed three-dimensional spoiled gradient-echo FLASH MR imaging in the detection of patello-femoral articular cartilage abnormalities. Radiology 1996;198(1):209–12.
5. Buckwalter JA, Mankin HJ. Articular cartilage. Part I: Tissue design and chondrocyte-matrix interactions. J Bone Joint Surg Am 1997;79(4):600–11.
6. Bullough PG. The pathology of osteoarthritis. In: Moskowitz RW, Howell DS, Goldberg VM, et al,

editors. Osteoarthritis, diagnosis and medical/ surgical management. 2nd edition. Philadelphia: W.B. Saunders; 1992. p. 39–69.

7. Mow VC, Ratcliffe A, Poole AR. Cartilage and diarthrodial joints as paradigms for hierarchical materials and structures. Biomaterials 1992;13(2):67–97.

8. Yao JQ, Seedhom BB. Mechanical conditioning of articular cartilage to prevalent stresses. Br J Rheumatol 1993;32(11):956–65.

9. Thambyah A, Nather A, Goh J. Mechanical properties of articular cartilage covered by the meniscus. Osteoarthr Cartil 2006;14(6):580–8.

10. Hultkrantz W. Ueber die Spaltrichtungen der Gelenkknorpel. Verh Anat Ges 1898;12:248–56 [in German].

11. ap Gwynn I, Wade S, Kaab MJ, et al. Freeze-substitution of rabbit tibial articular cartilage reveals that radial zone collagen fibres are tubules. J Microsc 2000;197(Pt 2):159–72.

12. Clark JM. The organization of collagen in cryofractured rabbit articular cartilage: a scanning electron microscopic study. J Orthop Res 1985;3:17–29.

13. Clark JM. Variation of collagen fiber alignment in a joint surface: a scanning electron microscope study of the tibial plateau in dog, rabbit, and man. J Orthop Res 1991;9:246–57.

14. Jeffery AK, Blunn GW, Archer CW, et al. Three-dimensional collagen architecture in bovine articular cartilage. J Bone Joint Surg Br 1991;73(5):795–801.

15. Goodwin DW, Wadghiri YZ, Zhu H, et al. Macroscopic structure of articular cartilage of the tibial plateau: influence of a characteristic matrix architecture on MRI appearance. AJR Am J Roentgenol 2004;182(2):311–8.

16. Goodwin DW, Wadghiri YZ, Dunn JF. Micro-imaging of articular cartilage: T2, proton density and the magic angle effect. Acad Radiol 1998;5:790–8.

17. Mlynarik V, Degrassi A, Toffanin R, et al. Investigation of laminar appearance of articular cartilage by means of magnetic resonance microscopy. Magn Reson Imaging 1996;14(4):435–42.

18. Xia Y, Farquhar T, Burton-Wurster N, et al. Origin of cartilage laminae in MRI. J Magn Reson Imaging 1997;7:887–94.

19. Rubenstein JD, Kim JK, Morova-Protzner I, et al. Effects of collagen orientation on MR imaging characteristics of bovine articular cartilage. Radiology 1993;188(1):219–26.

20. Fullerton GD, Cameron IL, Ord VA. Orientation of tendons in the magnetic field and its effect on T2 relaxation times. Radiology 1985;155:433–5.

21. Henkelman RM, Stanisz GJ, Kim JK, et al. Anisotropy of NMR properties of tissues. Magn Reson Med 1994;32:592–601.

22. Rubenstein J, Recht M, Disler DG, et al. Laminar structures on MR images of articular cartilage. Radiology 1997;204(1):15–6.

23. Goodwin DW, Zhu H, Dunn JF. In vivo MR imaging of hyaline cartilage: correlation with scanning electron microscopy. AJR Am J Roentgenol 2000;174:405–9.

24. Goodwin DW, Lei H, Dunn JF. Vertical striations in the radial layer of MR images of hyaline cartilage are due to T2 effects. Paper presented at: 9th Annual Meeting, Proceedings of the International Society for Magnetic Resonance in Medicine. Glasgow (Scotland), April 21–27, 2001.

25. Disler DG, Peters TL, Muscoreil SJ, et al. Fat-suppressed spoiled GRASS imaging of knee hyaline cartilage: technique optimization and comparison with conventional MR imaging. AJR Am J Roentgenol 1994;163(4):887–92.

26. Henkelman RM, Stanisz GJ, Graham SJ. Magnetization transfer in MRI: a review. NMR Biomed 2001; 14(2):57–64.

27. Yao L, Gentili A, Thomas A. Incidental magnetization transfer contrast in fast spin-echo imaging of cartilage. J Magn Reson Imaging 1996;6(1):180–4.

28. Rubin DA, Harner CD, Costello JM. Treatable chondral injuries in the knee: frequency of associated focal subchondral edema. AJR Am J Roentgenol 2000;174(4):1099–106.

29. Rubenstein JD, Li JD, Majumdar S, et al. Image resolution and signal-to-noise ratio requirements for MR imaging of degenerative cartilage. AJR Am J Roentgenol 1997;169:1089–96.

30. Glaser C, Faber S, Eckstein F, et al. Optimization and validation of a rapid high-resolution T1-w 3D FLASH water excitation MRI sequence for the quantitative assessment of articular cartilage volume and thickness. Magn Reson Imaging 2001;19(2):177–85.

31. Hyhlik-Dürr A, Faber S, Burgkart R, et al. Precision of tibial cartilage morphometry with a coronal water-excitation MR sequence. Eur Radiol 2000;10(2): 297–303.

32. Erickson SJ, Prost R. Laminar structures on MR images of articular cartilage: reply. Radiology 1997;204:16–8.

33. Erickson SJ, Waldschmidt JG, Czervionke LF, et al. Hyaline cartilage: truncation artifact as a cause of trilaminar appearance with fat-suppressed three-dimensional spoiled gradient-recalled sequences. Radiology 1996;201:260–4.

34. Frank LR, Brossmann J, Buxton RB, et al. MR imaging truncation artifacts can create a false laminar appearance in cartilage. AJR Am J Roentgenol 1997;168(2):547–54.

Morphologic Imaging of Articular Cartilage

Colin D. Strickland, MD[a],*, Richard Kijowski, MD[b]

KEYWORDS

- Cartilage • MR imaging • Sequences • Osteoarthritis

Osteoarthritis is a highly prevalent chronic disease affecting millions of Americans and is one of the most common causes of disability in the United States.[1] The lifetime risk of developing osteoarthritis of the knee joint has been estimated at 45%[2] with an expected continued increase in prevalence caused by higher rates of obesity and the aging American population.[3] Osteoarthritis of the hip joint is also a common clinical problem, although the prevalence of the disease reported in the literature varies between 1% and 27%.[4] Acute cartilage injury is frequently seen following joint trauma and is a common cause of pain and disability in young and middle-aged patients.[5] With the enormous number of individuals in the United States suffering from the debilitating effects of osteoarthritis and acute cartilage injury, much research has been directed toward developing effective medical and surgical treatment options. Such endeavors require accurate and reproducible methods of cartilage assessment for both clinical and research applications.

Radiographs have been the traditional imaging modality used to evaluate patients with osteoarthritis and acute cartilage injury. However, radiographs can only assess joint space loss and osteophyte formation and are insensitive for detecting early cartilage degeneration.[6] For this reason, magnetic resonance (MR) imaging has become the imaging modality of choice for evaluating articular cartilage in both the clinical and research setting. Because of its high spatial resolution, multiplanar capability, and excellent tissue contrast, MR imaging can detect and characterize morphologic changes associated with cartilage degeneration and acute cartilage injury. Lack of exposure to ionizing radiation is an additional attractive feature of MR imaging, particularly in young patients. This article discusses the role of MR imaging in the evaluation of the articular cartilage of the knee and hip joints, which are the two joints most commonly affected by osteoarthritis and acute cartilage injury. The article also discusses the appearance of cartilage lesions on MR imaging and the advantages and limitations of currently available MR imaging techniques for evaluating cartilage morphology.

IMPORTANCE OF MORPHOLOGIC CARTILAGE ASSESSMENT

Accurate evaluation of articular cartilage in patients undergoing MR imaging of the knee and hip joints is clinically significant. Identifying focal and diffuse cartilage loss can explain the cause of joint pain in many symptomatic patients.[7] The pain and disability associated with osteoarthritis and acute cartilage injury can also be reduced through early diagnosis and appropriate treatment. Self-management activities such as weight control and physical activity may relieve symptoms and slow the progression of the disease process.[8] New medical therapies may soon become available for the treatment of patients with osteoarthritis and acute cartilage injury. The role of cytokines in the pathophysiology of osteoarthritis has led to the investigation of a multitude of pathways to explain symptoms and structural changes associated with the disease. Numerous agents, including interleukin (IL)-1

[a] Department of Radiology, University of Colorado Denver, Leprino Building, 12401 East 17th Avenue, Mail Stop L954, Aurora, CO 80045, USA
[b] Department of Radiology, University of Wisconsin School of Medicine and Public Health, 600 Highland Avenue, Madison, WI 53792, USA
* Corresponding author.
E-mail address: colin.strickland@ucdenver.edu

Magn Reson Imaging Clin N Am 19 (2011) 229–248
doi:10.1016/j.mric.2011.02.009
1064-9689/11/$ – see front matter © 2011 Elsevier Inc. All rights reserved.

receptor antagonist protein, tumor necrosis factor (TNF)-α blockers, calcitonin, and anabolic cytokines, have been evaluated as potential treatment options for patients with osteoarthritis.[9,10] Early intra-articular administration of hyaluronic acid has also been shown to reduce chondrocyte death and increase proteoglycan content of articular cartilage following acute traumatic injury.[11] Although no pharmaceutical agents are currently approved by the United States Food and Drug Administration for treatment of patients with osteoarthritis or acute cartilage injury, the development of disease-modifying drugs remains an important goal and an area of ongoing research.

Several surgical interventions are currently being used in clinical practice to treat degenerative and posttraumatic cartilage lesions within the knee and hip joints. Surgical procedures such as debridement, microfracture, bone marrow stimulation,[12] autologous osteochondral mosaicplasty,[13–15] and autologous chondrocyte transplantation[12,16,17] have been shown to provide significant pain relief in patients with acute cartilage injury and early osteoarthritis of the knee joint. During the past decade, conditions such as femoroacetabular impingement[18–20] and acetabular dysplasia[21,22] have been gaining increased attention as causes of premature osteoarthritis of the hip joint in young patients. Surgical interventions such as labral repair or debridement[23–25] along with femoral and acetabular osteochondroplasty[23,24] and acetabular osteotomy[25–27] are currently available to treat these patients. However, performing these procedures before the development of advanced joint degeneration is essential for their long-term success.[28,29] Thus, early detection of degenerative and posttraumatic cartilage loss within the knee and hip joints with MR imaging can help identify patients who may benefit from early surgical intervention.

APPEARANCE OF DEGENERATIVE AND POSTTRAUMATIC CARTILAGE LESIONS ON MR IMAGING

Normal articular cartilage has a smooth contour and multilaminar appearance owing to the presence of several layers with varying amounts of collagen, proteoglycans, and chondrocytes.[30] Degenerative changes within articular cartilage have characteristic features that correlate with the degree of disease severity. Initial changes associated with early cartilage degeneration include foci of fibrillation, fissuring, and surface irregularity (**Fig. 1**). Diffuse cartilage thinning and cartilage delamination are manifestations of advancing osteoarthritis (**Fig. 2**). As the disease

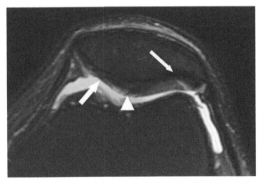

Fig. 1. A 41-year-old woman with knee pain. Axial, two-dimensional, fat-saturated, T2-weighted FSE image of the knee joint shows several morphologic abnormalities of early cartilage degeneration. A deep cartilage fissure (*small arrow*) is noted on the lateral patellar facet. Cartilage fibrillation (*arrowhead*) is present along the median ridge of the patella. A superficial partial-thickness cartilage lesion (*large arrow*) with obtuse margins is also seen on the medial patellar facet.

progresses, partial and full-thickness cartilage defects are commonly seen on opposing articular surfaces. Cartilage defects in the setting of osteoarthritis tend to have obtuse margins and may show increased T2 signal in the underlying subchondral bone marrow (**Fig. 3**). Additional findings of advanced osteoarthritis include subchondral sclerosis, subchondral cysts, and osteophyte formation, which are all well depicted by MR imaging.

Increased T2 signal resembling bone marrow edema is often seen adjacent to degenerative cartilage lesions and has received attention as an important component in the generation of pain in patients with osteoarthritis. These areas of subchondral bone marrow signal abnormality can be seen adjacent to 5% to 54% of cartilage lesions depending on their size and depth.[31] Although evidence of edema has been found on histologic analysis, additional marrow changes, including alterations in trabecular bone architecture, bone marrow fibrosis, necrosis, and hemorrhage, have been shown, suggesting that edema may play only a minor role in this imaging appearance.[32,33] For this reason, areas of increased T2 signal adjacent to degenerative cartilage lesions are referred to as the subchondral bone marrow edema pattern.[34] The clinical significance of the subchondral bone marrow edema pattern is controversial. However, recent studies have shown that these areas of signal abnormality correlate with pain[35] and progression of cartilage loss[36–38] in patients with osteoarthritis. Subchondral sclerosis and bone attrition are also commonly seen in association with advanced degenerative cartilage

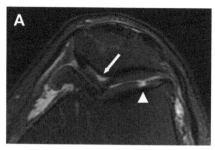
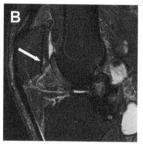

Fig. 2. A 56-year-old man with knee pain. (*A*) Axial, two-dimensional, fat-saturated, T2-weighted FSE image of the knee joint shows a large focus of cartilage delamination (*arrow*) on the medial patellar facet. Also note the deep partial-thickness cartilage lesion (*arrowhead*) on the lateral femoral trochlea. (*B*) Corresponding sagittal, two-dimensional, fat-saturated, T2-weighted FSE image of the knee joint shows the same focus of cartilage delamination (*arrow*) on the medial patellar facet.

loss and may reflect osseous remodeling related to altered stress.[39] Loss of mineralized trabecular bone has also been recently recognized as an additional osseous manifestation of advanced osteoarthritis.[40]

Traumatic cartilage lesions tend to have a different appearance than degenerative cartilage lesions on MR imaging and are characterized by sharp and acutely angulated margins (**Fig. 4**). In addition, traumatic cartilage lesions are often solitary and are found in characteristic locations according to the pattern of injury. Traumatic cartilage lesions are especially common in the knee joint and are the result of tangential, rotational, or shearing forces on the articular surface. The appearance of traumatic cartilage lesions on MR imaging depends on the mechanism of injury.

Tangential and rotational forces on articular cartilage secondary to injuries such as anterior cruciate ligament tear result in osteochondral impaction injuries. These impaction injuries are secondary to a pivot shift mechanism and manifest as areas of high T2 signal within the subchondral bone marrow of the anterior lateral femoral condyle and posterior tibial plateau with occasional depression of the articular surface and trabecular fracture lines (**Fig. 5**). These areas of bone marrow signal abnormality correlate with areas of significantly increased (*P*<.05) water and unsaturated lipid content and significantly decreased (*P*<.05) saturated lipid content on MR imaging spectroscopy.[41] Detection of high T2 signal within the subchondral bone marrow in the setting of acute joint injury should lead to careful scrutiny of the overlying articular cartilage. At MR imaging and arthroscopy, the articular cartilage overlying areas of subchondral bone marrow edema typically appears normal. However, biochemical changes of acute cartilage injury may be detected on histologic analysis[42] or when using advanced imaging techniques such as delayed gadolinium-enhanced MR imaging[43] and T1-rho imaging.[41,44] Areas of subchondral bone marrow edema may persist for several months following acute traumatic injury, although their long-term clinical significance remains unknown.[45]

Shearing forces on articular cartilage secondary to injuries such as transient patellar dislocation typically result in deep partial-thickness or

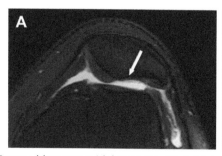
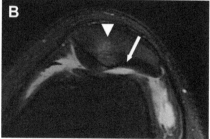

Fig. 3. A 47-year-old woman with knee pain. (*A*) Axial, two-dimensional, fat-saturated, T2-weighted FSE image of the knee joint shows a large deep partial-thickness cartilage lesion (*arrow*) with obtuse margins on the lateral patellar facet. (*B*) Axial, two-dimensional, fat-saturated T2-weighted FSE image of the knee joint obtained 18 months later shows progression of the cartilage lesion (*arrow*) with development of increased T2 signal (*arrowhead*) within the underlying bone marrow of patella. This area of signal abnormality within the bone marrow represents a combination of edema, trabecular microfracture, and vascular ingrowth.

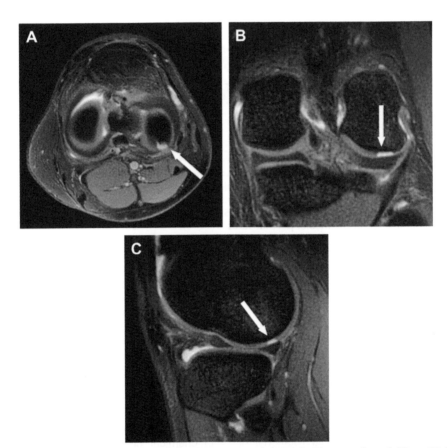

Fig. 4. A 32-year-old man with knee pain following trauma. (*A*) Axial, (*B*) coronal, and (*C*) sagittal VIPR-SSFP images of the knee joint shows a full-thickness cartilage lesion (*arrows*) on the lateral femoral condyle. Note that the cartilage lesion has sharply defined acute margins and is surrounded by normal cartilage, two characteristics suggesting an acute traumatic cause.

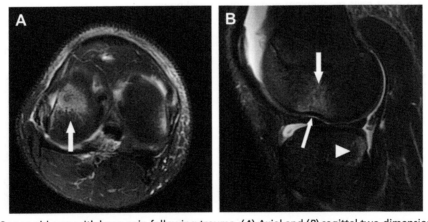

Fig. 5. An 18-year-old man with knee pain following trauma. (*A*) Axial and (*B*) sagittal two-dimensional, fat-saturated, T2-weighted FSE images of the knee joint show an osteochondral impaction fracture (*small arrow*) of the lateral femoral condyle with underlying subchondral bone marrow edema (*large arrows*). Also note the bone marrow edema (*arrowhead*) within the posterior lateral tibial plateau consistent with a posttraumatic contusion. This osteochondral injury pattern is typically of the pivot shift mechanism associated with anterior cruciate ligament tear.

full-thickness cartilage defects with acutely angulated margins that may also involve the underlying subchondral bone. Cartilage flap tears and cartilage delamination from the underlying subchondral bone plate may also occur. In the setting of transient patellar dislocation, the injury pattern is typically seen on the medial patellar facet and anterior lateral femoral condyle (**Fig. 6**). Cartilage shearing injuries are often unstable and may result in intra-articular cartilaginous or osteochondral loose bodies, which may lead to clinical symptoms such as locking that may mimic displaced meniscal tears.[46,47]

MORPHOLOGIC CARTILAGE IMAGING SEQUENCES

Techniques and approaches to MR imaging assessment of articular cartilage have changed rapidly in the past 2 decades. Various MR imaging pulse sequences have been successfully used to evaluate articular cartilage. These sequences include two-dimensional and three-dimensional fast spin echo sequences, three-dimensional gradient-echo sequences, dual echo in the steady-state (DESS) sequence, driven equilibrium Fourier transform sequence, and various steady-state free-precession sequences. The fact that so many MRI techniques exist for evaluating articular cartilage illustrates the challenges of accurate diagnosis and the inherent limitations of each imaging strategy.

Two-dimensional and Three-dimensional Fast Spin Echo Sequences

Two-dimensional fast spin echo (2D-FSE) sequences with intermediate-weighted and T2-weighted contrast are the most common sequences used in clinical practice to evaluate articular cartilage.[48–52] 2D-FSE sequences have high in-plane spatial resolution and can be used to evaluate the menisci, ligaments, and osseous structures in addition to articular cartilage. However, 2D-FSE sequences have thick slices and gaps between slices, which may limit visualization of small cartilage lesions secondary to partial volume averaging. Furthermore, T2-weighted 2D-FSE sequences create contrast between cartilage and synovial fluid at the expense of cartilage signal.[53] Although cartilage visibility on these sequences is partially limited by the magnetization transfer effect secondary to multiple off-resonance pulses, magnetization transfer contrast may also be clinically useful.[54,55] Intermediate-weighted 2D-FSE sequences have suboptimal contrast between cartilage and synovial fluid and suffer from image blurring caused by the acquisition of high spatial frequencies late in the echo train. However, contrast between cartilage and synovial fluid can be improved with the addition of fat suppression, whereas image blurring can be reduced with the use of short echo train lengths.

Recent research has brought attention to the use of three-dimensional fast spin echo (3D-FSE) sequences for evaluating articular cartilage such as fast spin echo Cube (FSE-Cube; GE Healthcare) and sampling perfection with application-oriented contrasts using different flip angle evolutions (SPACE, Siemens Medical Systems). 3D-FSE sequences use variable flip angle modulation to constrain T2 decay for an extended echo train, which allows intermediate-weighted images with bright synovial fluid to be acquired with minimal blurring. A major advantage of these sequences is their ability to acquire volumetric datasets with isotropic resolution, which allow articular cartilage

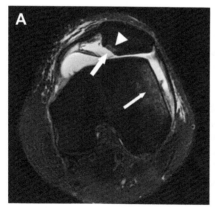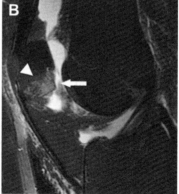

Fig. 6. A 24-year-old man with knee pain following trauma. (*A*) Axial and (*B*) sagittal two-dimensional fat-saturated T2-weighted FSE images of the knee joint show an osteochondral fracture (*large arrows*) of the medial patellar facet with underlying bone marrow edema (*arrowheads*). Also note the bone marrow edema (*small arrow*) within the anterior lateral femoral condyle consistent with a posttraumatic contusion. This osteochondral injury pattern is typically of transient lateral subluxation of the patella.

to be evaluated in any orientation following a single acquisition. 3D-FSE sequences can also be used to evaluate the menisci, ligament, and osseous structures in addition to articular cartilage.[56] 3D-FSE sequences have higher cartilage signal/noise ratio (SNR) but lower contrast between cartilage and synovial fluid compared with 2D-FSE sequences.[55,57] Magnetization transfer contrast is diminished on 3D-FSE sequences, which helps preserve cartilage signal but may potentially decrease the conspicuity of early cartilage degeneration. In-plane spatial resolution is also lower on 3D-FSE sequences compared with 2D-FSE sequences unless long acquisition times are used, which may also limit the detection of superficial cartilage lesions.

Three-dimensional Gradient-Echo Sequences

Gradient-echo sequences were the first three-dimensional sequences used for cartilage imaging. Gradient-echo sequences can be divided into dark fluid sequences and bright fluid sequences based on the signal intensity of synovial fluid. Dark fluid sequences include T1-weighted spoiled gradient-recalled echo (SPGR; GE Healthcare), fast low-angle shot (FLASH; Siemens Medical Systems), and T1 fast field echo (T1-FFE; Philips Healthcare). Bright fluid gradient-echo sequences include T2*-weighted gradient-recalled echo acquired in the steady state (GRASS; GE Healthcare), gradient-recalled echo (GRE; Siemens Medical Systems), and fast field echo (FFE; Philips Healthcare). Fat suppression is typically added to gradient-echo sequences to reduce chemical shift artifact and to optimize the overall dynamic contrast range of the image. Frequency-selective fat saturation is the most commonly used method to suppress fat signal.[7,58–60] However, gradient-echo images with higher SNR and greater contrast between cartilage and adjacent joint structures can be obtained using recently developed fat-suppression techniques such as water excitation[61,62] and iterative decomposition of water and fat with echo asymmetry and least squares estimates (IDEAL).[63–65]

Both dark fluid and bright fluid three-dimensional gradient-echo sequences have been successfully used to evaluate articular cartilage in clinical practice and to perform cartilage volume measurements in osteoarthritis research studies.[7,58–60,66,67] However, the main disadvantage of using dark fluid sequences for clinical cartilage imaging is the low signal intensity of synovial fluid, which may decrease the conspicuity of superficial cartilage lesions (**Fig. 7**). Dark fluid sequences have lower contrast between articular cartilage and synovial fluid than bright fluid sequences.[68] In addition, the

surface properties of degenerative cartilage may influence the ability of three-dimensional sequences to detect superficial cartilage lesions. Superficial degeneration shortens the T2 relaxation time of cartilage. For dark fluid sequences, the T2 shortening of degenerative cartilage has no effect on its signal intensity and contrast relative to synovial fluid. However, for bright fluid sequences, the effect of T2 shortening is to decrease the signal intensity of degenerative cartilage and thus increase its contrast relative to synovial fluid, which may result in greater conspicuity of superficial cartilage lesions.[69]

Three-dimensional DESS Sequence

DESS is another three-dimensional sequence that has been used to evaluate articular cartilage. The DESS sequence acquires 2 gradient echoes separated by a refocusing pulse that are combined into a single image. Adding the 2 echoes enhances the T2*-weighting of the image and increases the signal intensity of both cartilage and synovial fluid.[70] Although the DESS sequence has primarily been performed with a flip angle of less than 60°, some investigators have proposed the use of a larger flip angle to further accentuate fluid signal and improve contrast between cartilage and synovial fluid.[71] Cartilage SNR and contrast between cartilage and synovial fluid can also be improved by an individualized weighting procedure instead of the conventional averaging of the 2 gradient-echo images.[72] In a recent study comparing multiple three-dimensional isotropic resolution sequences for evaluating the articular cartilage of the knee joint at 3.0T, a water-excitation DESS sequence with 0.5-mm isotropic resolution and an 8-minute scan time was found to have the highest contrast between cartilage and synovial fluid and the greatest overall performance on qualitative assessment.[73] A water-excitation DESS sequence with near isotropic resolution is also being used in the Osteoarthritis Initiative to evaluate the articular cartilage of the knee joint.[74]

Three-dimensional Driven Equilibrium Fourier Transform

Driven equilibrium Fourier transform (DEFT) and variants such as fast recovery fast spin echo and driven equilibrium (DRIVE) are additional three-dimensional cartilage imaging sequences. The DEFT sequence differs from other techniques in that a 90° pulse is used to return transverse magnetization to the z-axis which increases signal from tissues such as synovial fluid that have long T1 relaxation times.[62,75,76] The result is an image that is dependent on the ratio of T1/T2 signal rather

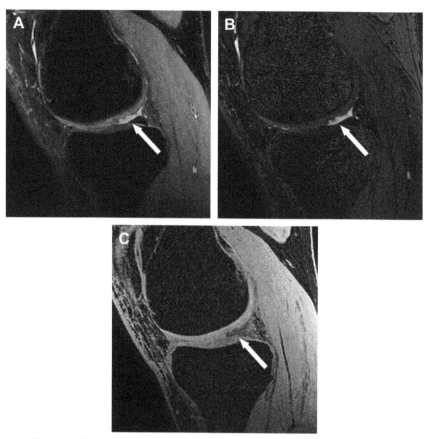

Fig. 7. A 46-year-old man with knee pain. (*A*) Sagittal fat-saturated FSE-Cube, (*B*) sagittal IDEAL-GRASS, and (*C*) sagittal IDEAL-SPGR images of the knee joint show a superficial partial-thickness cartilage lesion (*arrows*) on the medial femoral condyle. FSE-Cube and IDEAL-GRASS are examples of bright fluid sequences, which create an arthrogramlike effect within the knee joint, whereas IDEAL-SPGR is an example of a dark fluid sequence. Note how the cartilage lesion is more conspicuous on the FSE-Cube and IDEAL-GRASS images than the IDEAL-SPGR image.

than traditional T1-weighting or T2-weighting. The DEFT sequence can create high-resolution three-dimensional images of the knee joint with bright synovial fluid when combined with a three-dimensional echo-planar readout. Cartilage signal is preserved by the use of a short echo time. The DEFT sequence has similar cartilage SNR to 2D-FSE and fat-suppressed SPGR sequences with as much as 4 times greater contrast between cartilage and synovial fluid.[76] The bright synovial fluid on DEFT images creates an arthrogramlike effect that may potentially increase the conspicuity of superficial cartilage lesions.

Three-dimensional Balanced Steady-state Sequences

Balanced steady-state free-precession (SSFP) sequences are additional three-dimensional sequences that have been used for evaluating articular cartilage. Balanced SSFP sequences include

commercially available sequences such as fast imaging using steady-state acquisition (FIESTA; GE Healthcare), true fast imaging with steady-state precession (true-FISP; Siemens Medical Systems), and balanced fast field echo imaging (balanced-FFE; Philips Healthcare), and variants such as fluctuating equilibrium magnetic resonance (FEMR),[77] vastly undersampled isotropic projection steady-state free precession (VIPR-SSFP),[78] and alternating repetition time vastly undersampled isotropic projection steady-state free precession (VIPR-ATR).[79] Balanced SSFP sequences can be combined with various methods of fat suppression such as water excitation,[80] linear combination,[81] intermittent frequency-selective fat saturation,[82] phase detection,[83] and IDEAL.[84] These sequences have higher cartilage SNR and higher contrast between cartilage and synovial fluid than 2D-FSE and three-dimensional fat-saturated SPGR sequences.[77,85–87] Balanced SSFP sequences also have highly versatile tissue contrast that can be used to evaluate the menisci, ligament, and osseous structures in addition to articular cartilage.[88,89]

The use of balanced SSFP sequences for evaluating articular cartilage has increased in recent years because of improvements in MR imaging technology that have reduced artifacts associated with eddy current–induced signal distortions and off-resonance effects.[90] However, banding artifacts caused by off resonance are still problematic when using long repetition times and high field strength scanners. To reduce banding artifacts, repetition times for balanced SSFP sequences are typically kept to less than 10 milliseconds, which ultimately limits spatial resolution. Balanced SSFP sequences with multiple acquisitions can be used to achieve higher resolution at the expense of additional scan time.[91]

The VIPR-SSFP sequence is a balanced SSFP variant that uses a highly SNR-efficient, dual-echo, radial k-space trajectory to improve spatial resolution while maintaining clinically feasible scan times. Unlike Cartesian methods, VIPR-SSFP sequence does not require phase encoding, slice encoding, or dephasing gradients, which allows for almost continuous acquisition of data. The sequence uses a linear combination method to separate signal from fat and water. At 1.5T, the optimal repetition time for linear combination fat-water separation is 2.4 milliseconds, which can be achieved while maintaining adequate time to allow for spatial encoding.[85] However, linear combination balanced SSFP sequences such as VIPR-SSFP are difficult to implement at 3.0T because of limitations on the time available for spatial encoding with the increase in magnetic field strength. At 3.0T, linear combination fat-water separation is performed by using a repetition time of 3.6 milliseconds and skipping a fat passband. The skipped passband increases the sensitivity to magnetic field inhomogeneity. However, the VIPR-SSFP sequence exploits the phase progression between the 2 half-echoes acquired within each repetition time to improve fat-water separation and reduce the sensitivity to off-resonance artifacts.[92] The VIPR-SSFP sequence can acquire multiplanar, fat-suppressed images of the knee joint with 0.5-mm isotropic resolution at 1.5T and 0.4-mm isotropic resolution at 3.0T following a single 5-minute acquisition.[85,92]

The VIPR-ATR sequence is another balanced SSFP variant that uses the highly SNR-efficient, dual-echo VIPR radial k-space trajectory. The VIPR-ATR sequence uses 2 different alternating length repetition times and radiofrequency phase cycling to create a null for off-resonance fat signal during the balanced SSFP acquisition. Compared with VIPR-SSFP, the VIPR-ATR sequence offers enhanced image quality with comparable fat suppression because its single k space acquisition allows for a reduction in undersampling artifact. Furthermore, the ability to image on-resonance avoids the image blurring associated with the VIPR-SSFP sequence when higher resolution requires longer data acquisition intervals. VIPR-ATR can acquire multiplanar, fat-suppressed images of the knee joint with 0.3-mm isotropic resolution at 3.0T following a single 8-minute acquisition (**Fig. 8**).[79] In contrast, the water-excitation DESS sequence used in the Osteoarthritis Initiative produces images of the knee joint with $0.4 \times 0.5 \times 0.7$-mm voxel size at 3.0T with an acquisition time of more than 10 minutes.[74]

DIAGNOSTIC PERFORMANCE OF MORPHOLOGIC CARTILAGE IMAGING SEQUENCES

Multiple previous studies with surgical correlation have documented the diagnostic performance of various MR imaging techniques for evaluating the articular cartilage of the knee joint on both 1.5T and 3.0T imaging systems.[7,48–52,56,75,88,89,93–96] The sensitivity and specificity of these sequences for detecting surgically confirmed cartilage lesions are summarized in **Table 1**. In most studies, diagnostic performance is highest on the thick articular surface of the patella and lowest on the lateral tibial plateau where the curved articular surface is more prone to partial volume averaging and imaging artifacts. Diagnostic performance is also higher for deep partial-thickness and full-thickness cartilage lesions than for superficial cartilage lesions. On 1.5T imaging systems, cartilage imaging sequences have sensitivity values ranging between 45% for water-excitation true-FISP[89] and 94% for 2D-FSE,[49] with specificity values ranging between 70%[50] and 99%.[49] On 3.0T imaging systems, these sequences have sensitivity values ranging between 66% for IDEAL-GRASS[94] to 80% for 2D-FSE,[51] with specificity values ranging between 80%[50] and 97%.[51] It is impossible to compare the sensitivity and specificity values of the various sequences used in previously published studies because of differences in MR imaging hardware, imaging parameters, patient populations, and reader experience.

Studies directly comparing various two-dimensional and three-dimensional sequences for evaluating the articular cartilage of the knee joint tend to show similar diagnostic performance for the differing techniques (**Fig. 9**). Duc and colleagues[95] found that water-excitation true-

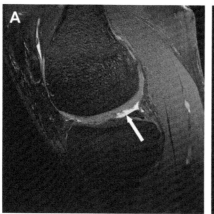
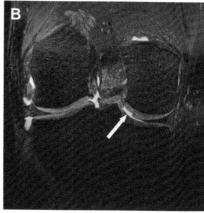

Fig. 8. A 47-year-old man with knee pain. (*A*) Sagittal and (*B*) coronal VIPR-ATR images of the knee joint show a superficial partial-thickness cartilage lesion (*arrows*) on the medial femoral condyle. Because of its highly SNR-efficient radial k-space trajectory, VIPR-ATR can acquire 0.3-mm isotropic resolution images of the knee joint with balanced SSFP tissue contrast in an 8-minute scan time.

Table 1
Diagnostic performance of various two-dimensional and three-dimensional sequences for detecting surgically confirmed cartilage lesions within the knee joint

Sequence	Field Strength	Voxel Size (mm)	Number of Subjects	Sensitivity (%)	Specificity (%)
2D fast spin echo[52]	1.5T	0.3×0.6×3.5	88	87	94
2D fast spin echo[49]	1.5T	0.5×0.7×4.0	130	94	99
2D fast spin echo[48]	1.5T	0.3×0.6×4.0	54	59–74	87–91
2D fast spin echo[93]	1.5T	0.6×0.6×4.0	26	91	98
2D fast spin echo[95]	1.5T	0.4×0.7×3.0	30	63–67	88–94
2D fast spin echo[50]	1.5T	0.5×0.6×3.0	100	61–74	70–90
2D fast spin echo[51]	1.5T	0.5×0.6×3.0	26	59–74	92–97
Water excitation SPGR[95]	1.5T	0.4×0.4×1.7	30	62–74	78–89
Fat-saturated SPGR[7]	1.5T	0.5×0.9×1.5	114	75–85	94–97
Water excitation true-FISP[95]	1.5T	0.4×0.7×1.7	30	58–64	80–94
Water excitation true-FISP[89]	1.5T	0.6×0.6×0.6	30	45–63	82–83
VIPR-SSFP[88]	1.5T	0.5×0.5×0.5	95	77	92
Water excitation FLASH[93]	1.5T	0.6×0.6×2.0	26	46	92
DESS[96]	1.5T	0.6×0.8×1.4	80	83	97
Water excitation DESS[95]	1.5T	0.4×0.7×1.7	30	56–72	78–95
DEFT[75]	1.5T	0.3×0.8×3.0	24	69	93
2D fast spin echo[50]	3.0T	0.4×0.6×3.0	100	70–71	80–93
2D fast spin echo[51]	3.0T	0.4×0.6×3.0	26	67–80	92–97
IDEAL-GRASS[94]	3.0T	0.4×0.7×1.0	95	66–71	93–94
Fat-saturated FSE-Cube[56]	3.0T	0.7×0.7×0.7	100	73	89

Ranges are for multiple readers in some studies.

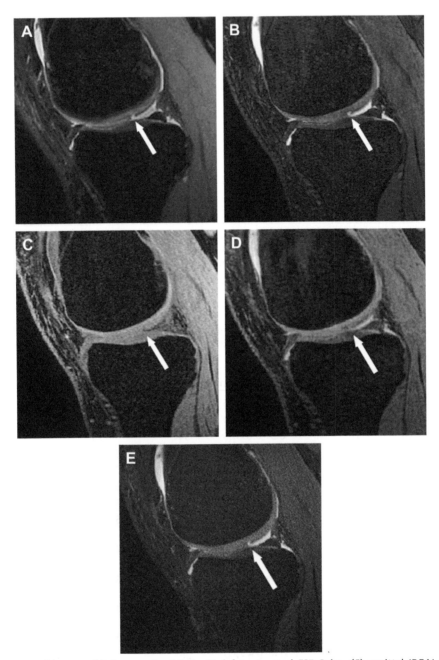

Fig. 9. A 44-year-old man with knee pain. (*A*) Sagittal fat-saturated FSE-Cube, (*B*) sagittal IDEAL-GRASS, (*C*) sagittal IDEAL-SPGR, (*D*) sagittal water-excitation DESS, and (*E*) sagittal VIPR-SSFP images of the knee joint show a superficial cartilage fissure (*arrows*) on the medial femoral condyle.

FISP, fat-saturated intermediate-weighted 2D-FSE, water-excitation DESS, and fat-saturated FLASH sequences had similar sensitivity and specificity for detecting surgically confirmed cartilage lesions in 30 patients at 1.5T. Kijowski and colleagues[88] found that an isotropic resolution VIPR-SSFP sequence had similar sensitivity and significantly higher (*P*<.05) specificity than a routine MR imaging protocol consisting of multiplanar fat-saturated, intermediate-weighted, and T2-weighted 2D-FSE sequences for detecting surgically confirmed cartilage lesions in 95 patients at 1.5T. In a study performed on 26 patients with surgical correlation at 1.5T, Mohr[93] found that a fat-saturated, intermediate-weighted 2D-FSE sequence had significantly higher (*P*<.05) sensitivity and similar specificity as a water-excitation FLASH sequence for detecting cartilage lesions. In a comparison of fat-saturated intermediate-weighted 2D-FSE, water-excitation DESS, and water-excitation SPACE sequences for detecting histologically confirmed cartilage lesions in 10 cadaveric patellar specimens at 1.5T, Schaefer and colleagues[97] found results comparable with earlier reports with superior performance of the 2D-FSE sequence. In 2 separate studies performed at 3.0T on 100 patients with surgical correlation, Kijowski and colleagues[56,94] found that fat-saturated FSE-Cube[56] and IDEAL-GRASS[94] sequences had sensitivity and specificity for detecting cartilage lesions that were similar to those of a routine MR imaging protocol consisting of multiplanar fat-saturated intermediate-weighted and T2-weighted 2D-FSE

sequences. There is little evidence to suggest that newly developed three-dimensional cartilage imaging sequences outperform currently used 2D-FSE sequences for evaluating the articular cartilage of the knee joint in clinical practice.

Most cartilage imaging has focused on the knee joint. Few previous studies have documented the diagnostic performance of MR imaging for evaluating the articular cartilage of the hip joint. Accurate cartilage assessment within the hip joint is challenging because of the thin articular cartilage and spherical surface geometry of the femoral head and acetabulum. Furthermore, the need for a large field of view and the absence of specialized coils for evaluating the hip joint result in images with low spatial resolution. The sensitivity of MR imaging for detecting surgically confirmed

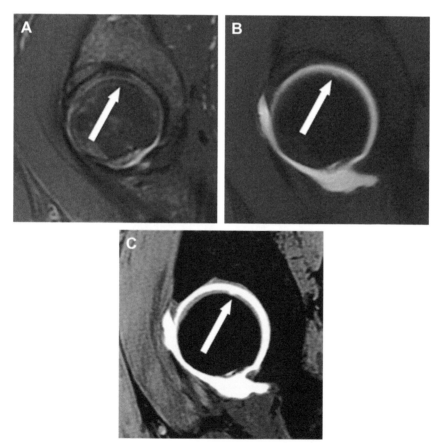

Fig. 10. A 46-year-old woman with a surgically confirmed, deep, partial-thickness cartilage lesion on the posterior superior femoral head. (A) Sagittal, two-dimensional, fat-saturated, intermediate-weighted FSE image of the hip joint from an MR imaging examination shows normal-appearing articular cartilage (arrow) on the posterior superior femoral head. (B) Sagittal, two-dimensional, fat-saturated, T1-weighted FSE image and (C) sagittal IDEAL-SPGR image of the hip joint from an MR arthrogram examination performed 2 weeks later show a small, contrast-filled, deep, partial-thickness cartilage defect (arrow) on the posterior superior femoral head. The cartilage lesion is more conspicuous on the IDEAL-SPGR images because of distension of the joint with contrast and use of a thinner volumetric acquisition. (From Kijowski R. Clinical cartilage imaging of the knee and hip joint. Am J Roentgenol 2010;195(3):625; with permission.)

cartilage lesions within the hip joint range between 49% for fat-saturated SPGR sequences[98] and 93% for 2D-FSE sequences,[99] with specificity values ranging between 76% and 89%. Because of the limitations of MR imaging, MR arthrography has become the imaging modality of choice for evaluating patients with suspected hip joint degeneration (**Fig. 10**). However, the diagnostic performance of MR arthrography is not much better than MR imaging, with sensitivity values for detecting surgically confirmed cartilage lesions ranging between 41% and 79% and specificity values ranging between 77% and 100%.[100,101] Future development of more SNR-efficient sequences and specialized multichannel coils

may allow images with higher spatial resolution and thinner slices to be obtained in clinically feasible scan times, which may improve the ability of MR imaging and MR arthrography to evaluate the articular cartilage of the hip joint.

LIMITATIONS OF CARTILAGE IMAGING SEQUENCES

MR imaging techniques face several limitations that may become particularly problematic when applied to cartilage imaging. Articular cartilage is a thin structure with complex geometry. Both the articular surface and the interface between cartilage and subchondral bone are important sites of

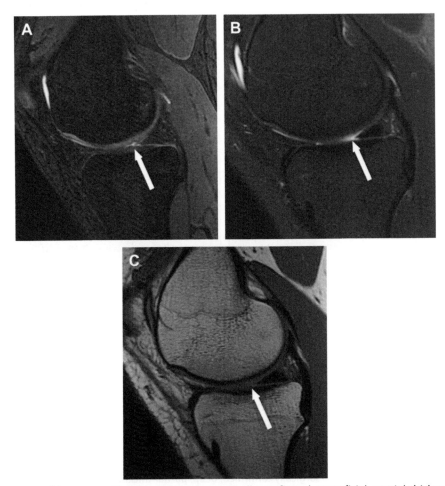

Fig. 11. A 20-year-old woman with knee pain and a surgically confirmed, superficial, partial-thickness cartilage lesion on the medial femoral condyle. (*A*) Sagittal VIPR-SSFP image of the knee joint shows a superficial partial-thickness cartilage lesion (*arrows*) on the medial femoral condyle. (*B*) Sagittal, two-dimensional, fat-saturated, T2-weighted FSE image and (*C*) sagittal, two-dimensional, intermediate-weighted FSE image of the knee joint show normal articular cartilage (*arrows*) on the medial femoral condyle. The cartilage lesion could not be visualized on the fat-saturated, T2-weighted FSE image because of partial volume averaging secondary to the thick slices and gaps between slices and could not be visualized on the intermediate-weighted FSE image because of suboptimal contrast between articular cartilage and synovial fluid.

injury that may be partially obscured because of limited spatial resolution and artifact. Of particular interest in clinical cartilage imaging is the detection and characterization of superficial cartilage lesions. Traditionally, it has been in this role that morphologic cartilage imaging sequences have been least accurate. In multiple studies with surgical correlation, the sensitivity of various two-dimensional and three-dimensional sequences for detecting superficial cartilage lesions range between 44% and 75% for the knee joint,[49,50,56,75,94] and are as low as 22% for the hip joint.[102]

The low sensitivity of MR imaging for detecting superficial cartilage lesions may be the result of secondary suboptimal tissue contrast,[69] partial volume averaging,[103] and the inability to evaluate cartilage in multiple planes (**Fig. 11**).[49] However, the main factor that limits the ability of currently available MR imaging techniques to identify early

cartilage degeneration is suboptimal spatial resolution. In-plane spatial resolution of 0.3 mm has been shown to be necessary to detect superficial morphologic changes of articular cartilage such as fibrillation and pitting, which is beyond the capability of most clinically available sequences.[104] Occasionally, superficial cartilage lesions can be identified on T2-weighted 2D-FSE sequences as areas of increased signal intensity within articular cartilage (**Fig. 12**).[105,106] The increased signal intensity is presumably secondary to increased water content and altered collagen ultrastructure of degenerative cartilage, which can be detected using the high fluid sensitivity and magnetization transfer contrast of T2-weighted 2D-FSE sequences.[54,107] However, signal intensity changes within articular cartilage are nonspecific findings and may also be the result of imaging artifacts such as truncation[108] and magic angle effect.[109]

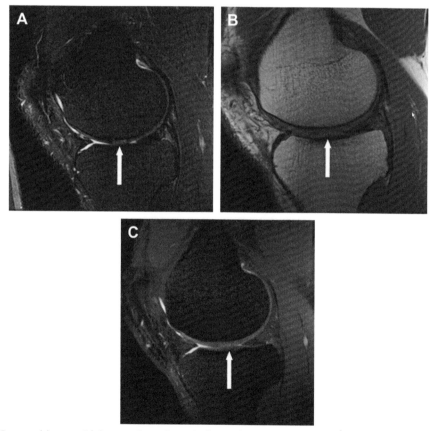

Fig. 12. A 43-year-old man with knee pain and surgically confirmed superficial cartilage fibrillation on the medial femoral condyle. (*A*) Sagittal, two-dimensional, fat-saturated, T2-weighted FSE image of the knee joint shows an area of high signal intensity within the articular cartilage (*arrow*) of the medial femoral condyle. (*B*) Sagittal, two-dimensional, intermediate-weighted FSE image and (*C*) sagittal VIPR-SSFP image of the knee joint show normal articular cartilage (*arrows*) on the medial femoral condyle. Superficial cartilage fibrillation could not be visualized on the intermediate-weighted FSE and VIPR-SSFP images because of decreased fluid sensitivity and lack of magnetization transfer effect compared with the fat-saturated T2-weighted FSE image.

In addition, the signal intensity of articular cartilage on T2-weighted 2D-FSE images is also influenced by the degree of articular surface compression.[110]

HIGH FIELD STRENGTH CARTILAGE IMAGING

The use of high field strength 3.0T MR imaging systems is becoming widespread in clinical practice and has the potential to improve cartilage imaging. 3.0T systems can produce images of articular cartilage with higher spatial resolution and decreased slice thickness compared with 1.5T systems without reducing SNR or prolonging acquisition time. 3.0T systems can also create images with greater contrast between cartilage and adjacent joint structures.[111,112] The improvement in spatial resolution, slice thickness, and tissue contrast made possible by the use of 3.0T

MR imaging systems may allow for better detection and characterization of cartilage lesions in patients with joint pain.

Experimental studies comparing 1.5T and 3.0T MR imaging systems for detecting cartilage lesions in animal and human cadaver models have shown an improved diagnostic performance of 3.0T systems.[111,113–116] Two clinical studies have also compared the diagnostic performance of multiplanar fat-saturated 2D-FSE sequences performed at 1.5T and 3.0T for detecting cartilage lesions within the knee joint (**Fig. 13**). Kijowski and colleagues[50] compared the diagnostic performance of 2D-FSE sequences performed at 1.5T and 3.0T on 2 different patient populations each consisting of 100 individuals with surgical correlation. The sequences had significantly higher ($P<.05$) specificity and accuracy and similar

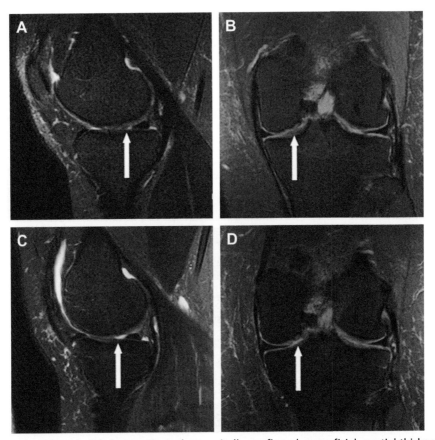

Fig. 13. A 36-year-old man with knee pain and a surgically confirmed, superficial, partial-thickness cartilage lesion on the medial femoral condyle. (*A*) Sagittal and (*B*) coronal two-dimensional fat-saturated T2-weighted FSE images of the knee joint from a 1.5T MR imaging examination show subtle irregularity of the articular cartilage (*arrows*) on the medial femoral condyle. (*C*) Sagittal and (*D*) coronal two-dimensional, fat-saturated, T2-weighted FSE images of the knee joint from a 3.0T MR imaging examination performed 3 weeks later show a focal, superficial, partial-thickness cartilage defect (*arrows*) on the medial femoral condyle. (*From* Kijowski R. Clinical cartilage imaging of the knee and hip joint. Am J Roentgenol 2010;195(3):624; with permission.)

sensitivity for detecting cartilage lesions at 3.0T than at 1.5T.[50] In a second study performed on 26 patients with surgical correlation who were evaluated on both 1.5T and 3.0T systems, Wong and colleagues[51] found that 2D-FSE sequences had significantly higher ($P<.05$) sensitivity and similar specificity and accuracy for detecting cartilage lesions at 3.0T. In both studies, the 2D-FSE sequences had significantly higher ($P<.05$) accuracy of grading cartilage lesions at 3.0T. These studies clearly document an improved diagnostic performance of 2D-FSE sequences for detecting and characterizing cartilage lesions within the knee joint at 3.0T rather than at 1.5T. Diagnostic performance can be further improved at 3.0T if specialized three-dimensional cartilage imaging sequences are used along with 2D-FSE sequences to evaluate articular cartilage.[117]

Ultrahigh field strength MR imaging is an emerging technology that has the potential to further improve cartilage imaging. An increase in magnetic field strength from 3.0T to 7.0T results in an increase in SNR by a factor of 2.3.[118] Although SNR may be significantly improved with increasing field strength to more than 3.0T, certain limitations become more problematic. Drawbacks of ultrahigh field strength MR imaging include an increase in susceptibility, pulsation, and chemical shift artifacts.[119] To compensate for greater chemical shift artifact, the receiver bandwidth needs be increased, which causes a reduction in SNR. In addition, energy deposition in tissue increases with increasing magnetic field strength, and limitations of the specific absorption rate on ultrahigh field strength MR imaging systems may prohibit the use of certain types of sequences, especially those that require multiple refocusing pulses.[120] Physiologic sensations such as vertigo and light flashes also become more disturbing on ultrahigh field strength MR imaging systems, reflecting an increased sensitivity to motion in the higher magnetic field.[121]

Despite the potential drawbacks of ultrahigh field strength MR imaging systems, the promise of increased SNR makes it an attractive technology for evaluating articular cartilage. The feasibility of evaluating articular cartilage on ultrahigh field strength systems has been shown in healthy volunteers.[122,123] In addition, Stahl and colleagues[124] compared image quality and diagnostic confidence of fat-saturated intermediate-weighted 2D-FSE, SPGR, and FIESTA sequences performed at 3.0T and 7.0T on 10 patients with osteoarthritis of the knee joint. For the intermediate-weighted 2D-FSE sequence, limitations of the specific absorption rate required modification of the imaging parameters yielding incomplete coverage of the knee joint,

extensive chemical shift and pulsation artifacts, and suboptimal fat suppression. However, the SPGR and FIESTA sequences were found to be well suited for evaluating articular cartilage at 7.0T. Both sequences had significantly higher ($P<.05$) cartilage SNR at 7.0T than at 3.0T, and the FIESTA sequence had significantly higher ($P<.05$) contrast between cartilage and synovial fluid at 7.0T. Despite improvements in image quality for the SPGR and FIESTA sequences at 7.0T, there was no statistically significant difference in the sensitivity or diagnostic confidence of the sequences at 3.0T and 7.0T for detecting cartilage lesions within the knee joint. Additional studies are needed to document an advantage of using ultrahigh field strength MR imaging systems for evaluation of articular cartilage in clinical practice and osteoarthritis research studies.

SUMMARY

MR imaging remains the imaging modality of choice for morphologic evaluation of articular cartilage. Accurate detection and characterization of cartilage lesions is necessary to guide medical and surgical therapy and remains a primary role of imaging of the musculoskeletal system. The variety of MR imaging techniques available for evaluating articular cartilage underscores the challenges of providing accurate noninvasive diagnosis of cartilage lesions. Limited spatial resolution, suboptimal tissue contrast, and artifacts remain major hurdles in the development of clinically useful sequences. Recent work using 3.0T MR imaging systems shows promise in improving the detection and characterization of cartilage lesions in patients with joint pain. In the future, the use ultrahigh field strength MR imaging systems, multichannel coils, and more SNR-efficient sequences may allow images of articular cartilage to be obtained with even higher spatial resolution and greater tissue contrast in clinically feasible scan times. The improved image quality may allow for better evaluation of articular cartilage and earlier detection of degenerative and posttraumatic cartilage lesions in symptomatic patients.

REFERENCES

1. Arthritis: meeting the challenge. At-A-Glance. Atlanta (GA): Centers for Disease Control and Prevention. Atlanta (GA), 2010.
2. Murphy LB, Helmick CG, Schwartz TA, et al. Lifetime risk of symptomatic knee osteoarthritis. Arthritis Rheum 2008;59(9):1207–13.
3. Zhang Y, Jordan JM. Epidemiology of osteoarthritis. Rheum Dis Clin North Am 2008;34(3): 515–29.

4. Dagenais S, Garbedian S, Wai EK. Systematic review of the prevalence of radiographic primary hip osteoarthritis. Clin Orthop Relat Res 2009; 467(3):623–37.

5. Buckwalter JA, Brown TD. Joint injury, repair, and remodeling: roles in post-traumatic osteoarthritis. Clin Orthop Relat Res 2004;(423):7–16.

6. Hellio Le Graverand MP, Mazzuca S, Duryea J, et al. Radiographic-based grading methods and radiographic measurement of joint space width in osteoarthritis. Radiol Clin North Am 2009;47(4):567–79.

7. Disler DG, McCauley TR, Kelman CG, et al. Fat-suppressed three-dimensional spoiled gradient-echo MR imaging of hyaline cartilage defects in the knee: comparison with standard MR imaging and arthroscopy. AJR Am J Roentgenol 1996; 167(1):127–32.

8. Jackson DW, Simon TM, Aberman HM. Symptomatic articular cartilage degeneration: the impact in the new millennium. Clin Orthop Relat Res 2001;(Suppl 391):S14–25.

9. Malemud CJ. Anticytokine therapy for osteoarthritis: evidence to date. Drugs Aging 2010;27(2): 95–115.

10. Hellio Le Graverand-Gastineau MP. OA clinical trials: current targets and trials for OA. Choosing molecular targets: what have we learned and where we are headed? Osteoarthritis Cartilage 2009;17(11):1393–401.

11. Kaplan LD, Lu Y, Snitzer J, et al. The effect of early hyaluronic acid delivery on the development of an acute articular cartilage lesion in a sheep model. Am J Sports Med 2009;37(12):2323–7.

12. Bedi A, Feeley BT, Williams RJ 3rd. Management of articular cartilage defects of the knee. J Bone Joint Surg Am 2010;92(4):994–1009.

13. Hangody L, Fules P. Autologous osteochondral mosaicplasty for the treatment of full-thickness defects of weight-bearing joints: ten years of experimental and clinical experience. J Bone Joint Surg Am 2003;85-A(Suppl 2):25–32.

14. Muller S, Breederveld RS, Tuinebreijer WE. Results of osteochondral autologous transplantation in the knee. Open Orthop J 2010;4:111–4.

15. Gudas R, Kalesinskas RJ, Kimtys V, et al. A prospective randomized clinical study of mosaic osteochondral autologous transplantation versus microfracture for the treatment of osteochondral defects in the knee joint in young athletes. Arthroscopy 2005;21(9):1066–75.

16. Gikas PD, Aston WJ, Briggs TW. Autologous chondrocyte implantation: where do we stand now? J Orthop Sci 2008;13(3):283–92.

17. Brittberg M, Lindahl A, Nilsson A, et al. Treatment of deep cartilage defects in the knee with autologous chondrocyte transplantation. N Engl J Med 1994;331(14):889–95.

18. Clohisy JC, Beaule PE, O'Malley A, et al. AOA symposium. Hip disease in the young adult: current concepts of etiology and surgical treatment. J Bone Joint Surg Am 2008;90(10):2267–81.

19. Leunig M, Beaule PE, Ganz R. The concept of femoroacetabular impingement: current status and future perspectives. Clin Orthop Relat Res 2009; 467(3):616–22.

20. Ganz R, Parvizi J, Beck M, et al. Femoroacetabular impingement: a cause for osteoarthritis of the hip. Clin Orthop Relat Res 2003;(417):112–20.

21. Jacobsen S. Adult hip dysplasia and osteoarthritis. Studies in radiology and clinical epidemiology. Acta Orthop Suppl 2006;77(324):1–37.

22. Lievense AM, Bierma-Zeinstra S, Schouten B, et al. Influence of hip dysplasia on the development of osteoarthritis of the hip. Ann Rheum Dis 2004; 63(6):621–6.

23. Philippon MJ, Briggs KK, Yen YM, et al. Outcomes following hip arthroscopy for femoroacetabular impingement with associated chondrolabral dysfunction: minimum two-year follow-up. J Bone Joint Surg Br 2009;91(1):16–23.

24. Brunner A, Horisberger M, Herzog RF. Sports and recreation activity of patients with femoroacetabular impingement before and after arthroscopic osteoplasty. Am J Sports Med 2009; 37(5):917–22.

25. Beck M, Leunig M, Parvizi J, et al. Anterior femoroacetabular impingement: part II. Midterm results of surgical treatment. Clin Orthop Relat Res 2004;(418):67–73.

26. Sanchez-Sotelo J, Trousdale RT, Berry DJ, et al. Surgical treatment of developmental dysplasia of the hip in adults: I. Nonarthroplasty options. J Am Acad Orthop Surg 2002;10(5):321–33.

27. Siebenrock KA, Schoeniger R, Ganz R. Anterior femoro-acetabular impingement due to acetabular retroversion. Treatment with periacetabular osteotomy. J Bone Joint Surg Am 2003;85-A(2):278–86.

28. Sambandam SN, Hull J, Jiranek WA. Factors predicting the failure of Bernese periacetabular osteotomy: a meta-regression analysis. Int Orthop 2009; 33(6):1483–8.

29. Clohisy JC, St John LC, Schutz AL. Surgical treatment of femoroacetabular impingement: a systematic review of the literature. Clin Orthop Relat Res 2010;468(2):555–64.

30. Waldschmidt JG, Rilling RJ, Kajdacsy-Balla AA, et al. In vitro and in vivo MR imaging of hyaline cartilage: zonal anatomy, imaging pitfalls, and pathologic conditions. Radiographics 1997;17(6): 1387–402.

31. Kijowski R, Lu A, Block W, et al. Subchondral bone marrow edema in patients with degeneration of the articular cartilage of the knee joint. Radiology 2006;238(3):943–9.

32. Link TM. Correlations between joint morphology and pain and between magnetic resonance imaging, histology, and micro-computed tomography. J Bone Joint Surg Am 2009;91(Suppl 1): 30–2.

33. Zanetti M, Bruder E, Romero J, et al. Bone marrow edema pattern in osteoarthritic knees: correlation between MR imaging and histologic findings. Radiology 2000;215(3):835–40.

34. Saadat E, Jobke B, Chu B, et al. Diagnostic performance of in vivo 3-T MRI for articular cartilage abnormalities in human osteoarthritic knees using histology as standard of reference. Eur Radiol 2008;18(10):2292–302.

35. Felson DT, Chaisson CE, Hill CL, et al. The association of bone marrow lesions with pain in knee osteoarthritis. Ann Intern Med 2001;134(7):541–9.

36. Davies-Tuck ML, Wluka AE, Forbes A, et al. Development of bone marrow lesions is associated with adverse effects on knee cartilage while resolution is associated with improvement–a potential target for prevention of knee osteoarthritis: a longitudinal study. Arthritis Res Ther 2010;12(1):R10.

37. Roemer FW, Guermazi A, Javaid MK, et al. Change in MRI-detected subchondral bone marrow lesions is associated with cartilage loss: the MOST Study. A longitudinal multicentre study of knee osteoarthritis. Ann Rheum Dis 2009;68(9):1461–5.

38. Neogi T, Felson D, Niu J, et al. Cartilage loss occurs in the same subregions as subchondral bone attrition: a within-knee subregion-matched approach from the Multicenter Osteoarthritis Study. Arthritis Rheum 2009;61(11):1539–44.

39. Roemer FW, Neogi T, Nevitt MC, et al. Subchondral bone marrow lesions are highly associated with, and predict subchondral bone attrition longitudinally: the MOST study. Osteoarthritis Cartilage 2010;18(1):47–53.

40. Bolbos RI, Zuo J, Banerjee S, et al. Relationship between trabecular bone structure and articular cartilage morphology and relaxation times in early OA of the knee joint using parallel MRI at 3 T. Osteoarthritis Cartilage 2008;16(10):1150–9.

41. Li X, Ma BC, Bolbos RI, et al. Quantitative assessment of bone marrow edema-like lesion and overlying cartilage in knees with osteoarthritis and anterior cruciate ligament tear using MR imaging and spectroscopic imaging at 3 Tesla. J Magn Reson Imaging 2008;28(2):453–61.

42. Johnson DL, Urban WP Jr, Caborn DN, et al. Articular cartilage changes seen with magnetic resonance imaging-detected bone bruises associated with acute anterior cruciate ligament rupture. Am J Sports Med 1998;26(3):409–14.

43. Tiderius CJ, Olsson LE, Nyquist F, et al. Cartilage glycosaminoglycan loss in the acute phase after an anterior cruciate ligament injury: delayed gadolinium-enhanced magnetic resonance imaging of cartilage and synovial fluid analysis. Arthritis Rheum 2005;52(1):120–7.

44. Bolbos RI, Link TM, Ma CB, et al. T1rho relaxation time of the meniscus and its relationship with T1rho of adjacent cartilage in knees with acute ACL injuries at 3 T. Osteoarthritis Cartilage 2009; 17(1):12–8.

45. Davies NH, Niall D, King LJ, et al. Magnetic resonance imaging of bone bruising in the acutely injured knee–short-term outcome. Clin Radiol 2004;59(5):439–45.

46. Recht MP, Goodwin DW, Winalski CS, et al. MRI of articular cartilage: revisiting current status and future directions. AJR Am J Roentgenol 2005; 185(4):899–914.

47. Rubin DA. Magnetic resonance imaging of chondral and osteochondral injuries. Top Magn Reson Imaging 1998;9(6):348–59.

48. Sonin AH, Pensy RA, Mulligan ME, et al. Grading articular cartilage of the knee using fast spin-echo proton density-weighted MR imaging without fat suppression. AJR Am J Roentgenol 2002; 179(5):1159–66.

49. Bredella MA, Tirman PF, Peterfy CG, et al. Accuracy of T2-weighted fast spin-echo MR imaging with fat saturation in detecting cartilage defects in the knee: comparison with arthroscopy in 130 patients. AJR Am J Roentgenol 1999;172(4): 1073–80.

50. Kijowski R, Blankenbaker DG, Davis KG, et al. Comparison of 1.5- and 3.0-T MR imaging for evaluating the articular cartilage of the knee joint. Radiology 2009;250(3):839–48.

51. Wong S, Steinbach L, Zhao J, et al. Comparative study of imaging at 3.0 T versus 1.5 T of the knee. Skeletal Radiol 2009;38(8):761–9.

52. Potter HG, Linklater JM, Allen AA, et al. Magnetic resonance imaging of articular cartilage in the knee. An evaluation with use of fast-spin-echo imaging. J Bone Joint Surg Am 1998;80(9):1276–84.

53. Gold GE, Chen CA, Koo S, et al. Recent advances in MRI of articular cartilage. AJR Am J Roentgenol 2009;193(3):628–38.

54. Yao L, Gentili A, Thomas A. Incidental magnetization transfer contrast in fast spin-echo imaging of cartilage. J Magn Reson Imaging 1996;6(1):180–4.

55. Gold GE, Busse RF, Beehler C, et al. Isotropic MRI of the knee with 3D fast spin-echo extended echo-train acquisition (XETA): initial experience. AJR Am J Roentgenol 2007;188(5):1287–93.

56. Kijowski R, Davis KW, Woods MA, et al. Knee joint: comprehensive assessment with 3D isotropic resolution fast spin-echo MR imaging–diagnostic performance compared with that of conventional MR imaging at 3.0 T. Radiology 2009;252(2): 486–95.

57. Notohamiprodjo M, Horng A, Pietschmann MF, et al. MRI of the knee at 3T: first clinical results with an isotropic PDfs-weighted 3D-TSE-sequence. Invest Radiol 2009;44(9):585–97.

58. Recht MP, Kramer J, Marcelis S, et al. Abnormalities of articular cartilage in the knee: analysis of available MR techniques. Radiology 1993;187(2): 473–8.

59. Recht MP, Piraino DW, Paletta GA, et al. Accuracy of fat-suppressed three-dimensional spoiled gradient-echo FLASH MR imaging in the detection of patellofemoral articular cartilage abnormalities. Radiology 1996;198(1):209–12.

60. Disler DG, McCauley TR, Wirth CR, et al. Detection of knee hyaline cartilage defects using fat-suppressed three-dimensional spoiled gradient-echo MR imaging: comparison with standard MR imaging and correlation with arthroscopy. AJR Am J Roentgenol 1995;165(2):377–82.

61. Hardy PA, Recht MP, Piraino DW. Fat suppressed MRI of articular cartilage with a spatial-spectral excitation pulse. J Magn Reson Imaging 1998; 8(6):1279–87.

62. Yoshioka H, Alley M, Steines D, et al. Imaging of the articular cartilage in osteoarthritis of the knee joint: 3D spatial-spectral spoiled gradient-echo vs. fat-suppressed 3D spoiled gradient-echo MR imaging. J Magn Reson Imaging 2003;18(1): 66–71.

63. Siepmann DB, McGovern J, Brittain JH, et al. High-resolution 3D cartilage imaging with IDEAL SPGR at 3 T. AJR Am J Roentgenol 2007;189(6):1510–5.

64. Chen CA, Lu W, John CT, et al. Multiecho IDEAL gradient-echo water-fat separation for rapid assessment of cartilage volume at 1.5 T: initial experience. Radiology 2009;252(2):561–7.

65. Kijowski R, Tuite M, Passov L, et al. Cartilage imaging at 3.0T with gradient refocused acquisition in the steady-state (GRASS) and IDEAL fat-water separation. J Magn Reson Imaging 2008;28(1): 167–74.

66. Marshall KW, Mikulis DJ, Guthrie BM. Quantitation of articular cartilage using magnetic resonance imaging and three-dimensional reconstruction. J Orthop Res 1995;13(6):814–23.

67. Peterfy CG, van Dijke CF, Janzen DL, et al. Quantification of articular cartilage in the knee with pulsed saturation transfer subtraction and fat-suppressed MR imaging: optimization and validation. Radiology 1994;192(2):485–91.

68. Kijowski RB, Reeder R, Takami S, et al. SPGR and imaging of the knee at 3T with water excitation and 2D autocalibrating parallel imaging. In: Proceedings of the 16th Annual Scientific Meeting of the International Society of Magnetic Resonance in Medicine. Toronto, 2008.

69. Mosher TJ, Pruett SW. Magnetic resonance imaging of superficial cartilage lesions: role of contrast in lesion detection. J Magn Reson Imaging 1999;10(2):178–82.

70. Hardy PA, Recht MP, Piraino D, et al. Optimization of a dual echo in the steady state (DESS) free-precession sequence for imaging cartilage. J Magn Reson Imaging 1996;6(2):329–35.

71. Moriya S, Miki Y, Yokobayashi T, et al. Three-dimensional double-echo steady-state (3D-DESS) magnetic resonance imaging of the knee: contrast optimization by adjusting flip angle. Acta Radiol 2009;50(5):507–11.

72. Deimling M, Jellus V, Horger W, et al. Self weighted combination of SSFP echoes with a double-echo steady state (DESS) sequence. In: Proceedings of the 13th Annual Scientific Meeting of International Society of Magnetic Resonance in Medicine. South Beach, Miami (FL), 2005.

73. Friedrich KM, Reiter G, Kaiser B, et al. High-resolution cartilage imaging of the knee at 3T: Basic evaluation of modern isotropic 3D MR-sequences. Eur J Radiol 2010. [Epub ahead of print].

74. Peterfy CG, Schneider E, Nevitt M. The Osteoarthritis Initiative: report on the design rationale for the magnetic resonance imaging protocol for the knee. Osteoarthritis Cartilage 2008; 16(12):1433–41.

75. Gold GE, Fuller SE, Hargreaves BA, et al. Driven equilibrium magnetic resonance imaging of articular cartilage: initial clinical experience. J Magn Reson Imaging 2005;21(4):476–81.

76. Hargreaves BA, Gold GE, Lang PK, et al. MR imaging of articular cartilage using driven equilibrium. Magn Reson Med 1999;42(4):695–703.

77. Gold GE, Hargreaves BA, Vasanawala SS, et al. Articular cartilage of the knee: evaluation with fluctuating equilibrium MR imaging–initial experience in healthy volunteers. Radiology 2006;238(2): 712–8.

78. Lu A, Barger AV, Grist TM, et al. Improved spectral selectivity and reduced susceptibility in SSFP using a near zero TE undersampled three-dimensional PR sequence. J Magn Reson Imaging 2004;19(1):117–23.

79. Klaers JL, Brodsky EK, Block WF, et al. Knee joint assessment: 3D radial fat-suppressed alternating TR SSFP. In: Proceedings of the 18th Annual Scientific Meeting of International Society of Magnetic Resonance in Medicine. Stockholm (Sweden), 2010.

80. Kornaat PR, Doornbos J, van der Molen AJ, et al. Magnetic resonance imaging of knee cartilage using a water selective balanced steady-state free precession sequence. J Magn Reson Imaging 2004;20(5):850–6.

81. Vasanawala SS, Pauly JM, Nishimura DG. Linear combination steady-state free precession MRI. Magn Reson Med 2000;43(1):82–90.

82. Scheffler K, Heid O, Hennig J. Magnetization preparation during the steady state: fat-saturated 3D TrueFISP. Magn Reson Med 2001; 45(6):1075–80.

83. Vasanawala SS, Hargreaves BA, Pauly JM, et al. Rapid musculoskeletal MRI with phase-sensitive steady-state free precession: comparison with routine knee MRI. AJR Am J Roentgenol 2005; 184(5):1450–5.

84. Reeder SB, Pelc NJ, Alley MT, et al. Rapid MR imaging of articular cartilage with steady-state free precession and multipoint fat-water separation. AJR Am J Roentgenol 2003;180(2):357–62.

85. Kijowski R, Lu A, Block W, et al. Evaluation of the articular cartilage of the knee joint with vastly undersampled isotropic projection reconstruction steady-state free precession imaging. J Magn Reson Imaging 2006;24(1):168–75.

86. Duc SR, Koch P, Schmid MR, et al. Diagnosis of articular cartilage abnormalities of the knee: prospective clinical evaluation of a 3D water-excitation true FISP sequence. Radiology 2007; 243(2):475–82.

87. Gold GE, Reeder SB, Yu H, et al. Articular cartilage of the knee: rapid three-dimensional MR imaging at 3.0 T with IDEAL balanced steady-state free precession–initial experience. Radiology 2006; 240(2):546–51.

88. Kijowski R, Blankenbaker DG, Klaers JL, et al. Vastly undersampled isotropic projection steady-state free precession imaging of the knee: diagnostic performance compared with conventional MR. Radiology 2009;251(1):185–94.

89. Duc SR, Pfirrmann CW, Koch PP, et al. Internal knee derangement assessed with 3-minute three-dimensional isovoxel true FISP MR sequence: preliminary study. Radiology 2008;246(2):526–35.

90. Cukur T, Bangerter NK, Nishimura DG. Enhanced spectral shaping in steady-state free precession imaging. Magn Reson Med 2007;58(6):1216–23.

91. Bangerter NK, Hargreaves BA, Vasanawala SS, et al. Analysis of multiple-acquisition SSFP. Magn Reson Med 2004;51(5):1038–47.

92. Klaers J, Jashnani Y, Jung Y, et al. Dual half-echo phase correction for implementation of 3D radial SSFP at 3.0 T. Magn Reson Med 2010;63(2):282–9.

93. Mohr A. The value of water-excitation 3D FLASH and fat-saturated PDw TSE MR imaging for detecting and grading articular cartilage lesions of the knee. Skeletal Radiol 2003;32(7):396–402.

94. Kijowski R, Blankenbaker DG, Woods MA, et al. 3.0-T evaluation of knee cartilage by using three-dimensional IDEAL GRASS imaging: comparison with fast spin-echo imaging. Radiology 2010; 255(1):117–27.

95. Duc SR, Pfirrmann CW, Schmid MR, et al. Articular cartilage defects detected with 3D water-excitation true FISP: prospective comparison with sequences commonly used for knee imaging. Radiology 2007; 245(1):216–23.

96. Murphy BJ. Evaluation of grades 3 and 4 chondromalacia of the knee using T2*-weighted 3D gradient-echo articular cartilage imaging. Skeletal Radiol 2001;30(6):305–11.

97. Schaefer FK, Kurz B, Schaefer PJ, et al. Accuracy and precision in the detection of articular cartilage lesions using magnetic resonance imaging at 1.5 Tesla in an in vitro study with orthopedic and histopathologic correlation. Acta Radiol 2007;48(10):1131–7.

98. Nishii T, Nakanishi K, Sugano N, et al. Articular cartilage evaluation in osteoarthritis of the hip with MR imaging under continuous leg traction. Magn Reson Imaging 1998;16(8):871–5.

99. Mintz DN, Hooper T, Connell D, et al. Magnetic resonance imaging of the hip: detection of labral and chondral abnormalities using noncontrast imaging. Arthroscopy 2005;21(4):385–93.

100. Byrd JW, Jones KS. Diagnostic accuracy of clinical assessment, magnetic resonance imaging, magnetic resonance arthrography, and intra-articular injection in hip arthroscopy patients. Am J Sports Med 2004;32(7):1668–74.

101. Schmid MR, Notzli HP, Zanetti M, et al. Cartilage lesions in the hip: diagnostic effectiveness of MR arthrography. Radiology 2003;226(2):382–6.

102. Anderson LA, Peters CL, Park BB, et al. Acetabular cartilage delamination in femoroacetabular impingement. Risk factors and magnetic resonance imaging diagnosis. J Bone Joint Surg Am 2009;91(2):305–13.

103. Hargreaves BA, Gold GE, Beaulieu CF, et al. Comparison of new sequences for high-resolution cartilage imaging. Magn Reson Med 2003;49(4): 700–9.

104. Rubenstein JD, Li JG, Majumdar S, et al. Image resolution and signal-to-noise ratio requirements for MR imaging of degenerative cartilage. AJR Am J Roentgenol 1997;169(4):1089–96.

105. De Smet AA, Monu JU, Fisher DR, et al. Signs of patellar chondromalacia on sagittal T2-weighted magnetic resonance imaging. Skeletal Radiol 1992;21(2):103–5.

106. McCauley TR, Kier R, Lynch KJ, et al. Chondromalacia patellae: diagnosis with MR imaging. AJR Am J Roentgenol 1992;158(1):101–5.

107. Gray ML, Burstein D, Lesperance LM, et al. Magnetization transfer in cartilage and its constituent macromolecules. Magn Reson Med 1995; 34(3):319–25.

108. Frank LR, Brossmann J, Buxton RB, et al. MR imaging truncation artifacts can create a false laminar appearance in cartilage. AJR Am J Roentgenol 1997;168(2):547–54.

109. Rubenstein JD, Kim JK, Morova-Protzner I, et al. Effects of collagen orientation on MR imaging characteristics of bovine articular cartilage. Radiology 1993;188(1):219–26.

110. Shiomi T, Nishii T, Tanaka H, et al. Loading and knee alignment have significant influence on cartilage MRI T2 in porcine knee joints. Osteoarthritis Cartilage 2010;18(7):902–8.

111. Masi JN, Sell CA, Phan C, et al. Cartilage MR imaging at 3.0 versus that at 1.5 T: preliminary results in a porcine model. Radiology 2005; 236(1):140–50.

112. Kornaat PR, Reeder SB, Koo S, et al. MR imaging of articular cartilage at 1.5T and 3.0T: comparison of SPGR and SSFP sequences. Osteoarthritis Cartilage 2005;13(4):338–44.

113. Link TM, Sell CA, Masi JN, et al. 3.0 vs 1.5 T MRI in the detection of focal cartilage pathology–ROC analysis in an experimental model. Osteoarthritis Cartilage 2006;14(1):63–70.

114. Fischbach F, Bruhn H, Unterhauser F, et al. Magnetic resonance imaging of hyaline cartilage defects at 1.5T and 3.0T: comparison of medium T2-weighted fast spin echo, T1-weighted two-dimensional and three-dimensional gradient echo pulse sequences. Acta Radiol 2005;46(1):67–73.

115. Barr C, Bauer JS, Malfair D, et al. MR imaging of the ankle at 3 Tesla and 1.5 Tesla: protocol optimization and application to cartilage, ligament and tendon pathology in cadaver specimens. Eur Radiol 2007;17(6):1518–28.

116. Bauer JS, Krause SJ, Ross CJ, et al. Volumetric cartilage measurements of porcine knee at 1.5-T and 3.0-T MR imaging: evaluation of precision and accuracy. Radiology 2006;241(2):399–406.

117. Kijowski R, Blankenbaker DG, Woods M, et al. Clinical usefulness of adding 3D cartilage imaging sequences to a routine knee MR protocol. Am J Roentgenol 2011;196(1):159–67.

118. Krug R, Stehling C, Kelley DA, et al. Imaging of the musculoskeletal system in vivo using ultra-high field magnetic resonance at 7 T. Invest Radiol 2009;44(9):613–8.

119. Kuo R, Panchal M, Tanenbaum L, et al. 3.0 Tesla imaging of the musculoskeletal system. J Magn Reson Imaging 2007;25(2):245–61.

120. Regatte RR, Schweitzer ME. Ultra-high-field MRI of the musculoskeletal system at 7.0T. J Magn Reson Imaging 2007;25(2):262–9.

121. Weintraub MI, Khoury A, Cole SP. Biologic effects of 3 Tesla (T) MR imaging comparing traditional 1.5 T and 0.6 T in 1023 consecutive outpatients. J Neuroimaging 2007;17(3):241–5.

122. Krug R, Carballido-Gamio J, Banerjee S, et al. In vivo bone and cartilage MRI using fully-balanced steady-state free-precession at 7 tesla. Magn Reson Med 2007;58(6):1294–8.

123. Pakin SK, Cavalcanti C, La Rocca R, et al. Ultra-high-field MRI of knee joint at 7.0T: preliminary experience. Acad Radiol 2006;13(9):1135–42.

124. Stahl R, Krug R, Kelley DA, et al. Assessment of cartilage-dedicated sequences at ultra-high-field MRI: comparison of imaging performance and diagnostic confidence between 3.0 and 7.0 T with respect to osteoarthritis-induced changes at the knee joint. Skeletal Radiol 2009;38(8):771–83.

MR Imaging of Articular Cartilage Physiology

Jung-Ah Choi, MD, PhD[a,b], Garry E. Gold, MD[a,c,d],*

KEYWORDS

- MR imaging • Articular cartilage • Physiology
- Osteoarthritis

Osteoarthritis (OA) has become the most prevalent chronic disease of the elderly[1,2] and is an important cause of disability in our society, with increasing incidence not only in the United States[3] but in other parts of the world.[4–6] It is primarily a disease of the articular cartilage,[7–9] which may become pathologic by degeneration or acute injury.[10] Because the incidence of the disease is continually increasing, there is a need for accurate noninvasive evaluation before the onset of irreversible changes.[11,12] There are many diagnostic imaging methods for evaluation of the articular cartilage (**Table 1**). Conventional radiography has been used to detect secondary gross changes of the joint cartilage, manifested by the narrowing of the joint space distance,[13] and allows visualization of secondary changes, such as osteophyte formation,[10] but this imaging method only allows detection of later stage of the disease when changes are already irreversible. It does not allow direct visualization of the cartilage. Conventional or computed tomography arthrography has also been used to evaluate surface irregularities of the cartilage; however, it is limited in its invasiveness and provides limited evaluation.[14]

MR imaging has become the best imaging modality for assessment of the articular cartilage[15–19] because of its ability to manipulate contrast to highlight different tissue types.[10] Conventional MR imaging sequences that are currently used for evaluation of cartilage have the ability to depict mostly morphologic changes, such as fibrillation and partial-thickness or full-thickness defects[10]; however, they are limited in their capability for comprehensive assessment of cartilage, with limited spatial resolution[20] and limited information about cartilage physiology.

Commonly used conventional MR imaging methods include two-dimensional or multislice T1-weighted, proton density (PD)-weighted, and T2-weighted imaging with or without fat suppression.[10] New developments in imaging hardware and software include improved gradients and radiofrequency coils, fast or turbo spin echo imaging techniques such as water-only excitation.[10] Although spoiled gradient recalled (SPGR) and gradient echo (GRE) techniques have produced excellent images with high resolution ($0.3 \times 0.6 \times 1.5$ mm)[21] and three-dimensional (3D) SPGR is considered the current standard for morphologic imaging of cartilage,[22,23] these methods have the disadvantages of lack of reliable contrast between cartilage and fluid and long imaging times.[10]

Therefore, newer techniques have emerged for morphologic imaging of cartilage, some of which include dual-echo steady-state (DESS) imaging, driven equilibrium Fourier transform (DEFT) imaging, balanced steady-state free precession (SSFP) imaging with fat suppression and its variants, such as fluctuating equilibrium MR imaging (FEMR), linear combination (LC) SSFP,

[a] Department of Radiology, Stanford University, 300 Pasteur Drive, Stanford, CA 94305, USA
[b] Department of Radiology, Seoul National University Bundang Hospital, Seoul National University College of Medicine, 300 Gumi-dong, Bundang-gu, Seongnam, Gyeongido 463-707, Seoul, South Korea
[c] Department of Bioengineering, Stanford University, 300 Pasteur Drive, Stanford, CA 94305, USA
[d] Department of Orthopedic Surgery, Stanford University, 300 Pasteur Drive, Stanford, CA 94305, USA
* Corresponding author.
E-mail address: gold@stanford.edu

Magn Reson Imaging Clin N Am 19 (2011) 249–282
doi:10.1016/j.mric.2011.02.010
1064-9689/11/$ – see front matter © 2011 Elsevier Inc. All rights reserved.

Table 1
Pros and cons of various MR imaging methods for evaluating cartilage physiology

	Pros	Cons
Sodium imaging	High specificity for PG content. High contrast image without exogenous contrast agent	Requires special coils, high-field scanners, and long imaging times
T1ρ imaging	Sensitive to early PG depletion	Requires high RF power. SAR limits
dGEMRIC	High resolution and sensitivity	Delay before imaging. Need for contrast agent. Possibility of nephrogenic systemic fibrosis in patients with kidney problems
T2 mapping	Sensitive to collagen matrix, water content, and motion	May be less sensitive in detection of early degeneration
Ultrashort echo time imaging	Only technique to examine osteochondral junction	Technical challenges. Disadvantage of scan time. Difficulty in slice selection
Magnetization transfer	Improved contrast between cartilage and fluid; detection of localized cartilage lesions	Difficult quantification. SAR limits
Diffusion-weighted imaging	Postoperative evaluation	Low SNR and spatial resolution

Abbreviations: PG, proteoglycan; RF, radiofrequency; SAR, specific absorption rate; SNR, signal/noise ratio.

incremental decrease in end points through aggressive lipid lowering (IDEAL) SSFP, phase-sensitive SSFP, and vastly interpolated projection reconstruction (VIPR) imaging.[10] These newer methods based on SSFP, as well as advances in parallel technology with improved imaging times in 3D FSE imaging, have improved the contrast, resolution, and acquisition time of morphologic imaging of cartilage. However, these techniques are still limited in their ability to depict physiology and biochemistry of cartilage, although they allow time for the application of other sequences to explore cartilage physiology.[10]

To understand the principles of MR imaging of cartilage physiology, this article reviews some of the basic concepts of cartilage anatomy and physiology.

FUNCTIONAL ANATOMY AND PHYSIOLOGY OF CARTILAGE

Articular cartilage is hypocellular and composed of about 4% chondrocytes by wet weight.[24] The main component of the tissue is the extracellular matrix, which is 65% to 85% water, which decreases slightly with depth from the articular surface,[24] and solid components, which include type II collagen (15%–20%) and large aggregating molecules of proteoglycans (PGs) (3%–10%), which are called aggrecans.[25] Most of the extracellular water is associated with the aggrecan

molecules and freely exchangeable with synovial fluid,[24] whereas a small portion of water is bound in the interfibrillar space of the collagen fibrils (**Fig. 1A**).[26,27]

The biochemical properties of cartilage are strongly influenced by the content and structure of collagen and PGs in the matrix, which differ from bone interface to the articular surface.[25,28] The orientation and alignment of collagen matrix vary according to the depth from the articular surface as well as regionally within the joint.[24] At the most superficial aspect of the articular surface, there is a layer of dense collagen fibers, called the lamina splendens, which has a smooth surface, and PGs such as lubricin,[29] surface zone protein, and constituents of synovial fluid help reduce the friction of the articular surface. Underneath the lamina splendens, tropocollagen molecules, which are components of type II collagen, are organized into a leafletlike structure.[30] The superficial layer follows, where collagen fibrils have an orientation parallel to the articular surface. The transitional zone is the next layer, which thickens near the periphery of the articular surface.[31] In recent studies, the transitional zone has been shown to have anisotropy[32,33] with a preferential orientation oblique to the articular surface.[24] Deeper to the transition zone is the radial zone, where collagen fibrils have a radial or perpendicular orientation to the bone surface and chondrocytes are aligned in a columnlike pattern.[34] Collagen fibrils cross the

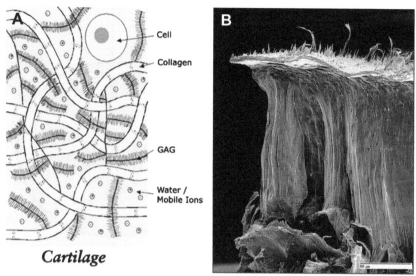

Fig. 1. (*A*) Cartilage is mostly acellular and avascular, and has a limited ability to heal. The extracellular matrix consists of water, collagen, and glycosaminoglycan. Several aggrecan molecules are attached to a central core fiber filament of hyaluronic acid, to which the aggrecan monomers are bound through a linking protein. A large number of carboxyl and sulfate residues on the GAG side chains are ionized in physiologic conditions and impart a negative charge density. (*B*) The collagen fibers have a unique zonal architecture, as shown on this freeze fracture image, with superficial, tangential, radial, and calcified zones. (*A: Courtesy of* Deb Burstein, BIDMC; and *B: Courtesy of* Doug Goodwin MD.)

bone/cartilage interface at the tidemark zone, anchoring the cartilage to the subchondral bone (see **Fig. 1B**).[24] The characteristic arrangement of collagen leads to the magic angle effect and laminar appearance on proton MR images.[35]

There are also regional differences in organization and composition of the collagen within the joint; weight-bearing regions that are frequently exposed to compressive load, such as the femorotibial joint, have a thicker radial zone and a thinner transitional zone[36] and are organized into thicker fibrils at regular intervals.[37] This pattern is not seen in areas that are not prone to habitual loading. The transitional zone is thicker near the periphery of the joint, where the cartilage is prone to shear stress, and the direction of the collagen fibers is the prevailing direction of shear strain.[31]

The aggrecans, which are large molecules of aggregating PGs, lie interposed amidst the meshwork of type II collagen fibrils and their concentration varies within the cartilage layer, with the highest levels in the middle section, which decrease near the bone interface and articular surface.[38,39] Aggrecan consists of a protein core with a long, extended domain to which many glycosaminoglycan (GAG) side chains are linked; these include chondroitin sulfate (CS) and keratan sulfate (KS), with CS as the predominant GAG molecule in cartilage.[35] In turn, several aggrecan molecules are attached to a central core fiber

filament of hyaluronic acid,[40] to which the aggrecan monomers are bound through a linking protein. A large number of carboxyl and sulfate residues on the GAG side chains are ionized in physiologic conditions and impart a negative charge density.[35] GAG chains are so densely packed that the concentration of negative charge can be as much as 150 mM to 300 mM in normal articular cartilage.[41] These negative charges allow the GAG molecules to be fixed to the matrix and are referred to as fixed charge, and the concentration of this fixed charge is referred to as fixed-charge density (FCD).[41] These negative ions attract positive counterions and water molecules and provide a strong electrostatic repulsive force between the PGs, which act together to produce the swelling pressure of cartilage.[35] However, swelling of the PGs is constrained by the surrounding collagen meshwork, which produces an interstitial fluid pressure of about 9 MPa,[42] and this contributes to the compressive stiffness of cartilage that is essential for normal cartilage function (**Fig. 2**).[24] Collagen II fibers, which are the predominant type of collagen in cartilage, provide a tensile force opposing the tendency of the PGs to expand the cartilage and also immobilize the PGs.[35]

The cartilage interface with the subchondral bone is important to normal cartilage function as well; this area is represented as the subchondral

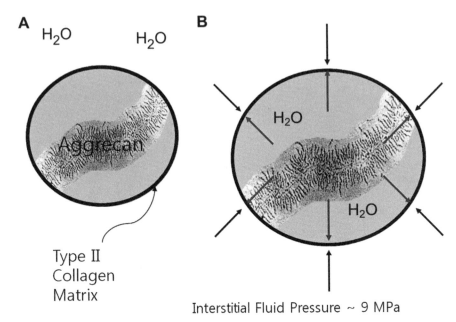

Fig. 2. (*A, B*) Negative ions attract positive counterions and water molecules and provide a strong electrostatic repulsive force between the proteoglycans, which contribute to the swelling pressure of cartilage; this swelling of the proteoglycans is constrained by the surrounding collagen meshwork, which produces an interstitial fluid pressure of about 9 MPa. (*Courtesy of* Timothy Mosher, MD, Hershey, PA.)

plate, which consists of the tidemark zone, the zone of calcified cartilage, lamellar subchondral cortical bone, and the underlying trabecular bone.[24] Type II collagen fibrils pass through the tidemark zone, ending in the zone of calcified cartilage,[43] and there is a potential cleavage plane between the zone of calcified cartilage and subchondral cortical bone in response to shear stress (**Fig. 3**).[44] The subchondral plate can remodel in response to altered biomechanics secondary to

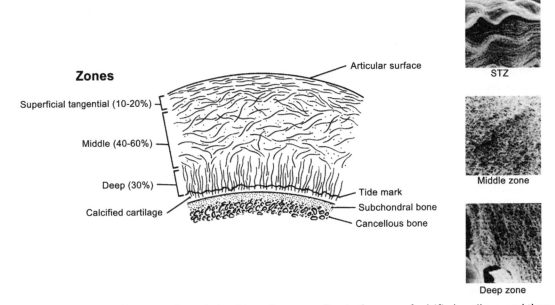

Fig. 3. Type II collagen fibrils pass through the tidemark zone, ending in the zone of calcified cartilage, and there is a potential cleavage plane between the zone of calcified cartilage and subchondral cortical bone in response to shear stress. (*Modified from* Mow VC, Hayes WC. Basic orthopedic biomechanics. 2nd edition. Lippincott Williams & Wilkins; 1997; with permission.)

joint injury or damage to overlying cartilage, and its thickness varies according to joint geometry and other patient factors, such as age, weight, and exercise.[45]

Stress is defined as the intensity of force imparted onto the articular surface per unit area, and the deformation of the tissue in response to such stress is called tissue strain.[24] The tissue strain that develops within tissue in response to applied stress varies with time, and such tissues possess viscoelastic properties,[24] which result from interaction between the 3 main components of cartilage, namely water, type II collagen matrix, and aggrecan.[46] The types of stress imposed on cartilage can be categorized as compression, tension, and shear.[24]

Compression causes cartilage to deform and produces a bulk flow of water through the extracellular matrix into the synovial space.[47] The ability of cartilage to resist compression is a result of the ability of the extracellular matrix to limit water permeability,[48] which is optimal in healthy cartilage in which the water flow is able to dissipate most of the energy imparted onto the tissue during compression (Fig. 4). This ability is lacking in degenerative cartilage, in which water movement becomes less restricted and more of the compression force is imparted to collagen and aggrecan matrix, which leads to degeneration.[24] Cartilage is stiffer near the bone[49] and most of the tissue deformation occurs in the superficial layer of cartilage.[24] Tension causes deformity of the contour of cartilage, which is resisted by the fibrillar type II collagen meshwork and hydrated aggrecans.[50]

Shear stress is produced when one articular surface passes over the other, and at the bone/cartilage interface, where differences in compressive stiffness of tissues result in shear strain during high compressive loading (Fig. 5).[24] In healthy normal cartilage, the smooth surface of the lamina splendens, superficial zone protein, lubricin, and synovial fluid act together to reduce shear strain.[24] Extensive tensile strain may produce cleavage or fractures within the collagen matrix, leading to cartilage fissures along the collagen leaves or flap-type tears at the junction of the transitional and radial cartilage zones.[24] High compressive forces transmitted to the deep layer of cartilage produce high shear strain in the tidemark zone at the cartilage/bone interface. When this shear strain exceeds the material properties of the tissue, cleavage between calcified cartilage and subchondral bone may occur, leading to cartilage delamination.[24]

OA is characterized by changes in the cartilage biochemistry and microstructure. The earliest changes include reduced PG concentration, possible changes in the size of collagen fibril and aggregation of PG, increased water content, and increased synthesis and degradation of matrix macromolecules,[35] with disorganization of the collagen network (Fig. 6).[51] These changes lead to breakdown and decreased content of the PG matrix, which in turn lead to ulceration with inflow of PG into the synovial fluid with decreased water content of the cartilage, making it less resistive to stress. As OA progresses, collagen, PG, and water content are reduced further and the collagen network becomes severely disrupted.[52]

MR IMAGING OF CARTILAGE BIOCHEMISTRY AND PHYSIOLOGY

Conventional MR imaging methods have shown mostly morphologic changes of cartilage, which probably represent progressed stages of OA. Such morphologic changes are preceded by

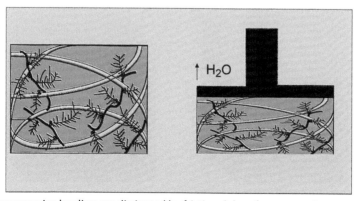

Fig. 4. Forces from compressive loading are dissipated by frictional drag forces as water moves through the extracellular matrix. (*Modified from* Mosher TJ, Mow VC, Hayes WC. Basic orthopedic biomechanics. 2nd edition. Lippincott Williams & Wilkins; 1997. p. 171; with permission.)

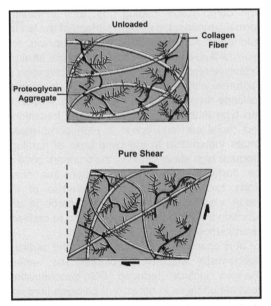

Fig. 5. Shear stress is produced when 1 articular surface passes over the other and at the bone/cartilage interface, where differences in compressive stiffness of tissues result in shear strain during high compressive loading. (*Modified from* Mosher TJ, Mow VC, Hayes WC. Basic orthopedic biomechanics. 2nd edition. Lippincott Williams & Wilkins; 1997. p. 171; with permission.)

commonly, on collagen content and orientation. Newer techniques have been developed to map various MR imaging parameters, assessing PG content, collagen content and orientation, water mobility, and regional cartilage compressibility. These techniques include sodium MR imaging, T1ρ, delayed gadolinium-enhanced MR imaging (dGEMRIC), T2 mapping, ultrashort echo time (UTE) imaging, MT, and diffusion-weighted imaging (DWI). Most of these have been studied in vitro using excised specimens; however, some of the techniques have been conducted in human studies.

MR imaging methods to measure PG depletion of cartilage, which is one of the earliest findings of OA, include sodium MR imaging, T1ρ mapping, and dGEMRIC.[41] Other methods, such as T2 mapping, UTE imaging, MT, and DWI, are mainly based on other biochemical and physiologic characteristics of cartilage, such as collagen content and orientation, water content and mobility, and regional cartilage compressibility.[10]

SODIUM MR IMAGING

Any atom with an odd number of protons and/or neutrons possesses a nuclear spin momentum and exhibits the MR phenomenon. Whereas conventional MR imaging methods have used H to generate signal, the atom ^{23}Na, which also has an odd number of protons or neutrons, can be used in cartilage imaging. The Larmor frequency of ^{23}Na is 11.262 MHz/T, compared with ^{1}H at 42.575 MHz/T, which means that at 1.5 T the resonant frequency of ^{23}Na is 16.9 MHz, compared with 63 MHz for ^{1}H.[53] In addition to the lower resonance frequency, the concentration of ^{23}Na is 320 μM (ie, lower than that of ^{1}H), with T2 relaxation times between 2 and 10 milliseconds,[54] often requiring imaging with a non-Cartesian trajectory.[55]

biochemical and structural changes in the extracellular matrix that change the biomechanical properties of the tissue.[10] Of the conventional MR imaging methods, T2-weighted images are highly sensitive to structural properties of cartilage, reflecting the T2 relaxation properties of type II collagen and water associated with it, exhibiting magnetization transfer (MT) and magic angle effects. Conventional methods have been based mostly on water content and, less

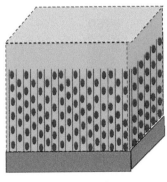

Normal

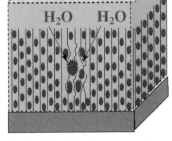

Early Matrix Degradation

Fig. 6. Maroudas Model of Early Cartilage Damage shows earliest changes including reduced PG concentration, possible changes in the size of collagen fibril, and increased water content. (*Courtesy of* Timothy Mosher, MD.)

Because of all of these factors, in vivo imaging using ^{23}Na is challenging and requires the use of special transmit and receive coils, which are not always available for clinical MR imaging systems, as well as long imaging times to obtain adequate signal/noise ratio (SNR) (**Fig. 7**).[53]

Sodium-23 atoms are associated with the negatively charged GAG side chains and thus the main component of the high fixed-charge density present in the PG sulfate and carboxylate groups[53] in the extracellular matrix[25,56] with spatial variation of concentration within the normal cartilage.[54] Loss of PG (and hence GAG and FCD) because of cartilage degeneration results in loss of sodium ions from the tissue, which results in lower FCD, thereby releasing positively charged sodium ions.[35] Sodium imaging has been shown to be sensitive to small changes in PG concentration in studies using in vitro cartilage specimens.[57–62] Studies have been published on obtaining quantitative measurements of sodium concentration in cartilage[54,63] and obtaining signal from sodium bound to macromolecules in the extracellular matrix.[35,57,64–69] With the use of higher field 3.0 T (**Fig. 8**) or 7.0 T (**Fig. 9**) MR imaging, better spatial resolution has been achieved and in vivo studies have been performed,[70–74] which suggest that Na imaging can be used for physiologic assessment of cartilage with potential application in postoperative patients as well.[74] Triple quantum filtered imaging,[75] use of 3D cones at high-field MR imaging,[73] 3D radial acquisition with UTEs,[72] and inversion recovery techniques[76] have been shown to be feasible with promising results (**Fig. 10**), but clinical application of ^{23}Na imaging is still limited in many aspects, including the specific absorption rate (SAR) limits.

However, because of its high specificity for PG content and ability to depict cartilage with high contrast without the requirement for exogenous contrast agents, such as in dGEMRIC,[77] and with developments in high-field MR imaging, advances in gradient technology and radiofrequency coil technology, and parallel imaging techniques,[78,79] sodium MR imaging has become more feasible[70–74] and may be used in the future to quantify early physiologic and molecular changes associated with OA.

T1ρ IMAGING

T1ρ imaging is possible when the magnetization is tipped into the transverse plane and then spin locked by a constant radiofrequency (RF) field. PG depletion, which is one of the earliest changes in OA, affects the physiochemical interactions within the macromolecular environment, and quantitative T1ρ imaging methods enable probing macromolecular slow motions at high static fields in cartilage.[51] Several studies have suggested that, with further GAG depletion, T1ρ reflects interaction of collagen with water.[80–82]

T1ρ imaging of cartilage to study cartilage degeneration was first suggested by Reddy and colleagues.[83] Earlier studies using phantom and specimens showed a strong correlation between T1ρ and cartilage PG content.[84–89] In a study by Akella and colleagues,[88] a strong correlation was shown between changes in PG and T1ρ, and, similar to T2 studies, T1ρ values also showed regional variations within cartilage, with the highest values in the superficial zone, decreasing in the middle zone, and increasing near the subchondral bone (**Fig. 11**).[88] Using sodium MR imaging,

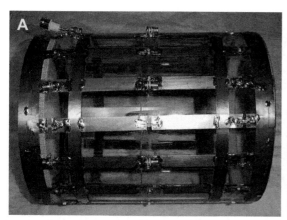
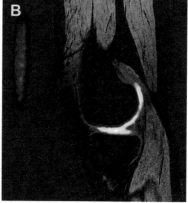

Fig. 7. (*A, B*) Sodium MR imaging requires high field strength and dedicated hardware; a dual-tuned ^{23}Na$^+$/^{1}H coil (*A*) allows direct measurement of GAG content (*B*). (*From* Staroswiecki E, Bangerter NK, Gurney PT, et al. In vivo sodium imaging of human patellar cartilage with a 3D cones sequence at 3T and 7T. J Magn Reson Imaging 2010;32(2):446–51; with permission.)

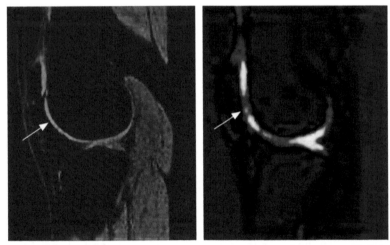

Fig. 8. Sodium MR imaging is sensitive to cartilage glycosaminoglycan. Advances in coil design and high field have made this a potential clinical tool. A patient with a prior anterior cruciate ligament tear shows areas of focal cartilage glycosaminoglycan loss (*left*) despite a normal proton MR imaging (*right*).

a strong correlation was found between T1ρ and FCD.[89] A study of cartilage specimens from patients undergoing total knee arthroplasty suggested T1ρ to be more sensitive to cartilage degeneration compared with T2 mapping (Fig. 12).[90]

Although there have been few in vivo studies, some have shown increased cartilage T1ρ values in subjects with OA compared with controls,[91,92] which further suggested the potential application of T1ρ imaging for evaluating cartilage. Studies on T1ρ and T2 have suggested that the values may be complementary and T1ρ may not only reflect PG content but other biochemical changes that occur in cartilage degeneration,[80,82,93] and may have a dependence on the angular orientation

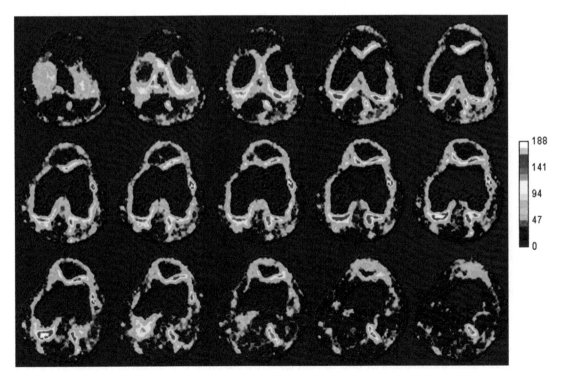

Fig. 9. Sodium MR imaging at 7.0 T shows direct measurement of cartilage glycosaminoglycan in a healthy volunteer's knee. (*Courtesy of* Ravinder Reddy, University of Pennsylvania.)

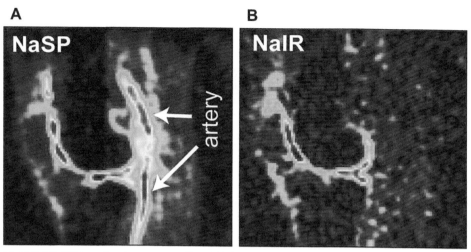

Fig. 10. (*A*, *B*) 7.0 T MR imaging improves sodium MR imaging resolution and SNR. An inversion recovery technique (*B*) is used to suppress signal from the popliteal artery (*A*). (*From* Madelin G, Lee JS, Inati S, et al. Sodium inversion recovery MRI of the knee joint in vivo at 7T. J Magn Reson 2010;207:42–52; with permission.)

of collagen fibers.[51] Several studies have suggested that the average T1ρ, which has a larger dynamic range, may be a more sensitive indicator of cartilage degeneration than T2.[94,95]

T1ρ imaging is a potentially useful technique that is sensitive to early PG depletion, one of the earliest changes in OA (**Fig. 13**).[94,96,97] Initial application of T1ρ in humans was limited to single-slice acquisition[98]; however, recent advances in T1ρ imaging techniques have included multislice and 3D acquisitions,[96,97,99,100] as well as rapid Cartesian acquisition strategies at 3.0 T.[101,102] However, a disadvantage of the T1ρ technique is the large RF power that is applied during the spin-locking preparation pulse, which may result in heating of tissue and problems with SAR; this should be overcome with development of new techniques and is not a significant problem at clinical MR imaging up to 3.0 T.[10] Implementations of parallel imaging techniques have enabled reduction of imaging times to 5 to 10 minutes.[101,103] Further studies are needed on T1ρ imaging to confirm its reliability in larger patient populations; however, it is a promising technique for investigation of cartilage degeneration and OA.

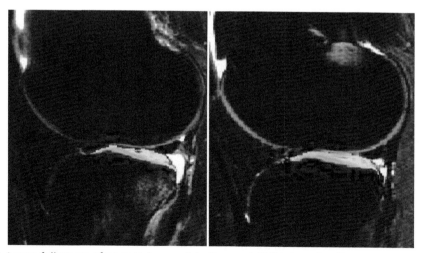

Fig. 11. T1ρ: 1-year follow-up after anterior cruciate ligament (ACL) tear. Baseline measurements (*left*) and measurements at 1 year after ACL reconstruction (*right*) show persistent cartilage damage despite resolution of bone marrow edemalike lesions. (*From* Li X. ISMRM 2007; with permission.)

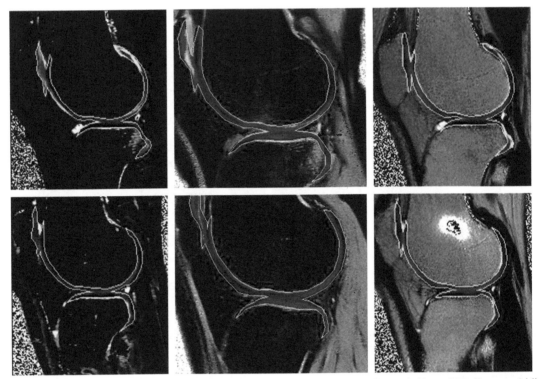

Fig. 12. Measurements of T1ρ (*upper left, middle*), dGEMRIC (*upper right, lower left*), and T2 (*lower middle, right*) before (*upper left, right, lower middle*) and 4 months after surgery (*upper middle, lower left, right*) show T1ρ and dGEMRIC to be more sensitive than T2. (*Courtesy of* Dan Thedens, University of Iowa.)

CONTRAST-ENHANCED IMAGING: dGEMRIC

As described earlier, the PG components of cartilage have GAG side chains with abundant negatively charged carboxyl and sulfate groups. The negative fixed charge on the cartilage macromolecules is balanced by the net charge of the mobile ions within the extracellular fluid (ECF). The ECF has a lower concentration of anions and a higher concentration of cations than blood or synovial

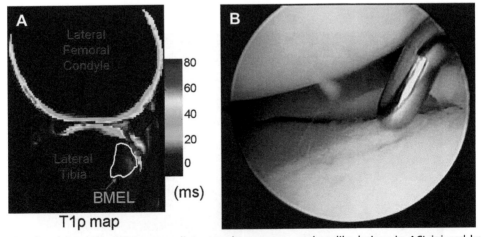

Fig. 13. (*A, B*) Increased T1ρ (*A*) is seen adjacent to bone marrow edemalike lesions in ACL-injured knee (*B*). (*Adapted from* Theologis AA, Kuo D, Cheng J, et al. Evaluation of bone bruises and associated cartilage in anterior cruciate ligament-injured and -reconstructed knees using quantitative t(1ρ) magnetic resonance imaging: 1-year cohort study. Arthroscopy 2011;27:65–76; with permission, and *From* Lozano JJ, Li X, Link TM, et al. Detection of posttraumatic cartilage injury using quantitative T1rho magnetic resonance imaging. A report of two cases with arthroscopic findings. Bone Joint Surg Am 2006;88:1349–52; with permission.)

fluid, and the difference between the concentrations of anions and cations in ECF equals the fixed-charged density (FCD).[41] GAG or FCD contribute significantly to load-bearing properties or compressive stiffness of cartilage,[104–106] so there is a substantial difference in the concentration of mobile ions between normal and GAG-depleted cartilage.[41] Many studies have attempted to measure GAG, including some of the first quantitative measurements of GAG distribution in relation to the depth from articular surface or topological position or with disease by Maroudas and colleagues.[107–110]

MR imaging enables noninvasive measurement of ion concentrations and simultaneously enables acquisition of spatial images.[41] One of the most common MR contrast agents, gadopentetate dimeglumine $Gd(DTPA)^{2-}$, is a clinically approved MR imaging contrast agent that can be used to indirectly measure FCD by allowing $Gd(DPTA)^{2-}$ to penetrate into cartilage and accumulate in high concentration in areas of cartilage with low GAG content.[111] Subsequent T1 mapping yields an image depicting GAG distribution, which is referred to as dGEMRIC with the delay meaning the time required for $Gd(DTPA)^{2-}$ to penetrate into cartilage.[111] Compared with sodium MR imaging, which entails a more direct measurement of FCD, the dGEMRIC technique using a contrast agent is an indirect method of measuring GAG content in articular cartilage.[112,113] Compared with sodium MR imaging, the advantages of dGEMRIC is a higher resolution and sensitivity; however, the disadvantages include the need for administration of a contrast agent and the need to convert T1 measurements into $Gd(DTPA)^{2-}$ concentration.[41] Areas of low GAG accumulate a higher concentration of the $Gd(DTPA)^{2-}$ with more rapid T1 relaxation of adjacent water protons.[10] After obtaining a series of images with different degrees of T1 weighting, a T1 map can be calculated to provide a regional assessment of relative $Gd(DPTA)^{2-}$ concentration that is inversely proportional to the regional GAG content.[114] dGEMRIC index refers to the acquisition of a single T1 map after administration of $Gd(DTPA)^{2-}$ and has been shown to be similar at both 1.5 T and 3.0 T field strengths.[114]

The dGEMRIC technique has been validated in both in vitro and in vivo studies as reflecting the GAG concentration of cartilage, with dGEMRIC measurements corresponding to gold standard measures for GAG.[114–116] Long-term in vitro studies have been conducted that enabled monitoring changes of GAG distribution in time with high resolution, allowing insight into the process of cartilage degradation, development, and repair.[41] For example, in a study by Allen and colleagues,[117] bovine cartilage plugs were monitored in time and it was found that chondrocytes could replenish GAG after trypsin depletion of GAG and after interleukin-1 (IL-1) treatment.[118] GAG measurements have been observed to correlate better in superficial layers of cartilage compared with deep layers where MR imaging can overestimate GAG.[119] Interobserver and intraobserver variability in the selection and calculation of regional T1 have not been shown to be significant sources of variation for this technique.[120]

In vivo studies have provided invaluable clinical insights into cartilage physiology and disease. Clinical studies have shown that the dGEMRIC images show lesions in cartilage not observed with administration of a nonionic contrast agent,[121] validating the correlation between dGEMRIC and distribution of GAG molecules. Several pilot clinical studies were done using dGEMRIC to evaluate the level of repair in cartilage implants.[122–124] Increased uptake of $Gd(DTPA)^{2-}$ has been observed in arthroscopically correlated regions of cartilage fibrillation and softening[125] and patellar chondrosis[126] and has been associated with joint space narrowing and malalignment within the femorotibial joint of the knee.[127] In a recent study, individuals exercising on a regular basis were shown to have higher dGEMRIC indices (ie, higher GAG concentrations) than sedentary subjects, correlating with the level of physical activity.[128] In another study, a change in dGEMRIC index was shown 4 months after a meniscal tear, corresponding to the amount of exercise.[129] This study provided an insight into the hypothesis that mechanical stimulation could change cartilage biochemistry (**Fig. 14**).[41]

The medial femorotibial compartment has been shown to have generally lower dGEMRIC index compared with the lateral femorotibial compartment of the knee,[130] consistent with previous biochemical studies, as well as possibly reflecting a response to different mechanical stresses, according to the location within the joint. Large variations in dGEMRIC were observed even when no joint space narrowing was observed on radiographs,[131] presumably representing biochemical changes preceding morphologic changes and actual loss of cartilage.[41] The dGEMRIC index also seems to be sensitive to cartilage-modifying injuries, as shown in studies of patients with anterior cruciate ligament (ACL)[132] or posterior cruciate ligament (PCL) injuries[133] who showed lower dGEMRIC values. In another study, cartilage lesions in patients with OA were more apparent using the dGEMRIC technique compared with the standard MR imaging

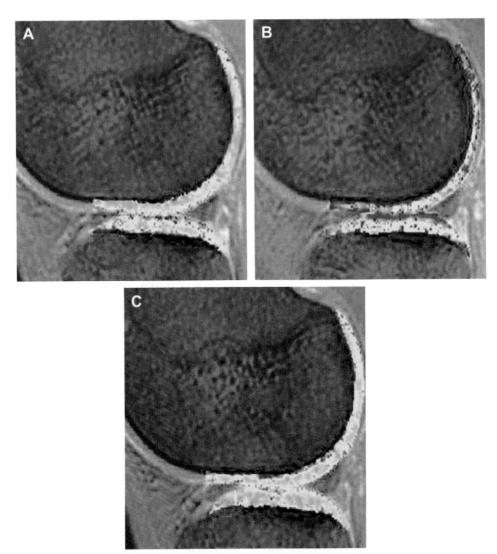

Fig. 14. (*A–C*) Temporal changes in the dGEMRIC index have been shown with physiologic events such as in an individual (*A*) before running a marathon, (*B*) 1 day after the marathon, and (*C*) 1 week after the marathon. (*Adapted from* Burstein D, Gray M, Mosher T, et al. Measures of molecular composition and structure in osteoarthritis. Radiol Clin N Am 2009;47:679; with permission.)

scans.[134] In a large cross-sectional study of patients with hip dysplasia, measures of severity of dysplasia and of pain correlated well with the dGEMRIC index but poorly with the radiological parameter of joint space narrowing.[135] dGEMRIC studies exploring the implication for planning and monitoring treatment have shown the dGEMRIC index to be the best predictor of failure[136] in osteotomy for hip dysplasia and increased dGEMRIC index in patients after surgery, suggesting the reversibility of cartilage injury (**Fig. 15**).[136]

dGEMRIC may provide a noninvasive way to depict the mechanical properties of cartilage by mapping the biochemical composition,[41] as shown in studies with good correlation between decreased GAG content, measured as increased dGEMRIC, and increased cartilage compressibility and site-matched stiffness measurements.[119,137–140] These studies showed results that could not be explained by GAG measurements alone, suggesting the need for combined GAG/collagen studies.[137–140] A preliminary study on osteochondral allografts also showed similar results of low GAG associated with indentation stiffness.[124] In a recent study, the in vivo effects of unloading and compression on T1-Gd relaxation times were investigated in healthy knee cartilage at 3.0 T, which again showed a relationship between biochemical load response and

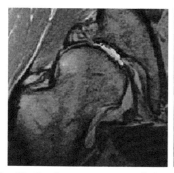
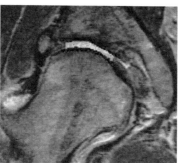
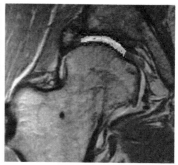

Fig. 15. Cartilage can potentially heal and result in an increase in the dGEMRIC index with intervention of osteotomy for hip dysplasia as depicted in preoperative (*left*), 20-month postoperative (*middle*), and 58-month postoperative (*right*) studies. (*Courtesy of* Deborah Burstein, BIDMC and Harvard University; with permission.)

biomechanical properties of articular cartilage (**Fig. 16**).[141] Recent studies have suggested a clinical application of dGEMRIC in the assessment of cartilage after repair (**Fig. 17**).[123,142–144] However, most of the results have shown heterogeneous uptake in repair tissue with time, and so one has to account for the baseline T1 of the tissue and Gd(DTPA)$^{2-}$ uptake being influenced not only by GAG content but also by water content and permeability of tissue; therefore, precontrast and postcontrast measurements of T1 are needed for accurate evaluation of the GAG content.[145,146] A recent study of autologous chondrocyte implantation with a fibrin-based scaffold in the knee showed dGEMRIC and T2 mapping to provide complementary information on the biochemical properties of repair tissue.[147]

Technical issues regarding optimization of the dGEMRIC technique for human clinical application have been investigated and reviewed.[77,148–150] Even though the contrast agent Gd(DTPA)$^{2-}$ has been approved for clinical use as an MR imaging

contrast agent, the dGEMRIC technique itself is an off-label application. The recommended dose for dGEMRIC studies is 0.2 mM/kg or twice the recommended clinical dose, but this should be corrected for body mass index.[151] Some investigators have advocated using a triple dose to improve sensitivity to small changes in GAG.[130] According to the dGEMRIC protocol as suggested by Burstein and colleagues,[77] the contrast agent is injected intravenously, the subject exercises the joint for about 10 minutes, and imaging is performed after 2 to 3 hours for the knee and 30 to 90 minutes for the hip; reproducibility of this technique was 10% to 15% for images taken 2 weeks to 2 months apart.[77]

Safety precautions must be taken when administering gadolinium-based contrast agents, because recently there have been reports linking gadolinium-based contrast media to nephrogenic systemic fibrosis, a highly debilitating condition similar to scleroderma that occurs in patients with moderate to severe renal impairment.[152–157]

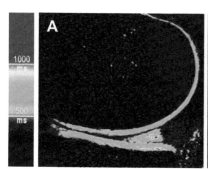
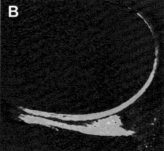
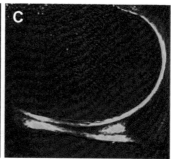

Fig. 16. Physiologic effects of mechanical loading. Sagittal dGEMRIC images of the knee joint, obtained at baseline (*A*), unloading (*B*), and compression (*C*) at identical window levels. Although there is no significant difference in T1-Gd relaxation times between baseline and unloading, there is a significant T1-Gd decrease between baseline and compression, and between unloading and compression. (*From* Mayerhoefer ME, Welsch GH, Mamisch TC, et al. The in vivo effects of unloading and compression on T1-Gd (dGEMRIC) relaxation times in healthy articular knee cartilage at 3.0 Tesla. Eur Radiol 2010;20:443–9; with permission.)

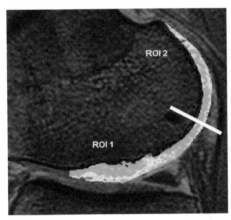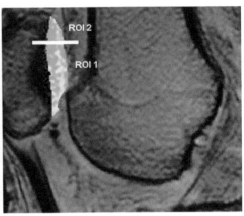

Fig. 17. dGEMRIC measurements in the knee after cartilage implants show dGEMRIC comparable with surrounding native cartilage 12 years after implant (ROI1, implant; ROI2, native). (*From* Vasiliadis HS, Danielson B, Ljungberg M, et al. Autologous chondrocyte implantation in cartilage lesions of the knee: long-term evaluation with magnetic resonance imaging and delayed gadolinium-enhanced magnetic resonance imaging technique. Am J Sports Med 2010;38:943–9; with permission.)

Even though the exact pathogenetic mechanism is still being investigated, it has been hypothesized that renal impairment leads to prolonged circulation of the contrast agent, leading to accumulation of free Gd^{3+} in tissue.[153] Because there is no cure for this potentially fatal condition, appropriate precautions and screening procedures should be undertaken when administering gadolinium-based contrast agents in all patients.[10]

Other limitations to the dGEMRIC technique include the delay period between injection and imaging and the long imaging time needed to acquire the series to T1-weighted images to calculate the T1 maps, necessitating correction for patient motion between acquisitions.[10] More recently, rapid 3D T1 mapping techniques have been developed to reduce acquisition time and improve spatial coverage.[145,148–151,158,159] These techniques still need to be validated further. As in all quantitative imaging techniques, there are assumptions and possible errors underlying the technique; in dGEMRIC, these include the conditions in which $Gd(DTPA)^{2-}$ fully penetrates cartilage; assumptions inherent in the conversion of T1 to $Gd(DPTA)^{2-}$ concentration; tissue cellularity in young or tissue-engineered samples, because $Gd(DPTA)^{2-}$ does not enter cells and cellular volume needs to be corrected for; and better T1 sequences that can cover the joint in a reasonable time frame.[111] In spite of these issues and limitations, the biophysical basis of this technique supported by validation studies in vitro and in vivo suggest that the dGEMRIC technique is a valuable tool in investigating cartilage status, disease, and repair and may contribute to understanding joint biomechanics in cartilage physiology as well as the role of loading and exercise in cartilage disorders.

T2 RELAXATION TIME MAPPING

One of the earliest physiologic changes in cartilage degeneration is increased permeability of the matrix, which leads to increased content and motion of water, resulting in increased stress on cartilage because the hydrodynamic pressure is not sustained by the matrix, which leads to PG-collagen matrix degeneration and, subsequently, morphologic changes in cartilage. The transverse relaxation time (T2) is constant for a given tissue at a given MR field strength,[160] unless altered by tissue damage or a contrast agent[160]; it is sensitive to slow-moving protons and is a function of the water content,[1,161–164] collagen content,[81,82,165–168] and orientation of the highly ordered anisotropic arrangement of collagen fibrils in the extracellular matrix (**Fig. 18**).[160,169–181] The immobilized water protons in the PG-collagen matrix promote T2

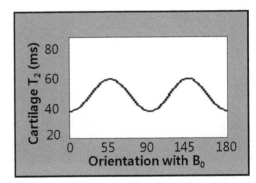

Fig. 18. The magic angle effect in cartilage. (*From* Xia Y, Moody JB, Alhadlaq H. Orientational dependence of T2 relaxation in articular cartilage: a microscopic MRI (microMRI) study. Magn Reson Med 2002;48: 460–9; with permission.)

decay and render the cartilage low in signal intensity (SI) on long echo time (TE) (T2-weighted) images, whereas the mobile water protons in synovial fluid maintain high SI.[51] As collagen and PG losses occur, the water molecules are increased in motion and content, manifesting high SI on T2-weighted images.[161,182] High SI in areas of damaged cartilage have been well depicted on conventional T2-weighted images with arthroscopic correlation.[183,184]

There is an orientation dependence of T2 in cartilage as a result of residual quadripolar relaxation mechanisms caused by the anisotropic arrangement of collagen fibrils,[68,81,185–190] and this is most pronounced in the radial zone where the fibers are aligned in a perpendicular direction to the bone, and also varies within the joint (Fig. 19).[36,172,173,180,191] Several studies have shed light on the significance of the orientation of the collagen matrix in cartilage disorders[192–196];

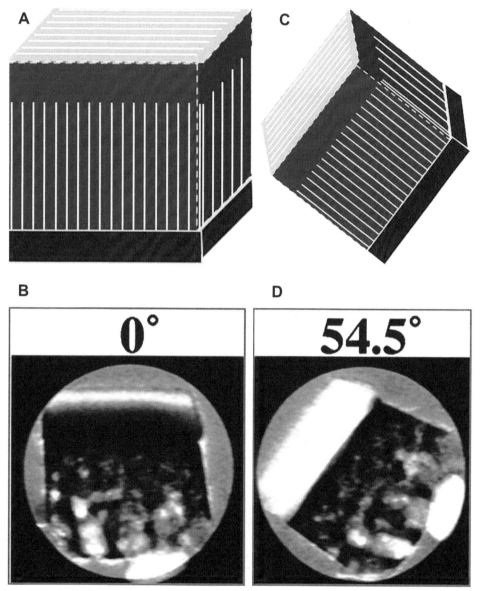

Fig. 19. (A–D) Dependence of cartilage T2 on collagen fibril orientation is shown on T2-weighted images (A, B) and the magic angle effects (C, D) as B0 increases approaching 54.5°. (B, D: From Xia Y, Moody JB, Alhadlaq H. Orientational dependence of T2 relaxation in articular cartilage: a microscopic MRI (microMRI) study. Magn Reson Med 2002;48:460–9; with permission; and A, C: Courtesy of Tim Mosher, MD, Penn State University; with permission.)

there have been studies suggesting a strong inverse relationship between cartilage T2 and collagen fiber anisotropy.[32,168,179,197,198] Such sensitivity to structural changes in collagen matrix, as well as changes in water content and motion, renders T2 mapping a useful technique to depict early changes in OA.[199] Loss of collagen matrix anisotropy has been observed to occur early in the disease process of OA and has been detected with T2 measurements (**Fig. 20**).[200] This disruption of collagen organization leads to increased permeability and water content of cartilage,[42,108] leading to increased compressibility of cartilage,[48] which in turn results in greater load-bearing stress on the solid components of the extracellular matrix,[201] which results in morphologic changes in the cartilage.

To accurately measure the T2 relaxation time, technical concerns are to be taken into account when selecting the MR technique.[202] Typically a multiecho spin echo technique is used with varying TEs and identical repetition times (TR), and signal levels are fitted to 1 or more decaying exponentials, depending on whether more than 1 distribution of T2 is believed to be within the sample[202]; T2 is defined as the time at which the signal decays to 37% of maximum.[51] For conventional MR imaging, a single exponential fit is usually adequate,[160] then an image of the T2 relaxation time is generated with either a color or gray-scale map. For accurate depiction of the depth-dependent spatial variation in cartilage T2, high-resolution T2 maps are needed, such that the resolution should ideally be in the range of

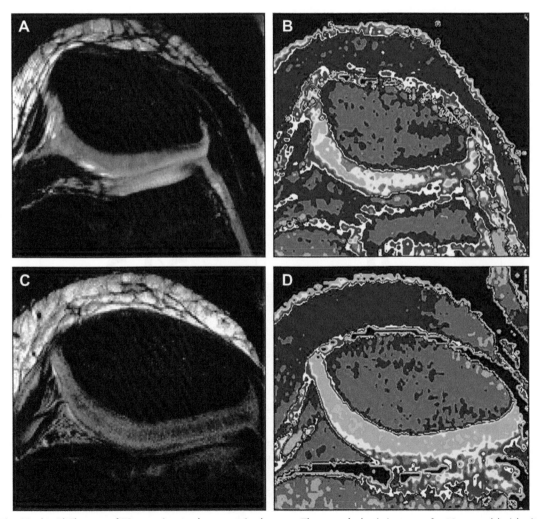

Fig. 20. (*A–D*) The use of T2 mapping to show matrix changes. The morphologic images of a 10-year-old girl with juvenile rheumatoid arthritis (*A*) and a healthy 10-year-old boy (*C*) and are both normal. The T2 maps (*B, D*) show large areas of collagen matrix disruption in the patient with juvenile rheumatoid arthritis (*B*). (*Courtesy of Bernard Dardzinski, Merck; with permission.*)

2% of total cartilage thickness for each pixel,[203] which is impossible with current technologies. However, there have been studies that attempted to decrease image acquisition time, using parallel imaging,[101] rapid T2 mapping sequences,[204] hybrid GRE/spin echo,[205] and GRE T2* mapping techniques.[206,207] Measurements of relaxation times have been shown to be anisotropic with respect to the main magnetic field.[169,171,187]

In vitro studies have been conducted to investigate the relationship between T2 measurements and biochemical composition of cartilage, with results showing a strong correlation between T2 and histologic indicators of cartilage degeneration in tissue samples and animal models.[80,140,168,208–212] Such studies showed increased T2 not only in areas of cartilage damage but also in adjacent areas, suggesting exposure of additional hydrophilic sites leading to a more efficient T2 relaxation and greater MT effects.[10] Aside from these validation studies, mostly conducted in vitro, in vivo studies have been conducted in the human knee joint[202,204,213–216] (Fig. 21), hip,[217,218] ankle,[219] and the proximal interphalangeal joint of the hands.[220] High-resolution in vivo studies have shown a spatial variation within cartilage with shorter T2 values as the layers get close to the subchondral bone, and higher T2 values as the layers get more superficial closer to the articular surface.[181,214,221,222] Regional variation within the femorotibial joint have also been shown,[223] as well as greater entropy of T2 in osteoarthritic cartilage.[224] According to various studies, regional variation of T2 seems to be affected by age,[214,221,225,226] because aging is associated with reorganization and changes of the collagen matrix starting from the superficial layer at the articular surface[10]; more significant increases in T2 have been observed in older individuals according to depth[221,226] and in general throughout the

cartilage.[226] However, gender does not seem to have a great influence on regional variation of T2.[227]

In spite of the numerous validation studies of changes in T2 correlating with the biochemical changes in cartilage, there have been limited clinical application studies using quantitative T2 mapping in the evaluation of arthritis. Increased T2 values have been reported in subjects with radiographically evident OA of the knee[90,208,216,223,228]; however, the T2 values did not correlate well with the radiographic degree of OA.[223] Increased T2 values have been attributed to collagen matrix degeneration in early OA, which are not increased further with progression of the disease, so further investigations are needed to determine the significance of T2 changes and their relationship to disease progression and treatment response.[10] However, T2 relaxation time may still provide an insight into the heterogeneous and complex process of cartilage degeneration in OA.

There have been studies investigating the relationship between cartilage morphology and T2, showing an inverse relationship between cartilage T2 and thickness,[223,229] higher cartilage T2 with greater loss of volume,[230] increase in mean cartilage T2 at longitudinal follow-up after 12 months in OA groups,[229] and increased T2 with cartilage defect regardless of unloading of the knee.[231] The study by Apprich and colleagues[231] also explored the effects of biomechanical stress on cartilage, which has also been a topic of interest in recent studies.

The effects of joint position and alignment have been investigated in several animal[232] and human studies,[233] with increased T2 values in knee flexion[232] and varus alignment.[233] There have been other studies exploring the relationship between T2 values and cartilage biomechanics; in initial feasibility studies, decrease in T2 was

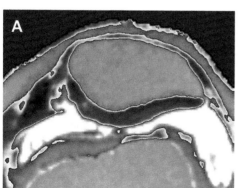
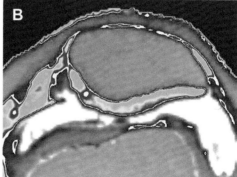

Fig. 21. (A, B) Heat scale and color scale T2 maps of a 26-year-old woman who had arthroscopic surgery for meniscal tear. (Courtesy of Tim Mosher, MD, Penn State University; with permission.)

observed when static compression was applied to the cartilage,[234–236] confirming a strong correlation between change in collagen fiber orientation and T2 values.[10] Quantitative T2 mapping in cartilage plugs showed zone-specific changes during compressive loading.[197] In a study from the Osteoarthritis Initiative, physically active individuals had more knee abnormalities and higher patellar T2 values.[237] In a recent study by Mosher and colleagues,[238] effect of age and training on knee cartilage were evaluated in response to running. Running resulted in decrease in cartilage thickness and T2 values in the superficial cartilage consistent with greater compressibility in the superficial layer, whereas age and level of physical activity did not affect the T2 changes in running; the changes in the superficial layer were concordant with results from an earlier study (**Figs. 22** and **23**).[239] Thus, T2 mapping may be a valuable technique in investigating the role of cartilage biomechanics in cartilage physiology.

T2 mapping has also been used to evaluate cartilage repair tissue after treatment.[139,147,168,212,240–249] In a study by White and colleagues,[244] repair tissue from osteochondral transplantation was shown to have the normal spatial variation of T2 values, which was absent in repair tissue from autologous chondrocyte implantation or microfracture techniques (**Fig. 24**). In a study by Domayer and colleagues,[147] T2 mapping and dGEMRIC provided complementary information on the biochemical properties of repair tissue after autologous chondrocyte implantation with a fibrin-based scaffold in the knee, which resulted in repair tissue with spatial variation of T2 values similar to normal articular cartilage

(**Fig. 25**). Another study evaluated cartilage repair tissue using T2 and T2* mapping after matrix-associated autologous chondrocyte transplantation on 3.0 T MR imaging and showed zonal variation.[246] In a study by Mamisch and colleagues,[247] differences in response to unloading were evaluated in control and cartilage repair tissue of the knee using T2 mapping, and the results showed differences in early and late unloading T2 values between normal healthy and repaired cartilage. Although many of these studies are initial or preliminary studies, the results suggest that T2 may be a potentially useful technique in postoperative evaluation of repaired cartilage.

UTE IMAGING

With the higher TEs ($\geq$10 milliseconds) used in most conventional T2-weighted sequences on conventional clinical scanners, MR signal from musculoskeletal tissues with short T2 characteristics, such as cortical bone, tendons, ligaments, menisci, and deep radial and calcified layers of cartilage, decay rapidly and produce little or no signal.[250,251] With UTE MR imaging, signal from tissues with predominantly short T2 (and T2*) can be detected[250,252–254] using TEs that are 20 to 50 times or even 100 to 1000 times shorter than those used in conventional imaging sequences,[250,255–257] enabling visualization of layers that are not normally depicted well on conventional sequences. The hyaline articular cartilage layer has been depicted as 2 layers on subtraction images, consisting of a high-signal layer and a low-signal superficial layer.[253] The region of the osteochondral junction consisting of the calcified cartilage layer and

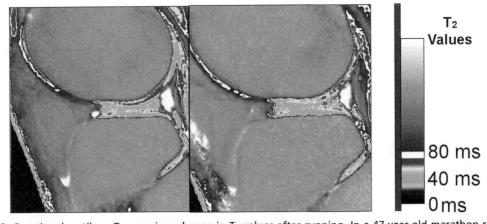

Fig. 22. Functional cartilage T_2 mapping: change in T_2 values after running. In a 47-year-old marathon runner, a T2 map after running show areas of T2 decrease, which may correspond with loss of cartilage water caused by compression.

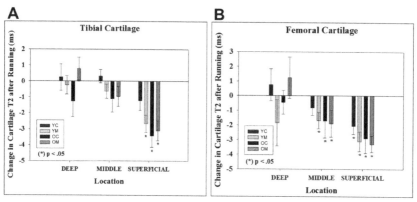

Fig. 23. (*A, B*) Functional cartilage T2 mapping: evaluating local tissue response to running. Change in cartilage T2 values after 30 minutes of running show statistically significant decrease in T2 values of superficial femoral and tibial cartilage, but no change in T2 near the bone/cartilage interface. OC, old (45–55 years) sedentary control; OM, old marathoner; YC, young (18–30 years) control; YM, young marathoner. (*Reproduced from* Mosher TJ, Liu Y, Torok CM. Functional cartilage MRI T2 mapping: evaluating the effect of age and training on knee cartilage response to running. Osteoarthritis Cartilage 2010;18:358–64; with permission.)

subchondral bone, which is important for solute transport between the vasculature and articular cartilage,[258] has been implicated to be important in the pathogenesis of OA,[251] with changes beginning in the calcified layer affecting the more superficial cartilage and subsequently causing cartilage degeneration.[259–265] However, the calcified layer of cartilage, because of rapid signal decay, produces little or no signal and is difficult to evaluate with conventional MR imaging sequences. In a study by Gold and colleagues,[256] projection reconstruction spectroscopic imaging (PRSI) technique and non-Cartesian k-space trajectory 3D cones techniques were used to depict articular cartilage at high resolution in vivo at scan times of 5 to 10 minutes. A recent study by Bae and

colleagues,[251] which used 2 complementary UTE techniques, suggested that the presence of the calcified layer as well as the deepest layer of uncalcified cartilage, with their short T2 values, contributed to the UTE signal without contribution from the subchondral bone (**Fig. 26**).

Technical challenges related to UTE imaging include distortion of the slice profile, errors in the radial k-space trajectories, and off resonance, which could be improved by gradient calibration, off-resonance correction, efficient long T2 water, and fat suppression (**Figs. 27–29**).[266–268] In spite of the technical challenges and disadvantage of scan time and difficulty in slice selection, UTE imaging may allow evaluation of the calcified layer of cartilage in OA.[269] UTE imaging may also be

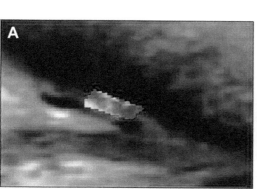
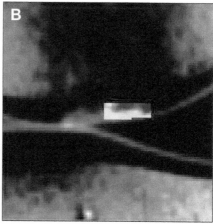

Fig. 24. (*A, B*) T2 mapping can be used to follow cartilage repair clinically and shows that a microfracture or fibrocartilage repair has lower T2 values than an osteochondral repair with hyaline cartilage. (*Courtesy of* Lawrence White, University of Toronto; with permission.)

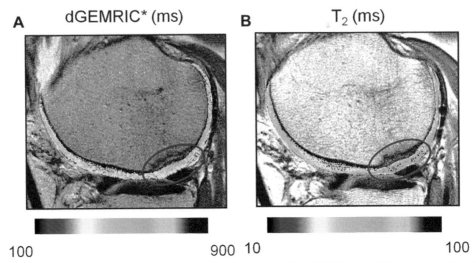

Fig. 25. (*A*, *B*) Autologous chondrocyte implantation followed with dGEMRIC and T2 mapping. The dGEMRIC study showed increasing GAG in the repair site (*A*), indicating formation of hyaline cartilage. (*Courtesy of* Miika Nieminen, University of Oulu and Oulu University Hospital, Oulu, Finland; with permission.)

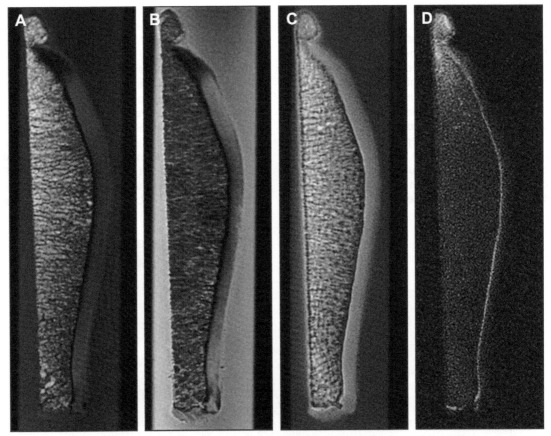

Fig. 26. (*A–D*) UTE MR imaging can be used to probe the deepest layer of cartilage, the calcified zone. Conventional MR imaging shows a signal void from this zone on T1-weighted (*A*) and PD-weighted images (*B*), but UTE MR imaging (*C*) and UTE MR imaging with long T2 suppression (*D*) show signal from the calcified zone. This zone may be important in the development of OA. (*Courtesy of* Christine Chung and Graeme Bydder, UCSD; with permission.)

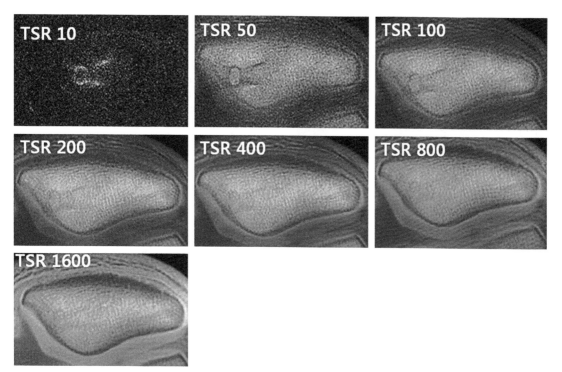

Fig. 27. Images acquired at 7 points with a saturation recovery times (TSR) ranging from 10 to 1600 milliseconds, where the region of interest was placed in a region of normal appearing calcified cartilage. In these volunteer images, excellent tissue signal saturation at TSR 10 and best visualization of the calcified layer at TSR 200 to 800 are noted. (*Courtesy of* Christine Chung and Graeme Bydder, UCSD; with permission.)

useful for postoperative assessment of cartilage repair, in which the removal of the calcified layer has been reported to improve surgical outcome,[270] and may be the only imaging method thus far that allows examination of the region of osteochondral junction.

MT

MT effect is present in any multislice MR imaging technique and is seen in cartilage,[169,271] especially prominent in the radial zone near the bone/cartilage interface.[272] It is prominently seen in turbo spin echo (TSE) sequences and can be a source

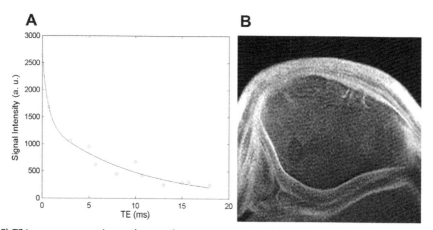

Fig. 28. (*A, B*) T2* measurement in a volunteer by constant TR-variable TE method. (*Courtesy of* Christine Chung, UCSD).

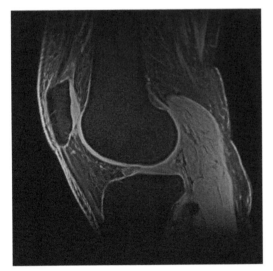

Fig. 29. High-resolution (300 mm) UTE MR imaging at 3.0 T shows the calcified zone well. (*Courtesy of* Christine Boada.)

of error in quantitative mapping techniques such as T1 or T2 mapping when multislice TSE sequences are used.[273–276] In contrast, GRE sequences exhibit less MT and, by applying an off-resonance RF pulse immediately before the GRE sequence, an MT contrast image[10] can be obtained, and by subtracting images, an isolated contribution from MT can be obtained; however,

the resulting image is usually prone to artifacts and has poor SNR.[10] Higher SNR may be achieved using 3.0 T MR scanners.[277]

Because MT is affected by many factors, such as RF power, pulse profile, and offset frequency, quantification of MT is difficult.[170,278] Higher RF power accompanies the problem with SAR, so quantitative MT techniques have been studied in a limited number of human studies.[279–282] Therefore, most studies have been conducted using tissue samples[281,283–288] or animal models[289–291] and have shown that MT is affected mostly by the collagen content and changes in collagen-water interaction. In a study of bovine cartilage specimens, MT ratio (MTR) showed depth dependency and higher values in the radial zone compared with the superficial zone, which suggested that MTR may not only be dependent on collagen content but other parameters, such as the arrangement of macromolecules, high solid content, bound water fraction, and radial orientation (**Fig. 30**).[272] In spite of the limitations, the technique has been applied to improve contrast between cartilage and fluid and, therefore, improve detection of localized cartilage lesions (see **Fig. 30**).[279,292–295] In a study evaluating T1, T2, and MTRs in early diagnosis of patellar cartilage OA, MTRs were found to have limitations in early diagnosis of OA.[216] There have been also preliminary studies on postoperative cartilage repair tissue, one of which showed too-small

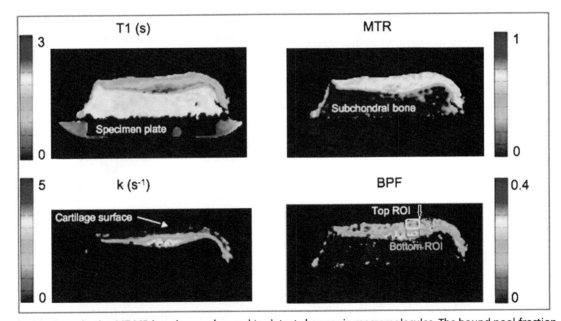

Fig. 30. Quantitative MT MR imaging can be used to detect changes in macromolecules. The bound pool fraction (*arrow*) correlates with cartilage glycosaminoglycan in its top layer. (*Courtesy of* Stikov, Keenan, Pauly, et al. ISMRM 2010 #827; with permission.)

differences between damaged and repaired cartilage MTR but evolution toward normal MTR in repair tissue, especially after articular cartilage injury repair.[282] Another study showed contrasting results, suggesting MTR to be capable of detecting differences between normal cartilage and areas of cartilage repair and possibly a useful tool in imaging biochemical changes in cartilage after repair.[296] Further investigations are needed to validate such studies.

DWI

Water is abundant within normal cartilage, composing about 65% to 85% of the extracellular matrix, and imaging of water diffusion throughout the cartilage is possible with MR imaging. In vitro studies have shown DWI to be sensitive to early cartilage degeneration.[174,297] The apparent diffusion coefficient (ADC) decreases as diffusion times get longer and indicate restriction of the water molecules by solid components of the cartilage, usually the collagen network.[115] When diffusion-sensitizing gradients are applied, water gains a random amount of phase and does not refocus, which results in signal loss of the tissue undergoing diffusion.[111] The amount of diffusion weighting, expressed as the b-value, depends on the amplitude and timing of the diffusion-sensitizing gradients. A map of the amount of diffusion that has occurred is called the ADC map, which uses the term apparent because the values reflect only the bulk water and not the water protons restricted by tissue membranes.[111]

In vivo DWI of cartilage is difficult because, to maximize cartilage signal, TE must be short, but diffusion-sensitizing gradients increase the TE and render the technique sensitive to motion.[111] Single-shot techniques have been used for DWI, but they are limited by low SNR and spatial resolution[111]; multiple acquisitions improve the SNR and resolution, but motion correction is needed (**Fig. 31**).[298] In an in vivo study, ADC measurements of articular cartilage in healthy volunteers showed comparable results with a study using cartilage specimens.[299]

DWI has also been evaluated in postoperative cartilage repair tissue. In a study by Mamisch and colleagues,[300] repaired cartilage after matrix-associated autologous chondrocyte transplantation at 3.0 T using a fast imaging with steady-state precession (FSIP) technique called reversed fast imaging with steady-state free precession (PSIF) showed higher ADC values in the repaired cartilage and a decrease in values at a later time point after surgery. In another study using high-field MR imaging, a dedicated multichannel coil, and sophisticated sequences, DWI showed higher ADC values in the repair tissue and was shown to provide additional information than T2 and T2* mapping about cartilage ultrastructure and cartilage repair tissue in the ankle joint.[248] In another study, DWI was able to differentiate between healthy cartilage and cartilage repair tissue in both microfracture therapy and matrix-associated autologous chondrocyte transplantation, with good correlation between ADC values and clinical scoring.[249] In another recent study, DWI detected

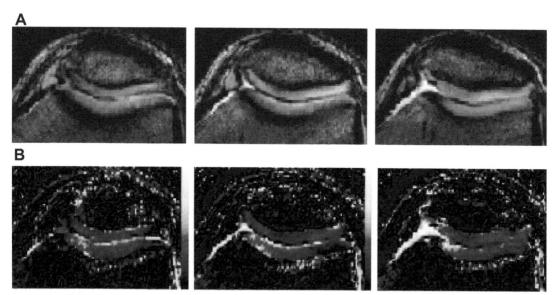

Fig. 31. (*A, B*) 3D SSFP cartilage diffusion imaging. (*From* Miller KL, Hargreaves BA, Gold GE, et al. Steady-state diffusion-weighted imaging of in vivo knee cartilage. Magn Reson Med 2004;51:394–8; with permission.)

changes of diffusion within cartilage repair tissue up to 2 years after surgery, which then became stabilized with zonal variations.[301] Although the results of most of these studies are preliminary, they suggest DWI to be a potentially useful technique in the evaluation of the biochemical and physiologic changes in postoperative cartilage repair tissue.

SUMMARY

Although conventional MR imaging methods were able to depict morphologic changes when the disease was already at a progressed state, the newer MR imaging methods are more based on cartilage physiology. Sodium imaging is highly specific for changes in PG content without the need for an exogenous contrast agent, but requires special transmit and receive coils, long imaging times, and is limited by SAR problems. T1ρ imaging is sensitive to early PG depletion but, again, is limited by SAR problems because it requires high RF power during the spin-locking preparation pulse. dGEMRIC has high resolution and sensitivity but requires long imaging times, including a delay before imaging, and administration of an exogenous contrast agent, which accompanies a small risk of nephrogenic systemic fibrosis. T2 mapping is straightforward to perform and is sensitive to changes in collagen as well as water content, but may be less sensitive in early degeneration than other methods. UTE MR imaging may be the only technique to examine the osteochondral junction, but technical difficulties, such as scan time and difficulty in slice selection, make this challenging. MT provides improved contrast between cartilage and fluid, allowing detection of localized cartilage lesions, but is difficult to quantify and may have SAR problems. Diffusion-weighted imaging may be a valuable tool in postoperative imaging but is limited by low SNR and spatial resolution. There remains more to be investigated the MR imaging of cartilage physiology, but these promising methods can give researchers important insights into the initiation, progression, and eventual treatment of OA.

REFERENCES

1. Liess C, Lusse S, Karger N, et al. Detection of changes in cartilage water content using MRI T2-mapping in vivo. Osteoarthritis Cartilage 2002;10:907–13.
2. Felson DT, Zhang Y, Hannan MT, et al. The incidence and natural history of knee osteoarthritis in the elderly. The Framingham Osteoarthritis Study. Arthritis Rheum 1995;38(10):1500–5.
3. Lawrence RC, Felson DT, Helmick CG, et al. National Arthritis Data W. Estimates of the prevalence of arthritis and other rheumatic conditions in the United States. Part II. Arthritis Rheum 2008; 58(1):26–35.
4. Kim I, Kim HA, Seo YI, et al. The prevalence of knee osteoarthritis in elderly community residents in Korea. J Korean Med Sci 2010;25(2):293–8.
5. Yoshimura N. Progress of research in osteoarthritis. Epidemiology of osteoarthritis in Japanese population. The Road Study. Clin Calcium 2009;19(11): 1572–7.
6. Kang X, Fransen M, Zhang Y, et al. The high prevalence of knee osteoarthritis in a rural Chinese population: the Wuchuan Osteoarthritis Study. Arthritis Rheum 2009;61(5):641–7.
7. Poole AR. An introduction to the pathophysiology of osteoarthritis. Front Biosci 1999;4:D662–70.
8. Roos H, Adalberth T, Dahlberg L, et al. Osteoarthritis of the knee after injury to the anterior cruciate ligament or meniscus: the influence of time and age. Osteoarthritis Cartilage 1995;3:261–7.
9. van den Berg WB. Pathophysiology of osteoarthritis. Joint Bone Spine 2000;67:555–6.
10. Gold GE, Mosher TJ. New MRI techniques for osteoarthritis. In: Bruno MA, Mosher TJ, Gold GE, editors. Arthritis in color: advanced imaging of arthritis. Philadelphia: Elsevier Saunders; 2009. p. 153–92.
11. Helmick CG, Felson DT, Lawrence RC, et al. Estimates of the prevalence of arthritis and other rheumatic conditions in the United States. Part I. Arthritis Rheum 2008;58(1):15–25.
12. Lawrence RC, Helmick CG, Arnett FC, et al. Estimates of the prevalence of arthritis and selected musculoskeletal disorders in the United States. Arthritis Rheum 1998;41(5):778–99.
13. Boegard T, Rudling O, Petersson IF, et al. Correlation between radiographically diagnosed osteophytes and magnetic resonance detected cartilage defects in the tibiofemoral joint. Ann Rheum Dis 1998;57:401–7.
14. Coumas JM, Palmer WE. Knee arthrography: evolution and current status. Radiol Clin North Am 1998;36:703–28.
15. Disler DG, McCauley TR. Clinical magnetic resonance imaging of articular cartilage. Top Magn Reson Imaging 1998;9:360–76.
16. Gold GE, McCauley TR, Gray ML, et al. What's new in cartilage? Radiographics 2003;23:1227–42.
17. Hodler J, Resnick D. Current status of imaging of articular cartilage. Skeletal Radiol 1996;25:703–9.
18. McCauley TR, Disler DG. Magnetic resonance imaging of articular cartilage of the knee. J Am Acad Orthop Surg 2001;9:2–8.
19. Recht MP, Resnick D. Magnetic resonance imaging of articular cartilage: an overview. Top Magn Reson Imaging 1998;9:328–36.

20. Rubenstein JD, Li JG, Majumdar S, et al. Image resolution and signal-to-noise ratio requirements for MR imaging of degenerative cartilage. AJR Am J Roentgenol 1997;169:1089–96.

21. Reeder SB, Hargreaves BA, Yu H, et al. Homodyne reconstruction and IDEAL water-fat decomposition. Magn Reson Med 2005;54:586–93.

22. Cicuttini F, Forbes A, Asbeutah A, et al. Comparison and reproducibility of fast and conventional spoiled gradient-echo magnetic resonance sequences in the determination of knee cartilage volume. J Orthop Res 2000;18:580–4.

23. Eckstein F, Westhoff J, Sittek H, et al. In vivo reproducibility of three-dimensional cartilage volume and thickness measurements with MR imaging. AJR Am J Roentgenol 1998;170:593–7.

24. Mosher TJ. Functional anatomy and structure of the "osteochondral unit". In: Bruno MA, Mosher TJ, Gold GE, editors. Arthritis in color: advanced imaging of arthritis. Philadelphia: Elsevier Saunders; 2009. p. 23–32.

25. Venn M, Maroudas A. Chemical composition and swelling of normal and osteoarthrotic femoral head cartilage. I. Chemical composition. Ann Rheum Dis 1977;36:121–9.

26. Torzilli PA. Influence of cartilage conformation on its equilibrium water partition. J Orthop Res 1985;3: 473–83.

27. Maroudas A, Schneiderman R. "Free" and "exchangeable" or "trapped" and "non-exchangeable" water in cartilage. J Orthop Res 1987;5: 133–8.

28. Guilak F, Meyer BC, Ratcliffe A, et al. The effects of matrix compression on proteoglycan metabolism in articular cartilage explants. Osteoarthritis Cartilage 1994;2:91–101.

29. Jay GD, Torres JR, Warman ML, et al. The role of lubricin in the mechanical behavior of synovial fluid. Proc Natl Acad Sci U S A 2007;104:6194–9.

30. Clark JM. The organization of collagen fibrils in the superficial zones of articular cartilage. J Anat 1990; 171:117–30.

31. Thompson AM, Stockwell RA. An ultrastructural study of the marginal transitional zone in the rabbit knee joint. J Anat 1983;136:701–13.

32. Xia Y, Moody JB, Burton-Wurster N, et al. Quantitative in situ correlation between microscopic MRI and polarized light microscopy studies of articular cartilage. Osteoarthritis Cartilage 2001; 9:393–406.

33. Clark JM. The organization of collagen in cryofractured rabbit articular cartilage: a scanning electron microscopic study. J Orthop Res 1985;3:17–29.

34. Clark JM. Variation in collagen fiber alignment in a joint surface: a scanning electron microscope study of the tibial plateau in dog, rabbit, and man. J Orthop Res 1991;9:246–57.

35. Borthakur A, Mellon E, Niyogi S, et al. Sodium and T1 rho MRI for molecular and diagnostic imaging of articular cartilage. NMR Biomed 2006;19: 781–821.

36. Moger CJ, Barrett R, Bleuet P, et al. Regional variations of collagen orientation in normal and diseased articular cartilage and subchondral bone determined using small angle X-ray scattering (SAXS). Osteoarthritis Cartilage 2007;15: 682–7.

37. Gomez S, Toffanin R, Bernstorff S, et al. Collagen fibrils are differently organized in weight-bearing and not-weight-bearing regions of pig articular cartilage. J Exp Zool 2000;287:346–52.

38. Franzen A, Inerot S, Hejderup SO, et al. Variations in the composition of bovine hip articular cartilage with distance from the articular surface. Biochem J 1981;195:535–43.

39. Bayliss MT, Venn M, Maroudas A, et al. Structure of proteoglycans from different layers of human articular cartilage. Biochem J 1983;209:387–400.

40. Roughley PJ. The structure and function of cartilage proteoglycans. Eur Cell Mater 2006;12:92–101.

41. Gray ML, Burstein D, Kim YJ, et al. Elizabeth Winston Lanier Award Winner. Magnetic resonance imaging of cartilage glycosaminoglycan: basic principles, imaging technique, and clinical applications. J Orthop Res 2007;26(3):281–91.

42. Maroudas AI. Balance between swelling pressure and collagen tension in normal and degenerative cartilage. Nature 1976;260:808–9.

43. Clark JM, Huber JD. The structure of the human subchondral plate. J Bone Joint Surg Br 1990;72: 866–73.

44. Otterness IG, Chang M, Burkhardt JE, et al. Histology and tissue chemistry of tidemark separation in hamsters. Vet Pathol 1999;36:138–45.

45. Doube M, Firth EC, Boyde A. Variations in articular calcified cartilage by site and exercise in the 18-month-old equine distal metacarpal condyle. Osteoarthritis Cartilage 2007;15:1283–92.

46. Mow VC, Huiskes R. Basic orthopaedic biomechanics & mechano-biology. Philadelphia: Lippincott Williams & Wilkins; 2005.

47. Lu XL, Mow VC. Biomechanics of articular cartilage and determination of material properties. Med Sci Sports Exerc 2008;40:193–9.

48. Armstrong CG, Mow VC. Variations in the intrinsic mechanical properties of human articular cartilage with age, degeneration, and water content. J Bone Joint Surg Am 1982;64:88–94.

49. Wong M, Carter DR. Articular cartilage functional histomorphology and mechanobiology: a research perspective. Bone 2003;33:1–13.

50. Schmidt MB, Mow VC, Chun LE, et al. Effects of proteoglycan extraction on the tensile behavior of articular cartilage. J Orthop Res 1990;8:353–63.

51. Blumenkrantz G, Majumdar S. Quantitative magnetic resonance imaging of articular cartilage in osteoarthritis. Eur Cell Mater 2007;13:75–86.

52. Dijkgraaf LC, deBont LG, Boering G, et al. The structure, biochemistry, and metabolism of osteoarthritis cartilage: a review of the literature. J Oral Maxillofac Surg 1995;53:1182–92.

53. Gold GE, Hargreaves BA, Stevens KJ, et al. Advanced MR imaging of articular cartilage. Orthop Clin North Am 2006;37(3):331–47, vi.

54. Shapiro EM, Borthakur A, Gougoutas A, et al. 23Na MRI accurately measures fixed charge density in articular cartilage. Magn Reson Med 2002;47(2):284–91.

55. Boada FE, Shen GX, Chang SY, et al. Spectrally weighted twisted projection imaging: reducing T2 signal attenuation effects in fast three-dimensional sodium imaging. Magn Reson Med 1997;38:1022–8.

56. Maroudas A, Muir H, Wingham J. The correlation of fixed negative charge with glycosaminoglycan content of human articular cartilage. Biochim Biophys Acta 1969;177:492–500.

57. Borthakur A, Hancu I, Boada FE, et al. In vivo triple quantum filtered twisted projection sodium MRI of human articular cartilage. J Magn Reson 1999; 141(2):286–90.

58. Borthakur A, Shapiro EM, Beers J, et al. Sensitivity of MRI to proteoglycan depletion in cartilage: comparison of sodium and proton MRI. Osteoarthritis Cartilage 2000;8(4):288–93.

59. Borthakur A, Shapiro EM, Akella SV, et al. Quantifying sodium in the human wrist in vivo by using MR imaging. Radiology 2002;224:598–602.

60. Insko EK, Kaufman JH, Leigh JS, et al. Sodium NMR evaluation of articular cartilage degradation. Magn Reson Med 1999;41:30–4.

61. Reddy R, Insko EK, Noyszewski EA, et al. Sodium MRI of human articular cartilage in vivo. Magn Reson Med 1998;39:697–701.

62. Wheaton AJ, Borthakur A, Dodge GR, et al. Sodium magnetic resonance imaging of proteoglycan depletion in an in vivo model of osteoarthritis. Acad Radiol 2004;11:21–8.

63. Shapiro EM, Borthakur A, Dandora R, et al. Sodium visibility and quantitation in intact bovine articular cartilage using high field (23)Na MRI and MRS. J Magn Reson 2000;142:24–31.

64. Choy J, Ling W, Jerschow A. Selective detection of ordered sodium signals via the central transition. J Magn Reson 2006;180:105–9.

65. Hancu I, van der Maarel JR, Boada FE. A model for the dynamics of spins 3/2 in biological media: signal loss during radiofrequency excitation in triple-quantum-filtered sodium MRI. J Magn Reson 2000;147:179–91.

66. Ling W, Jerschow A. Selecting ordered environments in NMR of spin 3/2 nuclei via frequency-sweep pulses. J Magn Reson 2005;176:234–8.

67. Ling W, Regatte RR, Schweitzer ME, et al. Behavior of ordered sodium in enzymatically depleted cartilage tissue. Magn Reson Med 2006;56:1151–5.

68. Navon G, Shinar H, Eliav U, et al. Multiquantum filters and order in tissues. NMR Biomed 2001;14:112–32.

69. Shinar H, Navon G. Multinuclear NMR and microscopic MRI studies of the articular cartilage nanostructure. NMR Biomed 2006;19:877–93.

70. Speer DP, Dahners L. The collagenous architecture of articular cartilage: correlation of scanning electron microscopy and polarized light microscopy observations. Clin Orthop Relat Res 1979;139:267–75.

71. Jeffery AK, Blunn GW, Archer CW, et al. Three-dimensional collagen architecture in bovine articular cartilage. J Bone Joint Surg Br 1991;73:795–801.

72. Wang L, Wu Y, Chang G, et al. Rapid isotropic 3D-sodium MRI of the knee joint in vivo at 7T. J Magn Reson Imaging 2009;30(3):606–14.

73. Staroswiecki E, Bangerter NK, Gurney PT, et al. In vivo sodium imaging of human patellar cartilage with a 3D cones sequence at 3T and 7T. J Magn Reson Imaging 2010;32(2):446–51.

74. Trattnig S, Welsch GH, Juras V, et al. 23Na MR imaging at 7T after knee matrix-associated autologous chondrocyte transplantation: preliminary results. Radiology 2010;257(1):175–84.

75. Hancu I, Boada FE, Shen GX. Three-dimensional triple-quantum-filtered (23)Na imaging of in vivo human brain. Magn Reson Med 1999;42:1146–54.

76. Rong P, Regatte RR, Jerschow A. Clean demarcation of cartilage tissue 23Na by inversion recovery. J Magn Reson 2008;193(2):207–9.

77. Burstein D, Velyvis J, Scott KT, et al. Protocol issues for delayed Gd(DTPA)$^{2-}$-enhanced MRI (dGEMRIC) for clinical evaluation of articular cartilage. Magn Reson Med 2001;45(1):36–41.

78. Pruessmann KP, Weiger M, Scheidegger MB, et al. SENSE: sensitivity encoding for fast MRI. Magn Reson Med 1999;42(5):952–62.

79. Sodickson DK, Manning WJ. Simultaneous acquisition of spatial harmonics (SMASH): fast imaging with radiofrequency coil arrays. Magn Reson Med 1997;38(4):591–603.

80. Mlynarik V, Trattnig S, Huber M, et al. The role of relaxation times in monitoring proteoglycan depletion in articular cartilage. J Magn Reson Imaging 1999;10:497–502.

81. Mlynarik V, Szomolanyi P, Toffanin R, et al. Transverse relaxation mechanisms in articular cartilage. J Magn Reson 2004;169:300–7.

82. Menezes NM, Gray ML, Hartke JR, et al. T2 and T1 rho MRI in articular cartilage systems. Magn Reson Med 2004;51:503–9.

83. Reddy R, Insko EK, Kaufman JH, et al. MR imaging of cartilage under spin-locking. In Proceedings of the International Society of Magnetic Resonance Medicine. Nice (France); 1995. p. 1535.

84. Regatte RR, Akella SV, Borthakur A, et al. Proteo-glycan depletion-induced changes in transverse relaxation maps of cartilage: comparison of T2 and T1rho. Acad Radiol 2002;9:1388–94.

85. Regatte RR, Akella SV, Borthakur A, et al. Proton spin-lock ratio imaging for quantitation of glycos-aminoglycans in articular cartilage. J Magn Reson Imaging 2003;17:114–21.

86. Duvvuri U, Kudchodkar S, Reddy R, et al. T1rho relaxation can assess longitudinal proteoglycan loss from articular cartilage in vitro. Osteoarthritis Cartilage 2002;10:838–44.

87. Duvvuri U, Reddy R, Patel SD, et al. T1rho-relaxa-tion in articular cartilage: effects of enzymatic degradation. Magn Reson Med 1997;38:863–7.

88. Akella SV, Regatte RR, Gougoutas AJ, et al. Proteo-glycan-induced changes in T1 rho-relaxation of articular cartilage at 4T. Magn Reson Med 2001; 46:419–23.

89. Wheaton AJ, Dodge GR, Borthakur A, et al. Detec-tion of changes in articular cartilage proteoglycan by T(1rho) magnetic resonance imaging. J Orthop Res 2005;23:102–8.

90. Regatte RR, Akella SV, Lonner JH, et al. T1 rho relaxation mapping in human osteoarthritis (OA) cartilage: comparison of T1rho with T2. J Magn Re-son Imaging 2006;23:547–53.

91. Li X, Han ET, Ma CB, et al. In vivo 3T spiral imaging based multi-slice T1 rho mapping of knee cartilage in osteoarthritis. Magn Reson Med 2005;54: 929–36.

92. Regatte RR, Akella SV, Wheaton AJ, et al. 3D-T1 rho-relaxation mapping of articular cartilage: in vivo assessment of early degenerative changes in symptomatic osteoarthritic subjects. Acad Radiol 2004;11:741–9.

93. Taylor C, Carballido-Gamio J, Majumdar S, et al. Comparison of quantitative imaging of cartilage for osteoarthritis: T2, T1rho, dGEMRIC and contrast-enhanced computed tomography. Magn Reson Imaging 2009;27(6):779–84.

94. Wheaton AJ, Casey FL, Gougoutas AJ, et al. Correlation of T1rho with fixed charge density in cartilage. J Magn Reson Imaging 2004;20: 519–25.

95. Majumdar S, Li X, Blumenkrantz G, et al. MR imaging and early cartilage degeneration and strategies for monitoring regeneration. J Musculoskelet Neuronal Interact 2006;6:382–4.

96. Regatte RR, Akella SV, Borthakur A, et al. In vivo proton MR three-dimensional T1rho mapping of human articular cartilage: initial experience. Radi-ology 2003;229:269–74.

97. Wheaton AJ, Borthakur A, Kneeland JB, et al. In vivo quantification of T1rho using a multislice spin-lock pulse sequence. Magn Reson Med 2004;52:1453–8.

98. Akella SV, Regatte RR, Borthakur A, et al. T1 rho MR imaging of the human wrist in vivo. Acad Radiol 2003;10:614–9.

99. Pakin SK, Schweitzer ME, Regatte RR. 3D-T1rho quantitation of patellar cartilage at 3.0T. J Magn Reson Imaging 2006;24:1357–63.

100. Borthakur A, Wheaton A, Charagundla SR, et al. Three-dimensional T1rho-weighted MRI at 1.5 Tesla. J Magn Reson Imaging 2003;17:730–6.

101. Zuo J, Li X, Banerjee S, et al. Parallel imaging of knee cartilage at 3 Tesla. J Magn Reson Imaging 2007;26:1001–9.

102. Witschey WR, Borthakur A, Elliott MA, et al. T1rho-prepared balanced gradient echo for rapid 3D T1rho MRI. J Magn Reson Imaging 2008;28: 744–54.

103. Pakin SK, Xu J, Schweitzer ME, et al. Rapid 3D-T1rho mapping of the knee joint at 3.0T with parallel imaging. Magn Reson Med 2006;56:563–71.

104. Maroudas A. Physicochemical properties of artic-ular cartilage. In: Freeman M, editor. Adult articular cartilage. 2nd edition. London: Pitman Medical; 1979. p. 215–90.

105. Eisenberg SR, Grodzinsky AJ. Swelling of articular cartilage and other connective tissues: electrome-chanochemical forces. J Orthop Res 1985;3:148–59.

106. Frank EH, Grodzinsky AJ, Koob TJ, et al. Streaming potentials: a sensitive index of enzymatic degrada-tion in particular cartilage. J Orthop Res 1987;5: 497–508.

107. Maroudas A, Bayliss MT, Venn MF. Further studies on the composition of human femoral head carti-lage. Ann Rheum Dis 1980;39:514–23.

108. Maroudas A, Venn M. Chemical composition and swelling of normal and osteoarthrotic femoral cartilage. II. Swelling. Ann Rheum Dis 1977;36: 399–406.

109. Ficat C, Maroudas A. Cartilage of the patella. Topo-graphical variation of glycosaminoglycan content in normal and fibrillated tissue. Ann Rheum Dis 1975;34:515–9.

110. Maroudas A, Evans H, Almeida L. Cartilage of the hip joint. Topographical variation of glycosamino-glycan content in normal and fibrillated tissue. Ann Rheum Dis 1973;32:1–9.

111. Gold GE, Burstein D, Dardzinski B, et al. MRI of articular cartilage in OA: novel pulse sequences and composition/functional markers. Osteoarthritis Cartilage 2006;14(Suppl A):A76–86.

112. Gray ML, Burstein D, Xia Y. Biochemical (and func-tional) imaging of articular cartilage. Semin Muscu-loskelet Radiol 2001;5:329–43.

113. Gray ML, Burstein D. Molecular (and functional) imaging of articular cartilage. J Musculoskeletal Neuronal Interact 2004;4:365–8.

114. Bashir A, Gray ML, Hartke J, et al. Nondestructive imaging of human cartilage glycosaminoglycan

concentration by MRI. Magn Reson Med 1999;41:857–65.

115. Burstein D, Gray ML, Hartman AL, et al. Diffusion of small solutes in cartilage as measured by nuclear magnetic resonance (NMR) spectroscopy and imaging. J Orthop Res 1993;11:465–78.

116. Trattnig S, Mlynarik V, Breitenseher M, et al. MRI visualization of proteoglycan depletion in articular cartilage via intravenous administration of Gd-DTPA. Magn Reson Imaging 1999;17:577–83.

117. Allen RG, Burstein D, Gray ML. Monitoring glycosaminoglycan replenishment in cartilage explants with gadolinium-enhanced magnetic resonance imaging. J Orthop Res 1999;17:430–6.

118. Williams A, Oppenheimer RA, Gray ML, et al. Differential recovery of glycosaminoglycan after IL-1-induced degradation of bovine articular cartilage depends on degree of degradation. Arthritis Res Ther 2003;5:R97–105.

119. Nieminen MT, Rieppo J, Silvennoinen J, et al. Spatial assessment of articular cartilage proteoglycans with Gd-DTPA-enhanced T1 imaging. Magn Reson Med 2002;48:640–8.

120. Tiderius CJ, Tjornstrand J, Akeson P, et al. Delayed gadolinium-enhanced MRI of cartilage (dGEMRIC): intra- and interobserver variability in standardized drawing of regions of interest. Acta Radiol 2004;45:628–34.

121. Bashir A, Gray ML, Boutin RD, et al. Glycosaminoglycan in articular cartilage: in vivo assessment with delayed Gd(DTPA)(2-)-enhanced MR imaging. Radiology 1997;205:551–8.

122. Hargreaves BA, Gold GE, Beaulieu CF, et al. Comparison of new sequences for high-resolution cartilage imaging. Magn Reson Med 2003;49:700–9.

123. Gillis A, Bashir A, McKeon B, et al. Magnetic resonance imaging of relative glycosaminoglycan distribution in patients with autologous chondrocyte transplants. Invest Radiol 2001;36:743–8.

124. Vasara AI, Nieminen MT, Jurvelin JS, et al. Indentation stiffness of repair tissue after autologous chondrocyte transplantation. Clin Orthop Relat Res 2005;433:233–42.

125. Tiderius CJ, Olsson LE, Leander P, et al. Delayed gadolinium-enhanced MRI of cartilage (dGEMRIC) in early knee osteoarthritis. Magn Reson Med 2003;49:488–92.

126. Nojiri T, Watanabe N, Namura T, et al. Utility of delayed gadolinium-enhanced MRI (dGEMRIC) for qualitative evaluation of articular cartilage of patellofemoral joint. Knee Surg Sports Traumatol Arthrosc 2006;14:718–23.

127. Williams A, Sharma L, McKenzie CA, et al. Delayed gadolinium-enhanced magnetic resonance imaging of cartilage in knee osteoarthritis: findings at different radiographic stages of disease and relationship to malalignment. Arthritis Rheum 2005;52:3528–35.

128. Tiderius CJ, Svensson J, Leander P, et al. dGEMRIC (delayed gadolinium-enhanced MRI of cartilage) indicates adaptive capacity of human knee cartilage. Magn Reson Med 2004;51:286–90.

129. Roos EM, Dahlberg L. Positive effects of moderate exercise on glycosaminoglycan content in knee cartilage: a four-month, randomized, controlled trial in patients at risk of osteoarthritis. Arthritis Rheum 2005;52:3507–14.

130. Tiderius CJ, Olsson LE, de Verdier H, et al. Gd-DTPA2-enhanced MRI of femoral knee cartilage: a dose-response study in healthy volunteers. Magn Reson Med 2001;46:1067–71.

131. Williams A, Gillis A, McKenzie C, et al. Glycosaminoglycan distribution in cartilage as determined by delayed gadolinium-enhanced MRI of cartilage (dGEMRIC): potential clinical applications. AJR Am J Roentgenol 2004;182:167–72.

132. Tiderius CJ, Olsson LE, Nyquist F, et al. Cartilage glycosaminoglycan loss in the acute phase after an anterior cruciate ligament injury: delayed gadolinium-enhanced magnetic resonance imaging of cartilage and synovial fluid analysis. Arthritis Rheum 2005;52:120–7.

133. Young AA, Stanwell P, Williams A, et al. Glycosaminoglycan content of knee cartilage following posterior cruciate ligament rupture demonstrated by delayed gadolinium-enhanced magnetic resonance imaging of cartilage (dGEMRIC). A case report. J Bone Joint Surg Am 2005;87:2763–7.

134. Stevens K, Hishioka H, Steines D, et al. Contrast enhanced MRI measurement of GAG concentrations in articular cartilage of knees with early osteoarthritis. In: Proceedings of the Radiological Society of North America 2001;275.

135. Kim YJ, Jaramillo D, Millis MB, et al. Assessment of early osteoarthritis in hip dysplasia with delayed gadolinium-enhanced magnetic resonance imaging of cartilage. J Bone Joint Surg Am 2003;85-A:1987–92.

136. Cunningham T, Jessel R, Zurakowski D, et al. Delayed gadolinium-enhanced magnetic resonance imaging of cartilage to predict early failure of Bernese periacetabular osteotomy for hip dysplasia. J Bone Joint Surg Am 2006;88:1540–8.

137. Samosky JT, Burstein D, Eric Grimson W, et al. Spatially-localized correlation of dGEMRIC-measured GAG distribution and mechanical stiffness in the human tibial plateau. J Orthop Res 2005;23:93–101.

138. Baldassarri M, Goodwin JS, Farley ML, et al. Relationship between cartilage stiffness and GAG content: correlation and prediction. J Orthop Res 2007;25:904–12.

139. Kurkijarvi JE, Nissi MJ, Kiviranta I, et al. Delayed gadolinium-enhanced MRI of cartilage (dGEMRIC) and T2 characteristics of human knee articular cartilage: topographical variation and relationships to mechanical properties. Magn Reson Med 2004; 52:41–6.

140. Nissi MJ, Toyras J, Laasanen MS, et al. Proteoglycan and collagen sensitive MRI evaluation of normal and degenerated articular cartilage. J Orthop Res 2004;22:557–64.

141. Mayerhoefer ME, Welsch GH, Mamisch TC, et al. The in vivo effects of unloading and compression on T1-Gd (dGEMRIC) relaxation times in healthy articular knee cartilage at 3.0 Tesla. Eur Radiol 2010;20:443–9.

142. Trattnig S, Mamisch TC, Pinker K, et al. Differentiating normal hyaline cartilage from post-surgical repair tissue using fast gradient echo imaging in delayed gadolinium-enhanced MRI (dGEMRIC) at 3 Tesla. Eur Radiol 2008;18:1251–9.

143. Kurkijarvi JE, Mattila L, Ojala RO, et al. Evaluation of cartilage repair in the distal femur after autologous chondrocyte transplantation using T2 relaxation time and dGEMRIC. Osteoarthritis Cartilage 2007;15:372–8.

144. Miyata S, Homma K, Numano T, et al. Assessment of fixed charge density in regenerated cartilage by Gd-DTPA-enhanced MRI. Magn Reson Med Sci 2006;5:73–8.

145. Trattnig S, Marlovits S, Gebetsroither S, et al. Three-dimensional delayed gadolinium-enhanced MRI of cartilage (dGEMRIC) for in vivo evaluation of reparative cartilage after matrix-associated autologous chondrocyte transplantation at 3.0T: preliminary results. J Magn Reson Imaging 2007;26:974–82.

146. Watanabe A, Wada Y, Obata T, et al. Delayed gadolinium-enhanced MR to determine glycosaminoglycan concentration in reparative cartilage after autologous chondrocyte implantation: preliminary results. Radiology 2006;239:201–8.

147. Domayer SE, Welsch GH, Nehrer S, et al. T2 mapping and dGEMRIC after autologous chondrocyte implantation with a fibrin-based scaffold in the knee: preliminary results. Eur J Radiol 2010;73(3): 636–42.

148. Andreisek G, White LM, Yang Y, et al. Delayed gadolinium-enhanced MR imaging of articular cartilage: Three-dimensional T1 mapping with variable flip angles and B1 correction. Radiology 2009; 252(3):865–73.

149. Studler U, White LM, Andreisek G, et al. Impact of motion on T1 mapping acquired with inversion recovery fast spin echo and rapid spoiled gradient recalled-echo pulse sequences for delayed gadolinium-enhanced MRI of cartilage (dGEMRIC) in volunteers. J Magn Reson Imaging 2010;32: 394–8.

150. Siversson C, Tiderius C-J, Neuman P, et al. Repeatability of T1-quantification in dGEMRIC for three different acquisition techniques: two-dimensional inversion recovery, three-dimensional look locker, and three-dimensional variable flip angle. J Magn Reson Imaging 2010;31:1203–9.

151. McKenzie CA, Williams A, Prasad PV, et al. Three-dimensional delayed gadolinium-enhanced MRI of cartilage (dGEMRIC) at 1.5T and 3.0T. J Magn Reson Imaging 2006;24:928–33.

152. Bellin MF, Van Der Molen AJ. Extracellular gadolinium-based contrast media: an overview. Eur J Radiol 2008;66:160–7.

153. Idee JM, Port M, Medina C, et al. Possible involvement of gadolinium chelates in the pathophysiology of nephrogenic systemic fibrosis: a critical review. Toxicology 2008;248:77–88.

154. Kallen AJ, Jhung MA, Cheng S, et al. Gadolinium-containing magnetic resonance imaging contrast and nephrogenic systemic fibrosis: a case-control study. Am J Kidney Dis 2008;51:966–75.

155. Marckmann P, Skov L, Rossen K, et al. Nephrogenic systemic fibrosis: suspected causative role of gadodiamide used for contrast-enhanced magnetic resonance imaging. J Am Soc Nephrol 2006;17:2359–62.

156. Nainani N, Panesar M. Nephrogenic systemic fibrosis. Am J Nephrol 2008;29:1–9.

157. Wiginton CD, Kelly B, Oto A, et al. Gadolinium-based contrast exposure, nephrogenic systemic fibrosis, and gadolinium detection in tissue. AJR Am J Roentgenol 2008;190:1060–8.

158. Li W, Scheidegger R, Wu Y, et al. Accuracy of T1 measurement with 3-D Look-Locker technique for dGEMRIC. J Magn Reson Imaging 2008;27: 678–82.

159. Kimelman T, Vu A, Storey P, et al. Three-dimensional T1 mapping for dGEMRIC at 3.0T using the Look Locker method. Invest Radiol 2006;41: 198–203.

160. Gold GE, Chen CA, Koo S, et al. Recent advances in MRI of articular cartilage. AJR Am J Roentgenol 2009;193:628–38.

161. Lehner KB, Rechl HP, Gmeinwieser JK, et al. Structure, function, and degeneration of bovine hyaline cartilage: assessment with MR imaging in vitro. Radiology 1989;170:495–9.

162. Lusse S, Claassen H, Gehrke T, et al. Evaluation of water content by spatially resolved transverse relaxation times of human articular cartilage. Magn Reson Imaging 2000;18:423–30.

163. Lusse S, Knauss R, Werner A, et al. Action of compression and cations on the proton and deuterium relaxation in cartilage. Magn Reson Med 1995;33:483–9.

164. Shapiro EM, Borthakur A, Kaufman JH, et al. Water distribution patterns inside bovine articular

cartilage as visualized by 1H magnetic resonance imaging. Osteoarthritis Cartilage 2001;9:533–8.

165. Fragonas E, Mlynarik V, Jellus V, et al. Correlation between biochemical composition and magnetic resonance appearance of articular cartilage. Osteoarthritis Cartilage 1998;6:24–32.

166. Nieminen MT, Toyras J, Rieppo J, et al. Quantitative MR microscopy of enzymatically degraded articular cartilage. Magn Reson Med 2000;43:676–81.

167. Watrin A, Ruaud JP, Olivier PT, et al. T2 mapping of rat patellar cartilage. Radiology 2001;219:395–402.

168. Watrin-Pinzano A, Ruaud JP, Cheli Y, et al. T2 mapping: an efficient MR quantitative technique to evaluate spontaneous cartilage repair in rat patella. Osteoarthritis Cartilage 2004;12:191–200.

169. Henkelman RM, Stanisz GJ, Kim JK, et al. Anisotropy of NMR properties of tissues. Magn Reson Med 1994;32:592–601.

170. Rubenstein JD, Kim JK, Morova-Protzner I, et al. Effects of collagen orientation on MR imaging characteristics of bovine articular cartilage. Radiology 1993;188:219–26.

171. Grunder W, Wagner M, Werner A. MR-microscopic visualization of anisotropic internal cartilage structures using the magic angle technique. Magn Reson Med 1998;39:376–82.

172. Xia Y, Farquhar T, Burton-Wurster N, et al. Diffusion and relaxation mapping of cartilage-bone plugs and excised disks using microscopic magnetic resonance imaging. Magn Reson Med 1994;31:273–82.

173. Xia Y. Relaxation anisotropy in cartilage by NMR microscopy (muMRI) at 14-micron resolution. Magn Reson Med 1998;39:941–9.

174. Xia Y, Farquhar T, Burton-Wurster N, et al. Origin of cartilage laminae in MRI. J Magn Reson Imaging 1997;7:887–94.

175. Goodwin DW, Dunn JF. High-resolution magnetic resonance imaging of articular cartilage: correlation with histology and pathology. Top Magn Reson Imaging 1998;9:337–47.

176. Mlynarik V, Degrassi A, Toffanin R, et al. A method for generating magnetic resonance microimaging T2 maps with low sensitivity to diffusion. Magn Reson Med 1996;35:423–5.

177. Kim DJ, Suh JS, Jeong EK, et al. Correlation of laminated MR appearance of articular cartilage with histology, ascertained by artificial landmarks on the cartilage. J Magn Reson Imaging 1999;10:57–64.

178. Xia Y. Heterogeneity of cartilage laminae in MR imaging. J Magn Reson Imaging 2000;11:686–93.

179. Nieminen MT, Rieppo J, Toyras J, et al. T2 relaxation reveals spatial collagen architecture in articular cartilage: a comparative quantitative MRI an polarized light microscopic study. Magn Reson Med 2001;46:487–93.

180. Xia Y, Moody JB, Alhadlaq H. Orientational dependence of T2 relaxation in articular cartilage: a microscopic MRI (microMRI) study. Magn Reson Med 2002;48:460–9.

181. Goodwin DW, Wadghiri YZ, Zhu H, et al. Macroscopic structure of articular cartilage of the tibial plateau: influence of a characteristic matrix architecture on MRI appearance. AJR Am J Roentgenol 2004;182:311–8.

182. Konig H, Sauter R, Delmling M, et al. Cartilage disorders: a comparison of spin-echo, CHESS, and FLASH sequence MR images. Radiology 1987;164:753–8.

183. Broderick L, Turner D, Renfrew D, et al. Severity of articular cartilage abnormality in patients with osteoarthritis: evaluation with fast spin-echo MR vs. arthroscopy. AJR Am J Roentgenol 1994;162:99–103.

184. Peterfy CG. Imaging of the disease process. Curr Opin Rheumatol 2002;14:590–6.

185. Shinar H, Seo Y, Ikoma K, et al. Mapping of the fiber orientation in articular cartilage at rest and under pressure studied by 2H double quantum filtered MRI. Magn Reson Med 2002;48:322–30.

186. Keinan-Adamsky K, Shinar H, Navon G. The effect of detachment of the articular cartilage from its calcified zone on the cartilage microstructure, assessed by 2H-spectroscopic double quantum filtered MRI. J Orthop Res 2005;23:109–17.

187. Xia Y. Magic-angle effect in magnetic resonance imaging of articular cartilage: a review. Invest Radiol 2000;35:602–21.

188. Krasnosselskaia LV, Fullerton GD, Dodd SJ, et al. Water in tendon: orientational analysis of the free induction decay. Magn Reson Med 2005;54:280–8.

189. Bydder M, Rahal A, Fullerton GD, et al. The magic angle effect: a source of artifact, determinant of image contrast, and technique for imaging. J Magn Reson Imaging 2007;25:290–300.

190. Cameron IL, Hunter KE, Ord VA, et al. Relationships between ice crystal size, water content and proton NMR relaxation times in cells. Physiol Chem Phys Med NMR 1985;17:371–86.

191. Xia Y. Averaged and depth-dependent anisotropy of articular cartilage by microscopic imaging. Semin Arthritis Rheum 2008;37:317–27.

192. Shirazi R, Shirazi-Adl A. Deep vertical collagen fibrils play a significant role in mechanics of articular cartilage. J Orthop Res 2008;26:608–15.

193. Korhonen RK, Julkunen P, Wilson W, et al. Importance of collagen orientation and depth-dependent fixed charge densities of cartilage on mechanical behavior of chondrocytes. J Biomech Eng 2008;130:021003.

194. Julkunen P, Korhonen RK, Nissi MJ, et al. Mechanical characterization of articular cartilage

by combining magnetic resonance imaging and finite-element analysis–a potential functional imaging technique. Phys Med Biol 2008;53: 2425–38.

195. Bae WC, Wong VW, Hwang J, et al. Wear-lines and split-lines of human patellar cartilage: relation to tensile biomechanical properties. Osteoarthritis Cartilage 2008;16:841–5.

196. Federico S, Herzog W. On the anisotropy and inhomogeneity of permeability in articular cartilage. Biomech Model Mechanobiol 2007;7:367–78.

197. Alhadlaq HA, Xia Y. The structural adaptations in compressed articular cartilage by microscopic MRI (microMRI) T(2) anisotropy. Osteoarthritis Cartilage 2004;12:887–94.

198. Xia Y. Averaged properties of articular cartilage from multidisciplinary microscopic imaging study. Conf Proc IEEE Eng Med Biol Soc 2005;3: 3161–4.

199. Mosher TJ, Dardzinski BJ. Cartilage MRI T2 relaxation time mapping: overview and applications. Semin Musculoskelet Radiol 2004;8:355–68.

200. Bi X, Yang X, Bostrom MP, et al. Fourier transform infrared imaging and MR microscopy studies detect compositional and structural changes in cartilage in a rabbit model of osteoarthritis. Anal Bioanal Chem 2007;387:1601–12.

201. Mow VC, Holmes MH, Lai WM. Fluid transport and mechanical properties of articular cartilage: a review. J Biomech 1984;17:377–94.

202. Smith HE, Mosher TJ, Dardzinski BJ, et al. Spatial variation in cartilage T2 of the knee. J Magn Reson Imaging 2001;14:50–5.

203. Xia Y. Resolution "scaling law" in MRI of articular cartilage. Osteoarthritis Cartilage 2007;15:363–5.

204. Van Breuseghem I, Bosmans HT, Elst LV, et al. T2 mapping of human femorotibial cartilage with turbo mixed MR imaging at 1.5 T: feasibility. Radiology 2004;233:609–14.

205. Quaia E, Toffanin R, Guglielmi G, et al. Fast T2 mapping of the patellar articular cartilage with gradient and spin-echo magnetic resonance imaging at 1.5 T: validation and initial clinical experience in patients with osteoarthritis. Skeletal Radiol 2008;37:511–7.

206. Bittersohl B, Hosalkar HS, Hughes T, et al. Feasibility of T2* mapping for the evaluation of hip joint cartilage at 1.5T using a three-dimensional (3D), gradient-echo (GRE) sequence: a prospective study. Magn Reson Med 2009;62(4):896–901.

207. Williams A, Qian A, Bear D, et al. Assessing degeneration of human articular cartilage with ultra-short echo time (UTE) T2* mapping. Osteoarthritis Cartilage 2010;18(4):539–46.

208. David-Vaudey E, Ghosh S, Ries M, et al. T2 relaxation time measurements in osteoarthritis. Magn Reson Imaging 2004;22:673–82.

209. Gahunia HK, Lemaire C, Cross AR, et al. Osteoarthritis in rhesus macaques: assessment of cartilage matrix quality by quantitative magnetic resonance imaging. Agents Actions Suppl 1993;39:255–9.

210. Gahunia HK, Babyn P, Lemaire C, et al. Osteoarthritis staging: comparison between magnetic resonance imaging, gross pathology and histopathology in the rhesus macaque. Osteoarthritis Cartilage 1995;3:169–80.

211. Spandonis Y, Heese FP, Hall LD. High resolution MRI relaxation measurements of water in the articular cartilage of the meniscectomized rat knee at 4.7T. Magn Reson Imaging 2004;22:943–51.

212. Watrin-Pinzano A, Ruaud JP, Cheli Y, et al. Evaluation of cartilage repair tissue after biomaterial implantation in rat patella using T2 mapping. MAGMA 2004;17:219–28.

213. Mosher TJ, Smith H, Dardzinski B, et al. MR imaging and T2 mapping of femoral cartilage: in vivo determination of the magic angle effect. AJR Am J Roentgenol 2001;177:665–9.

214. Dardzinski BJ, Laor T, Schmithorst VJ, et al. Mapping T2 relaxation time in the pediatric knee: feasibility with a clinical 1.5-T MR imaging system. Radiology 2002;225:233–9.

215. Dardzinski BJ, Mosher TJ, Li S, et al. Spatial variation of T2 in human articular cartilage. Radiology 1997;205:546–50.

216. Yao W, Qu N, Lu Z, et al. The application of T1 and T2 relaxation time and magnetization transfer ratios to the early diagnosis of patellar cartilage osteoarthritis. Skeletal Radiol 2009;38:1055–62.

217. Watanabe A, Boesch C, Siebenrock K, et al. T2 mapping of hip articular cartilage in healthy volunteers at 3T: a study of topographic variation. J Magn Reson Imaging 2007;26:165–71.

218. Nishii T, Tanaka H, Sugano N, et al. Evaluation of cartilage matrix disorders by T2 relaxation time in patients with hip dysplasia. Osteoarthritis Cartilage 2008;16:227–33.

219. Welsch GH, Mamisch TC, Weber M, et al. High-resolution morphological and biochemical imaging of articular cartilage of the ankle joint at 3.0T using a new dedicated phased array coil: in vivo reproducibility study. Skeletal Radiol 2008; 37:519–26.

220. Lazovic-Stojkovic J, Mosher TJ, Smith HE, et al. Interphalangeal joint cartilage: high-spatial-resolution in vivo MR T2 mapping—a feasibility study. Radiology 2004;233:292–6.

221. Mosher TJ, Dardzinski BJ, Smith MB. Human articular cartilage: influence of aging and early symptomatic degeneration on the spatial variation of T2-preliminary findings at 3 T. Radiology 2000; 214:259–66.

222. Dray N, Williams A, Prasad PV, et al. T2 in an OA population: Metrics for reporting data? [abstract

1995]. In: Proc Ann Meeting Int Soc Magn Resonance Med (ISMRM). Miami (FL); 2005.

223. Dunn TC, Lu Y, Jin H, et al. T2 relaxation time of cartilage at MR imaging: comparison with severity of knee osteoarthritis. Radiology 2004; 232:592–8.

224. Blumenkrantz G, Dunn TC, Carballido-Gamio J, et al. Spatial heterogeneity of cartilage T2 in osteoarthritic patients. Boston: OARSI; 2005.

225. Goebel JC, Watrin-Pinzano A, Bettembourg-Brault I, et al. Age-related quantitative MRI changes in healthy cartilage: preliminary results. Biorheology 2006;43:547–51.

226. Mosher TJ, Liu Y, Yang QX, et al. Age dependency of cartilage magnetic resonance imaging T2 relaxation times in asymptomatic women. Arthritis Rheum 2004;50:2820–8.

227. Mosher TJ, Collins CM, Smith HE, et al. Effect of gender on in vivo cartilage magnetic resonance imaging T2 mapping. J Magn Reson Imaging 2004;19:323–8.

228. Stahl R, Blumenkrantz G, Carballido-Gamio J, et al. MRI-derived T2 relaxation times and cartilage morphometry of the tibio-femoral joint in subjects with and without osteoarthritis during a 1-year follow-up. Osteoarthritis Cartilage 2007;15:1225–34.

229. Blumenkrantz G, Lindsey CT, Dunn TC, et al. A pilot, two-year longitudinal study of the interrelationship between trabecular bone and articular cartilage in the osteoarthritic knee. Osteoarthritis Cartilage 2004;12:997–1005.

230. Blumenkrantz G, Dunn TC, Ries MD, et al. Cartilage T2 as a marker of progression of osteoarthritis [abstract 2004]. In: Proc Ann Meet Am Coll Rheumatol. San Antonio (TX); 2004.

231. Apprich S, Welsch GH, Mamisch TC, et al. Detection of degenerative cartilage disease: comparison of high-resolution morphological MR and quantitative T2 mapping at 3.0 Tesla. Osteoarthritis Cartilage 2010;18(9):1211–7.

232. Shiomi T, Nishii T, Myoui A, et al. Influence of knee positions on T2, T2*, and dGEMRIC mapping in porcine knee cartilage. Magn Reson Med 2010; 64(3):707–14.

233. Friedrich KM, Shepard T, Chang G, et al. Does joint alignment affect the T2 values of cartilage in patients with knee osteoarthritis? Eur Radiol 2010; 20:1532–8.

234. Grunder W, Kanowski M, Wagner M, et al. Visualization of pressure distribution within loaded joint cartilage by application of angle-sensitive NMR microscopy. Magn Reson Med 2000;43: 884–91.

235. Alhadlaq HA, Xia Y. Modifications of orientational dependence of microscopic magnetic resonance imaging T(2) anisotropy in compressed articular cartilage. J Magn Reson Imaging 2005;22:665–73.

236. Nag D, Liney GP, Gillespie P, et al. Quantification of T(2) relaxation changes in articular cartilage with in situ mechanical loading of the knee. J Magn Reson Imaging 2004;19:317–22.

237. Stehling C, Liebl H, Krug R, et al. Patellar cartilage: T2 values and morphologic abnormalities at 3.0-T MR imaging in relation to physical activity in asymptomatic subjects from the Osteoarthritis Initiative. Radiology 2010;254(2):509–20.

238. Mosher TJ, Liu Y, Torok CM. Functional cartilage MRI T2 mapping: evaluating the effect of age and training on knee cartilage response to running. Osteoarthritis Cartilage 2010;18:358–64.

239. Mosher TJ, Smith HE, Collins C, et al. Change in knee cartilage T2 at MR imaging after running: a feasibility study. Radiology 2005;234:245–9.

240. Welsch GH, Mamisch TC, Domayer SE, et al. Cartilage T2 assessment at 3-T MR imaging: in vivo differentiation of normal hyaline cartilage from reparative tissue after two cartilage repair procedures—initial experience. Radiology 2008;247: 154–61.

241. Domayer SE, Kutscha-Lissberg F, Welsch G, et al. T2 mapping in the knee after microfracture at 3.0T: correlation of global T2 values and clinical outcome–preliminary results. Osteoarthritis Cartilage 2008;16:903–8.

242. Trattnig S, Mamisch TC, Welsch GH, et al. Quantitative T2 mapping of matrix-associated autologous chondrocyte transplantation at 3 Tesla: an in vivo cross-sectional study. Invest Radiol 2007;42:442–8.

243. Trattnig S, Millington SA, Szomolanyi P, et al. MR imaging of osteochondral grafts and autologous chondrocyte implantation. Eur Radiol 2007;17: 103–18.

244. White LM, Sussman MS, Hurtig M, et al. Cartilage T2 assessment: differentiation of normal hyaline cartilage and reparative tissue after arthroscopic cartilage repair in equine subjects. Radiology 2006;241:407–14.

245. Kangarlu A, Gahunia HK. Magnetic resonance imaging characterization of osteochondral defect repair in a goat model at 8T. Osteoarthritis Cartilage 2006;14:52–62.

246. Welsch GH, Trattnig S, Hughes T, et al. T2 and T2* mapping in patients after matrix-associated autologous chondrocyte transplantation: initial results on clinical use with 3.0-Tesla MRI. Eur Radiol 2010;20: 1515–23.

247. Mamisch TC, Trattnig S, Quirbach S, et al. Quantitative T2 mapping of knee cartilage: differentiation of healthy control cartilage and cartilage repair tissue in the knee with unloading—initial results. Radiology 2010;254(3):818–26.

248. Quirbach S, Trattnig S, Marlovits S, et al. Initial results of in vivo high-resolution morphological and biochemical cartilage imaging of patients after

matrix-associated autologous chondrocyte transplantation (MACT) of the ankle. Skeletal Radiol 2009;38(3):751–60.

249. Welsch GH, Trattnig S, Domayer S, et al. Multimodal approach in the use of clinical scoring, morphological MRI and biochemical T2-mapping and diffusion-weighted imaging in their ability to assess differences between cartilage repair tissue after microfracture therapy and matrix-associated autologous chondrocyte transplantation: a pilot study. Osteoarthritis Cartilage 2009;17(9):1219–27.

250. Robson MD, Gatehouse PD, Bydder M, et al. Magnetic resonance: an introduction to ultrashort TE (UTE) imaging. J Comput Assist Tomogr 2003; 27:825–46.

251. Bae WC, Dwek JR, Znamirowski R, et al. Ultrashort echo time MR imaging of osteochondral junction of the knee at 3T: identification of anatomic structures contributing to signal intensity. Radiology 2010; 254(3):837–45.

252. Bydder M, Du J, Takahashi AM, et al. Chemical shift artifact in center-out radial sampling: a potential pitfall in clinical diagnosis [abstract]. In: Proceedings of the Fifteenth Meeting of the International Society for Magnetic Resonance in Medicine. Berkeley (CA): International Society for Magnetic Resonance in Medicine; 2007. p. 1811.

253. Gatehouse PD, Thomas RW, Robson MD, et al. Magnetic resonance imaging of the knee with ultrashort TE pulse sequences. Magn Reson Imaging 2004;22:1061–7.

254. Gatehouse PD, Bydder GM. Magnetic resonance imaging of short T2 components in tissue. Clin Radiol 2003;58(1):1–19.

255. Gatehouse PD, He T, Puri BK, et al. Contrast-enhanced MRI of the menisci of the knee using ultrashort echo time (UTE) pulse sequences: imaging of the red and white zones. Br J Radiol 2004;77:641–7.

256. Gold GE, Thedens DR, Pauly JM, et al. MR imaging of articular cartilage of the knee: new methods using ultrashort TEs. AJR Am J Roentgenol 1998; 170:1223–6.

257. Filho GH, Du J, Pak BC, et al. Quantitative characterization of the Achilles tendon in cadaveric specimens: T1 and T2* measurements using ultrashort-TE MRI at 3T. AJR Am J Roentgenol 2009;192:W117–24.

258. Lyons TJ, Stoddart RW, McClure SF, et al. The tidemark of the chondro-osseous junction of the normal human knee joint. J Mol Histol 2005;36(3): 207–15.

259. Ferguson VL, Bushby AJ, Boyde A. Nanomechanical properties and mineral concentration in articular calcified cartilage and subchondral bone. J Anat 2003;203:191–9.

260. Li BH, Marshall D, Roe M, et al. The electron microscope appearance of the subchondral bone plate in the human femoral head in osteoarthritis and osteoporosis. J Anat 1999;195:101–10.

261. Burr DB. Anatomy and physiology of the mineralized tissues: role in the pathogenesis of osteoarthritis. Osteoarthritis Cartilage 2004;12:S20–30.

262. Martel-Pelletier J. Pathophysiology of osteoarthritis. Osteoarthritis Cartilage 2004;12:S31–3.

263. Muir P, McCarthy J, Radtke CL, et al. Role of endochondral ossification of articular cartilage and functional adaptation of the subchondral plate in the development of fatigue microcracking of joints. Bone 2006;38:342–9.

264. Squires GR, Okouneff S, Ionescu M, et al. The pathobiology of focal lesion development in aging human articular cartilage and molecular matrix changes characteristic of osteoarthritis. Arthritis Rheum 2003;48:1261–70.

265. Donohue JM, Buss D, Oegema TR, et al. The effects of indirect blunt trauma on adult canine articular cartilage. J Bone Joint Surg Am 1983;65:948–57.

266. Wansapura JP, Daniel BL, Pauly J, et al. Temperature mapping of frozen tissue using eddy current compensated half excitation RF pulses. Magn Reson Med 2001;46(5):985–92.

267. Noll DC, Pauly JM, Meyer CH, et al. Deblurring for non-2D Fourier transform magnetic resonance imaging. Magn Reson Med 1992;25(2):319–33.

268. Lu A, Daniel BL, Pauly KB. Improved slice excitation for ultrashort TE imaging with B0 and linear eddy current correction [abstract]. In: Proceedings of the Fourteenth Meeting of the International Society for Magnetic Resonance in Medicine. Berkeley (CA): International Society for Magnetic Resonance in Medicine; 2006. p. 2381.

269. Hwang J, Bae WC, Shieu W, et al. Increased hydraulic conductance of human articular cartilage and subchondral bone plate with progression of osteoarthritis. Arthritis Rheum 2008;58(12):3831–42.

270. Frisbie DD, Morisset S, Ho CP, et al. Effects of calcified cartilage on healing of chondral defects treated with microfracture in horses. Am J Sports Med 2006;34(11):1824–31.

271. Koskinen SK, Komu ME. Low-field strength magnetization transfer contrast imaging of the patellar cartilage. Acta Radiol 1993;34:124–6.

272. Regatte RR, Akella SV, Reddy R. Depth-dependent proton magnetization transfer in articular cartilage. J Magn Reson Imaging 2005;22:318–23.

273. Yao L, Gentili A, Thomas A. Incidental magnetization transfer contrast in fast spin-echo imaging of cartilage. J Magn Reson Imaging 1996;6:180–4.

274. Dixon WT, Engels H, Castillo M, et al. Incidental magnetization transfer contrast in standard multislice imaging. Magn Reson Imaging 1990;8:417–22.

275. Maier CF, Tan SG, Hariharan H, et al. T2 quantitation of articular cartilage at 1.5T. J Magn Reson Imaging 2003;17:358–64.

276. Watanabe A, Boesch C, Obata T, et al. Effect of multislice acquisition on T1 and T2 measurements of articular cartilage at 3T. J Magn Reson Imaging 2007;26:109–17.

277. Martirosian P, Boss A, Deimling M, et al. Systematic variation of off-resonance prepulses for clinical magnetization transfer contrast imaging at 0.2, 1.5, and 3.0 Tesla. Invest Radiol 2008;43:16–26.

278. Vahlensieck M, Traber F, Giesecke J, et al. Magnetization transfer contrast (MTC): optimizing off-resonance and on-resonance frequency MTC methods at 0.5 and 1.5T. Biomed Tech (Berl) 2001;46:10–7 [in German].

279. Peterfy CG, van Dijke CF, Janzen DL, et al. Quantification of articular cartilage in the knee with pulsed saturation transfer subtraction and fat-suppressed MR imaging: optimization and validation. Radiology 1994;192:485–91.

280. Hohe J, Faber S, Stammberger T, et al. A technique for 3D in vivo quantification of proton density and magnetization transfer coefficients of knee joint cartilage. Osteoarthritis Cartilage 2000;8:426–33.

281. Vahlensieck M, Dombrowski F, Leutner C, et al. Magnetization transfer contrast (MTC) and MTC-subtraction: enhancement of cartilage lesions and intracartilaginous degeneration in vitro. Skeletal Radiol 1994;23:535–9.

282. Palmieri F, De Keyzer F, Maes F, et al. Magnetization transfer analysis of cartilage repair tissue: a preliminary study. Skeletal Radiol 2006;35:903–8.

283. Kim DK, Ceckler TL, Hascall VC, et al. Analysis of water-macromolecule proton magnetization transfer in articular cartilage. Magn Reson Med 1993; 29:211–5.

284. Lattanzio PJ, Marshall KW, Damyanovich AZ, et al. Macromolecule and water magnetization transfer in articular cartilage. Magn Reson Med 2000;44: 840–51.

285. Seo GS, Aoki J, Moriya H, et al. Hyaline cartilage: in vivo and in vitro assessment with magnetization transfer imaging. Radiology 1996;201:525–30.

286. Toffanin R, Mlynarik V, Russo S, et al. Proteoglycan depletion and magnetic resonance parameters of articular cartilage. Arch Biochem Biophys 2001; 390:235–42.

287. Potter K, Butler JJ, Horton WE, et al. Response of engineered cartilage tissue to biochemical agents as studied by proton magnetic resonance microscopy. Arthritis Rheum 2000;43:1580–90.

288. Li W, Hong L, Hu L, et al. Magnetization transfer imaging provides a quantitative measure of chondrogenic differentiation and tissue development.

Tissue Eng Part C Methods 2010;16(6):1407–15. DOI:10.1089/ten.tec.2009.0777.

289. Laurent D, O'Byrne E, Wasvary J, et al. In vivo MRI of cartilage pathogenesis in surgical models of osteoarthritis. Skeletal Radiol 2006;35:555–64.

290. Laurent D, Wasvary J, O'Byrne E, et al. In vivo qualitative assessments of articular cartilage in the rabbit knee with high-resolution MRI at 3T. Magn Reson Med 2003;50:541–9.

291. Laurent D, Wasvary J, Yin J, et al. Quantitative and qualitative assessment of articular cartilage in the goat knee with magnetization transfer imaging. Magn Reson Imaging 2001;19:1279–86.

292. Wolff SD, Chesnick S, Frank JA, et al. Magnetization transfer contrast: MR imaging of the knee. Radiology 1991;179:623–8.

293. Niitsu M, Hirohata H, Yoshioka H, et al. Magnetization transfer contrast on gradient echo MR imaging of the temporomandibular joint. Acta Radiol 1995; 36:295–9.

294. Peterfy CG, Majumdar S, Lang P, et al. MR imaging of the arthritic knee: improved discrimination of cartilage, synovium, and effusion with pulsed saturation transfer and fat-suppressed T1-weighted sequences. Radiology 1994;191:413–9.

295. Mori R, Ochi M, Sakai Y, et al. Clinical significance of magnetic resonance imaging (MRI) for focal chondral lesions. Magn Reson Imaging 1999;17: 1135–40.

296. Welsch GH, Trattnig S, Scheffler K, et al. Magnetization transfer contrast and T2 mapping in the evaluation of cartilage repair tissue with 3T MRI. J Magn Reson Imaging 2008;28(4):979–86.

297. Kneeland JB. MRI probes biophysical structure of cartilage. Diagn Imaging (San Franc) 1996;18:36–40.

298. Butts K, Pauly J, de Crespigny A, et al. Isotropic diffusion-weighted and spiral-navigated interleaved EPI for routine imaging of acute stroke. Magn Reson Med 1997;38:741–9.

299. Xia Y, Farquhar T, Burton-Wurster N, et al. Self-diffusion monitors degraded cartilage. Arch Biochem Biophys 1995;323:323–8.

300. Mamisch TC, Menzel MI, Welsch GH, et al. Steady-state diffusion imaging for MR in-vivo evaluation of reparative cartilage after matrix-associated autologous chondrocyte transplantation at 3 tesla—preliminary results. Eur J Radiol 2008;65(1):72–9.

301. Friedrich KM, Mamisch TC, Plank C, et al. Diffusion-weighted imaging for the follow-up of patients after matrix-associated autologous chondrocyte transplantation. Eur J Radiol 2010;73(3):622–8.

Rapidly Progressive Osteoarthritis: Biomechanical Considerations

Eric A. Walker, MD[a,b,c], Derik Davis, MD[d],
Timothy J. Mosher, MD[a],*

KEYWORDS

- Osteoarthritis • Knee malalignment • Meniscal dysfunction
- Osteochondral unit injury

The American College of Rheumatology defines osteoarthritis (OA) as a heterogeneous group of conditions that leads to joint signs and symptoms that are associated with defective integrity of articular cartilage, and associated changes in the underlying bone and at the joint margins.[1] Although OA is a multifactorial disease process, early cartilage damage and ultimate loss of articular cartilage is a central feature and a significant contributor to clinical symptoms. The rate of progression of tissue damage and clinical symptoms can vary substantially between patients. A clinical challenge in managing patients with OA is differentiating individuals at risk for rapidly progressive disease. A potential role of imaging is identification of specific biomarkers that are prognostic of rapid OA progression. In clinical care such indicators could guide lifestyle changes or treatment recommendations in select patients at greatest risk for rapid onset of OA. In research, identifying subjects likely to have rapid OA progression would provide more efficient clinical trials by shortening the observation period or allowing for a smaller sample size.

It is difficult to identify specific features predictive of OA progression using radiographic methods. A systematic review of 1004 studies conducted prior to 2003 identified 37 studies meeting the inclusion criteria for quality and suggests that knee pain, radiologic severity at baseline, sex, quadriceps strength, knee injury, and regular sport activities are not related to OA progression.[2] For other factors, the evidence was limited or conflicting. The more recent use of magnetic resonance (MR) imaging in clinical studies of OA has the potential to provide additional imaging biomarkers that may be better predictors of OA progression. In a cohort of 43 subjects, Biswal and colleagues[3] found that anterior cruciate and meniscal tears along with focal chondral lesions in the central weight-bearing zones were predictive of more rapid OA progression. A recent report from the Multi-center Osteoarthritis Trial (MOST trial) identified high body mass index (BMI), meniscal damage, meniscal extrusion, and any high-grade MR imaging feature defined as a Whole-Organ Magnetic Resonance Imaging Score (WORMS) score of 2 or more as baseline risk factors for fast cartilage loss over a 30-month period.[4] However; because these features were present in both slow and rapid progressors, they did not predict the rate of OA

[a] Department of Radiology MC H066, Penn State University College of Medicine, Penn State Milton S. Hershey Medical Center, 500 University Drive, Hershey, PA 17033, USA
[b] Department of Radiology, Uniformed Services University of the Health Sciences, 4301 Jones Bridge Road, Bethesda, MD 20814, USA
[c] Department of Nuclear Medicine, Uniformed Services University of the Health Sciences, 4301 Jones Bridge Road, Bethesda, MD 20814, USA
[d] Department Diagnostic Radiology & Nuclear Medicine, University of Maryland Medical Center, 22 South Greene Street, Baltimore, MD 21201-1595, USA
* Corresponding author.
E-mail address: tmosher@psu.edu

Magn Reson Imaging Clin N Am 19 (2011) 283–294
doi:10.1016/j.mric.2011.02.008
1064-9689/11/$ – see front matter © 2011 Elsevier Inc. All rights reserved.

progression. Further study is needed to determine whether combination of imaging biomarkers or greater refinement of potential biomarkers will improve differentiation of those individuals who are likely to have rapidly progressive OA.

An underlying hypothesis for rapid cartilage loss in patients with OA is that perturbation from normal joint mechanics produces locally high biomechanical strains that exceed the material properties of the tissue, leading to rapid destruction. Several imaging findings are associated with focally high biomechanical forces and thus are potential candidates for predictive biomarkers of rapid OA progression. In this article, the authors focus on 3 aspects of knee biomechanics that have potential MR imaging correlates, and which may serve as prognostic biomarkers: knee malalignment, meniscal dysfunction, and injury of the osteochondral unit.

KNEE MALALIGNMENT

The causes of varus and valgus malalignment are multifactorial, and can lead to an imbalance in loading of knee articular cartilage. Local factors within the joint, such as loss of joint congruence through bone and cartilage injury, anterior cruciate ligament disruption, and meniscal degeneration and extrusion, play a role in determining alignment.[5] Other causes of acquired varus and valgus malalignment include osseous remodeling, osteophytes, and ligament and capsular damage resulting from chronic repetitive microtrauma and tissue remodeling.[6] Prior surgical procedures including osteotomy, meniscectomy, and meniscal debridement may also affect knee alignment.[7,8] Childhood malalignment has been proposed to have a high association with OA. In a natural history study by Schouten and colleagues,[9] patients with childhood varus or valgus malalignment had a fivefold increase in risk of OA. Deviation from neutral alignment at the hip, knee, or ankle will also affect load distribution at the knee.[10]

As illustrated in **Fig. 1**, static assessment of knee alignment can be made using the mechanical axis determined from full-length standing views of the lower extremities. The mechanical axis of the lower extremity is represented on radiographs by a line drawn from the center of the femoral head to the center of the talus. Mechanical axis deviation is measured by a perpendicular line drawn from the center of the knee to the mechanical axis on the anteroposterior radiograph. In a neutrally aligned limb, the mechanical axis passes just medial to the midpoint of the knee between the tibial spines. In a varus knee, the mechanical axis deviates medially, increasing the load on the medial

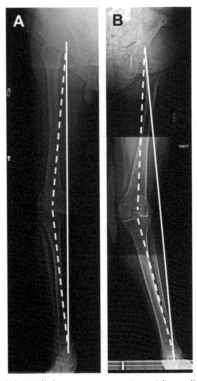

Fig. 1. (A) Medial compartment OA with medial deviation of the mechanical axis (*solid line*) and approximately 12° of varus malalignment of the knee (*dashed line*). (B) Lateral compartment OA with lateral deviation of the mechanical axis (*solid line*) and approximately 15° of valgus alignment (*dashed line*).

compartment. When the mechanical load-bearing axis passes lateral to the tibial spines, a valgus knee increases stress on the lateral compartment.

Knee alignment in the frontal plane is based on the relative angle between the mechanical axis of the femur and tibia. The mechanical axis of the femur passes from mid femoral head to center of the intracondylar notch. The mechanical axis of the tibia extends from the tibial spines to the mid talus. Measurement of knee alignment with the mechanical axis has been criticized for pelvic radiation exposure, higher cost, and the need for specialized equipment. A study by Kraus and colleagues[11] demonstrated a high correlation between the data obtained from full-limb measures of the mechanical axis and short-film measurements using the anatomic axis of the distal femur and proximal tibia. In the tibia, the mechanical and anatomic axes are the same, but they differ in the femur where the anatomic axis is defined by the line that bisects the distal femoral diaphysis. In this study, the anatomic axis measurement was offset a mean 4.2° valgus from the mechanical axis measurement (3.5° in women and 6.4° in men).

The average knee alignment in those who do not have OA has been shown to be approximately 1° to 2° varus.[11,12] In neutral alignment, the medial compartment bears 60% to 70% of the force across the knee during weight bearing.[13] It has been proposed that the greater degree of loading may predispose to medial tibiofemoral compartment OA,[10] which is 3 times more common than lateral compartment OA.[14]

A recent systematic review[15] found limited evidence for knee malalignment and incident knee OA; however, there was strong evidence that malalignment is an independent risk factor for progression of radiographic knee OA. With regard to incident OA, there are preliminary data to indicate that obese and overweight individuals with knee malalignment are at increased risk of developing knee OA compared with those with a normal BMI.[16]

In the presence of existing OA, malalignment is associated with more rapid structural damage in the compartment with increased compressive force. Varus and valgus alignment increases focal joint loading and risk of OA progression in the medial and lateral compartments, respectively.[10,17] The severity of malalignment at baseline showed a correlation with the magnitude of joint space narrowing and was linked to greater decline in physical function.[18] Varus malalignment has been shown to lead to a fourfold increase in medial knee OA progression. Valgus malalignment has been shown to predispose to a twofold to fivefold increase in lateral OA progression.[18,19] In an MR imaging study using quantitative assessment of cartilage in 251 knees, varus malalignment predicted medial tibial cartilage volume loss and tibial and femoral bone erosion, even after adjusting for other local factors such as meniscal damage, extrusion, and laxity.[20]

While there was an effect of malalignment at almost all stages of knee OA examined, the impact of varus or valgus malalignment on the probability of disease progression increased with baseline severity of OA. In knees with mild OA (Kellgren and Lawrence [K/L] grade 2: definite osteophytes and definite narrowing of joint space), the probability of 18-month progression in medial compartment OA was increased fourfold by varus alignment at baseline, and lateral progression increased twofold by valgus alignment (approaching statistical significance). In knees with moderate OA (K/L grade 3: moderate multiple osteophytes, definite narrowing of joint space, some sclerosis, and possible deformity of bone contour), the impact of malalignment in either the varus or valgus direction on OA progression over the subsequent 18 months demonstrated a tenfold

increase. The difference in impact between varus and valgus alignment on OA progression was less apparent in K/L grade 3 knees.[19,21]

Assessment of malalignment from standing radiographs provides only a static impression of the mechanical forces being imparted on the joint in the frontal plane. Dynamic assessment of limb biomechanics is complex, and is achieved through gait analysis and measurement of knee adduction moment, which requires dynamic measurement of the ground reaction force and lower extremity alignment. The knee adduction moment arm, which adducts the knee during the stance phase of normal gait, has been described as the best predictor of knee OA progression.[22] The mean maximum magnitude of the adduction moment during normal gait is approximately 3.3% body weight multiplied by height.[23] Data from Miyazaki and colleagues[22] found a significant relationship between adduction moment and the mechanical axis.[24]

Techniques for estimating knee alignment have been proposed using coronal MR images from the hip through the ankle in an unloaded state.[25] Although these techniques underestimate the degree of valgus malalignment, they have been shown to provide an accurate assessment of varus malalignment. Chronic high loading conditions can perturb the subchondral marrow signal and thus serve as an indirect marker of abnormal joint mechanics. As illustrated in **Fig. 2**, subchondral marrow changes with decreased T1-weighted signal intensity and increased T2-weighted signal intensity are frequently associated with increased biomechanical load. Areas of abnormal MR imaging signal have been shown to also have increased radionuclide uptake on bone scan,[26] suggesting they are associated with bone remodeling. Although frequently referred to as "bone marrow edema,"[26,27] when evaluated histologically these sites of abnormal signal intensity are associated with a combination of bone marrow necrosis, fibrosis, and trabecular abnormalities. The amount of true bone marrow edema was similar in marrow with abnormal signal and normal perifocal or control zones.[28] Although there is still variation in terminology, this finding is generally referred to as a bone marrow edema-like lesion (BML).

In patients with radiographic knee OA, those with subchondral BMLs are more likely to have knee pain than those without them.[29] Large BMLs are associated with both progression of cartilage defects in the tibiofemoral joint and more rapid lateral tibial cartilage loss.[30] The site of the BML is predictive of compartmental cartilage loss. Risk for medial progression was increased more than sixfold in patients with medial

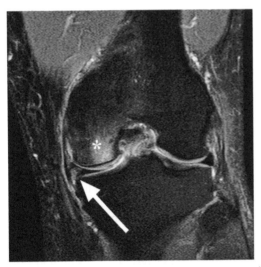

Fig. 2. Proton density (PD)-weighted fat-suppressed (FS) MR imaging (repetition time/echo time [TR/TE]: 3800 ms/28 ms) of a 44-year-old man with several-month history of medial knee pain demonstrates a peripheral tear of the medial meniscus (*arrow*) and hyperintense signal within the of the subchondral bone marrow of the medial femoral condyle (*asterisk*).

BMLs, and patients with lateral BMLs were at a similar risk for lateral progression.[26] Much of the relationship of BMLs with radiographic progression of OA is explained by their association with malalignment. Varus limbs have an extraordinarily high prevalence of medial BMLs, whereas lateral BMLs occurred preferentially in valgus aligned limbs. OA progression in patients with BMLs may be the consequence of the marrow lesions themselves, knee malalignment, or some combination of the two.[26] As discussed further in this article, BMLs are also associated with abnormal loading of subchondral bone resulting from meniscal injury and damage of the overlying articular cartilage.

MENISCAL DYSFUNCTION

Since the pioneering work of Fairbanks in the 1940s, the meniscus has been recognized as a critical component for normal knee function and biomechanics.[31] The meniscus plays a major role in load bearing and distribution, shock absorption, and knee proprioception, and it is also reported to play a role in knee stability and joint lubrication.[32,33] Menisci are wedge shaped in cross section, with capillaries and nerves that penetrate into the peripheral 10% to 30% of the outer edge of meniscus.[34,35] The lateral meniscus is more mobile in contradistinction to the medial

meniscus, which is firmly attached to the joint capsule. Under normal conditions the lateral meniscus is estimated to carry 70% of the load and the medial meniscus 50% of the load on their respective sides of the knee.[29] The load carried by the meniscus increases with knee flexion.[36]

The structural orientation of collagen in the meniscus contributes to the biomechanical properties of the tissue. Meniscal collagen is approximately 98% type I, which is tightly woven in a predominantly circumferential pattern.[37] Both menisci are attached to the tibia via anterior and posterior root ligaments, which anchor the circumferentially oriented hoop fibers.[38] The hoop fibers are stabilized with radially oriented tie fibers.[39] When the tibiofemoral joint is compressed, a portion of the compressive load is dissipated by converting the compressive force into tensile strain in the hoop fibers. The hoop strength of the collagen fiber orientation resists meniscal extrusion or subluxation. A damaged meniscus with disruption of the hoop fibers will be dislodged peripherally as axial load is applied, resulting in extrusion and joint space narrowing on radiograph.[40] Tears of the posterior insertional ligament illustrated in **Fig. 3** lead to loss of hoop strain, and from the standpoint of joint contact pressure are functionally similar to a complete meniscectomy.[41] Radial tears that transect the hoop fibers substantially decrease the contact area of the tibiofemoral joint, increase the compressive load on the articular cartilage, and synergistically act to concentrate high loads on a small region of the articular surface.[42] The absence of a functioning meniscus is reported to increase peak and average contact stresses in the medial compartment over a range of 40% to 700%.[43] As illustrated by the case presented in **Fig. 4**, locally high loading pressure can exceed the material properties of the tissue, resulting in rapid cartilage loss or osteochondral fracture.

Normal menisci are rarely present in knees with OA. Degenerative meniscal tears or maceration of the meniscus is often present suggesting a strong relation between OA and meniscal pathology.[44,45] In a study of middle-aged and elderly patients in Framingham, Massachusetts, 82% of knees with radiographic OA had meniscal damage and the prevalence increased with a higher K/L grade.[46] In many cases, it is difficult to determine whether meniscal damage or OA was first to develop. The meniscus and the articular surface are interdependent, and failure of one will lead to more rapid damage of the other by increased load.

Meniscal damage plays a significant role in progression of knee OA. Biswal and colleagues[3] demonstrated a higher rate of progression of

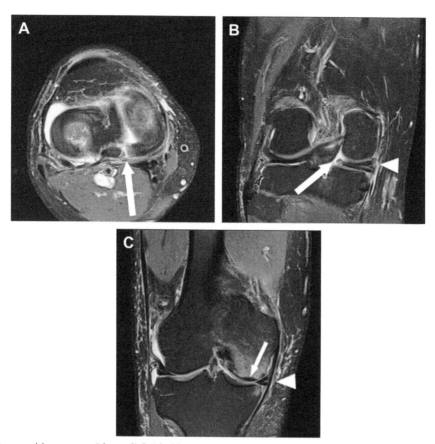

Fig. 3. A 52-year-old woman with medial-sided knee pain of several months' duration. (*A*) Axial PD-weighted FS MR imaging (TR/TE: 3300 ms/28 ms) demonstrates a radial tear of the posterior insertional root ligament of the medial meniscus (*arrow*). (*B*) Coronal PD-weighted FS MR imaging (TR/TE: 3800 ms/28 ms) demonstrates a radial root tear (*arrow*) with extrusion of the medial meniscus (*arrowhead*). (*C*) Coronal PD-weighted FS MR imaging of the mid tibiofemoral joint demonstrates medial meniscal extrusion (*arrowhead*) with subchondral fatigue fracture and surrounding marrow edema (*arrow*), due to focally elevated loading concentrated on the central tibiofemoral contact zone as a result of the dysfunctional meniscus.

cartilage loss in 26 of 43 patients with meniscal tears compared with a control group with intact menisci. In a study by Hunter and colleagues,[43] the most significant risk for cartilage loss was related to the WORMS meniscal damage variable. However, the WORMS grading system[47] does not specify the type of meniscal tear or the degree of meniscal extrusion. Another potential weakness of MR imaging for meniscal evaluation is that the lack of axial load on the knee may underestimate meniscal extrusion in the knee with OA. It remains uncertain as to what level of meniscal dysfunction related to loss of hoop strain must be lost before the risk of OA is increased.

In addition to removing displaced meniscal fragments that may cause symptoms of knee pain and locking, a goal of surgery in treatment of meniscal tears is to preserve meniscal function. Several methods of meniscal repair have been used over the years. The first reported operation was

a meniscal suturing by a British surgeon in 1883.[48] The same surgeon later recommended complete removal of the meniscus as preferable to repair. Total meniscectomy predominated for several years until it was shown to significantly increase the rate of OA progression. In 1948, Fairbank[31] compared preoperative and postoperative radiographs in 107 patients undergoing meniscectomy and demonstrated development of ridge formation on the femoral condyle, joint space narrowing, and flattening of the femoral condyle in the postoperative patients. Fairbank hypothesized that frequent radiographic changes found after total meniscectomy were caused by loss of the load-protective function of the menisci. Further studies confirmed an increased incidence of OA after total meniscectomy.[49–51] The most compelling argument against total meniscectomy was a 1998 study that reported a significant increase in risk for tibiofemoral OA over

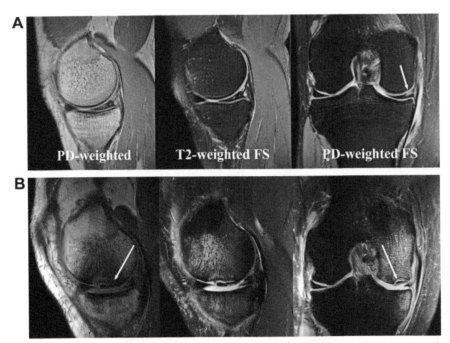

Fig. 4. A 52-year-old man with medial-sided knee pain. (*A*) Initial MR imaging examination demonstrated a complex tear of the posterior horn and body of the medial meniscus (*arrow*). (*B*) The patient developed acute worsening of knee pain 11 months following partial medial meniscectomy. Follow-up MR imaging examination demonstrates postsurgical changes from prior meniscectomy with an acute osteochondral fracture of the central medial femoral condyle (*arrow*).

a 21-year period following total meniscectomy when compared with a matched control group.[52] Total meniscectomy of the lateral compartment has been shown to have a worse outcome than medial meniscal resection,[53] possibly a result of the greater portion of load carried by the lateral meniscus than by the medial meniscus.

Arthroscopic partial meniscectomy has several advantages over total meniscectomy, and is presently the treatment of choice. This procedure involves a limited resection of only the damaged portion of the meniscus. Short-term benefits include decreased length of stay in the hospital and shorter rehabilitation time.[54] Long-term benefits include continued meniscal participation in load distribution, knee stability, and shock absorption if sufficient circumferentially oriented fibers are intact and hoop strength is sufficient to prevent extrusion.[55] Meniscal repair may be indicated for acute lesions in young patients if the lesion is in the outer one-third "red zone" of the meniscus with a vascular supply to allow healing. Meniscal transplants have been described,[56] but are preformed infrequently.

INJURIES OF THE OSTEOCHONDRAL UNIT

The primary function of articular cartilage is to provide a smooth transfer of force across joints.

As such it is useful to consider the cartilage and the underlying subchondral bone as a functional osteochondral unit that must withstand a combination of compressive, tensile, and shear stress. Failure of either the cartilage or subchondral bone component generally leads to failure of the other component. Chronic degeneration or acute injury of the osteochondral unit weakens the material properties of the tissue, which can lead to progressive damage when exposed to increased biomechanical loads.

The biochemical composition and structural organization of the osteochondral unit directly influence the ability of the tissue to sustain the high strains imparted on the tissue through activities of daily living, and help to predict the pattern of injuries when those strains exceed the material properties of the tissue. The principal components of articular cartilage are water, collagen, proteoglycans, and chondrocytes. Water is the major component of cartilage, making up between 75% and 80% of the tissue.[57] Cartilage is relatively acellular, with chondrocytes accounting for approximately 1% to 4% of the tissue. The negatively charged proteoglycans bind sodium and through osmotic force draw water into the extracellular matrix, causing the cartilage to swell. Type II collagen provides the major structural framework of the extracellular matrix and acts to constrain the swelling pressure of the hydrated proteoglycans.

Articular cartilage contains 4 histologically distinct zones: the superficial, middle, radial, and calcified cartilage layers. The orientation and concentration of collagen fibers differ for each zone. In general, collagen fibers are parallel to the articular surface in the superficial zone and oblique in the middle zone, while exhibiting a vertical orientation in the radial zone. The tidemark is a thin region where uncalcified cartilage transitions to calcified cartilage. The calcified cartilage zone interfaces with the subchondral bone. The different layers of the articular cartilage act together as a functional unit.[58–60]

The content and orientation of the type II collagen fibers in cartilage vary by location in the knee and reflect prevailing local biomechanical forces.[61] At the tibiofemoral articulation, the radial zone is thickest, and the superficial zone is thin in the central region uncovered by the meniscus, where compressive loading forces are high. At the periphery of the joint, covered by the meniscus, the cartilage experiences greater shear strain and the cartilage matrix is characterized by an oblique orientation of the collagen fibers along the primary orientation of the shear force. The orientation of the highly anisotropic collagen fibers of the radial zone results in a short T2 relaxation time of cartilage and results in lower signal intensity on T2-weighted or proton density (PD)-weighted images.[62] Sites of cartilage injury can be detected through an increase in cartilage T2 that occurs with disruption of the anisotropic collagen network and a focal increase in cartilage water content.

Two hypothetical models of chondral injury have been described. The first theory relates to chronic repetitive microtrauma leading to fatigue fractures of the collagen fibers.[63] Under normal conditions, the collagen meshwork constrains the swelling pressure produced by the highly charged proteoglycans that are within the interstices of the collagen meshwork. This swelling pressure and high viscosity of the extracellular matrix limits the mobility of cartilage water. When the healthy joint is loaded, much of the energy imparted on the osteochondral unit is dissipated through frictional drag forces of water as it is forced through the cartilage extracellular matrix. Very little energy is deposited in the solid extracellular matrix. When the collagen matrix is damaged, the proteoglycans are no longer constrained. As the proteoglycan swells and imbibes more water, there is an increase in both water content and the mobility of water in the matrix. No longer is energy dissipated in the cartilage water but instead the energy

is imparted on the solid cartilage matrix and subchondral bone, leading to structural damage and ultimately loss of tissue. This theory describes the progressive degenerative changes of OA.[64]

The second model of injury stems from an acute traumatic event, with axial, rotational, or tangential forces causing gross injury of the osteochondral unit. An important function of cartilage is to transfer the compressive force to the underlying bone, which is substantially stiffer. Cartilage demonstrates a depth-dependent difference in compressibility, with the cartilage becoming progressively stiffer toward bone. During physiologic loads most of the tissue deformation occurs in the superficial layer of cartilage, with very little compression occurring in the radial zone near the cartilage bone interface.[65] When the force exceeds the material properties of the tissue, gross fissures or tears can result in the cartilage. Articular cartilage is a viscoelastic material, indicating that the stiffness of the tissue is dependent on the rate at which the force is applied; this influences the location of the chondral injury. When the force is applied at high speed, fissures are produced along the articular cartilage surface. At low speed and low energy, splits initially occur in the deeper layers (**Fig. 5**).[66]

Differences in biomaterial properties of cartilage and bone can lead to high shear strain at the tidemark zone.[67] Compressive forces transmitted to the deep layers of cartilage from the articular surface are transferred into shear force as they reach the cartilage/bone interface. As demonstrated in **Fig. 6**, radial oriented collagen fibrils of the radial zone pass through the tidemark, terminating in the zone of calcified cartilage. Because the fibers do not pass into the subchondral cortex, there is a potential cleavage plane between the calcified cartilage and subchondral bone layers when the articular surface is exposed to a shearing force or compressive load. This pattern of injury is referred to as chondral delamination or debonding.[64] These lesions can occur in isolation, or may communicate with the articular surface through an associated deep fissure or cleft.[59,64,68,69] On MR imaging, fluid signal at the tidemark zone running parallel to the articular surface between the subchondral bone and articular cartilage indicates delamination (**Fig. 7**).

In the knee, delamination injuries are frequently found at the femoral condyle in association with a posterior horn of the medial meniscus injury, or at the patellar or femoral trochlear articular cartilage in association with shear or blunt injury (**Fig. 8**).[69] Delamination injury can lead to altered biomechanics, due to related dysfunction of the osteochondral unit.

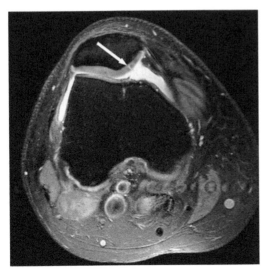

Fig. 5. A 34-year-old man with intermittent anterior knee pain. PD-weighted FS MR imaging (TR/TE: 3300 ms/28 ms) illustrates a full-thickness vertically oriented fissure of the medial patellar facet (*arrow*).

Large focal full-thickness articular cartilage defects can result from a chondral fracture. A biomechanical load related to sheer stress or compression from a traumatic event can acutely produce these lesions. All layers of articular cartilage are involved with disruption of the bonds between the uncalcified and calcified cartilage, resulting in intra-articular displacement of the chondral fragment. Fluid signal fills the void created by the defect on MR imaging. Sharp margins indicate an acute injury whereas obtuse, rounded, or irregular margins favor a chronic process.

Focal articular cartilage defects that involve fracture through subchondral bone are osteochondral lesions. These defects may arise from acute traumatic injury from an abnormal biomechanical load, or may stem from osteonecrosis or subchondral insufficiency fracture related to chronic repetitive microtrauma. MR imaging findings are variable, and depend on the extent of demarcation between the osteochondral lesion and the underlying subchondral bone. The most common sign of instability of the osteochondral fragment is a well-defined line of fluid signal dividing the lesion from the adjacent bone marrow on MR imaging. Signal intensity other than fluid signal at the demarcation zone denotes partial separation, healing, or chronic degeneration. Several criteria have been described that are predictive of osteochondral lesion instability.[59,69] Displaced osteochondral fragments create a deep fluid-filled void at the articular surface. Osteochondral lesions can lead to the development of OA, particularly in skeletally mature patients.[70,71] Prakash and Learmonth[70] conducted a retrospective review of outcomes following isolated osteochondral lesions of the femoral condyle that did not receive surgical management. MR imaging at the time of diagnosis and on follow-up was reviewed for 15 knees involving 12 patients, age range 9 to 46 years. For patients with symptoms before the age of 18, 6 out of the 7 knees had healed osteochondral lesions on follow-up, with one persistent defect. In comparison, skeletally mature subjects demonstrated signs of OA in 6 of 8 knees involved, with only 2 healing.

As with joint malalignment and meniscal injuries that lead to overloading of subchondral bone, BMLs are seen with focal chondral and osteochondral injuries. Subchondral cyst-like lesions are another potential osseous manifestation of

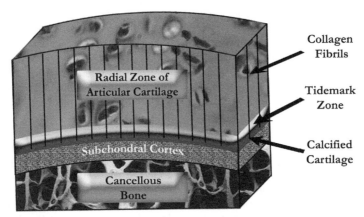

Fig. 6. Schematic illustration of the osteochondral junction. Vertically oriented collagen fibers from the cartilage radial zone pass through the tidemark zone, terminating in the zone of calcified cartilage. This process produces a potential cleavage plane between the subchondral cortex and the zone of calcified cartilage that is a site of chondral delamination injury.

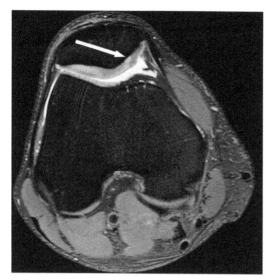

Fig. 7. A 28-year-old professional hockey player with anterior knee pain. PD-weighted FS MR imaging (TR/TE: 3300 ms/28 ms) illustrates focally elevated T2-weighted signal intensity at the osteochondral junction and deep radial zone of the medial patellar facet (*arrow*) consistent with a delamination injury of the osteochondral junction.

a chronic chondral injury. The presence of subchondral cysts is a stronger predictor of progressive cartilage loss and subsequent joint replacement than BMLs alone.[72] Two theories explain their formation. The first model relates to trauma as a direct consequence of bone necrosis resulting from excessive compressive load between two impacting articular surfaces. The second theory suggests that synovial fluid is infused into subchondral bone through full-thickness defects in articular cartilage as a result of hydraulic force.[73] Histologically, these lesions do not have an epithelial lining and are not true cysts. A recent longitudinal analysis of subjects enrolled in the MOST trial indicates the presence of BMLs is predictive of subchondral cyst development even after correction for full-thickness cartilage loss, supporting the theory that cysts represent focal sites of osseous necrosis arising from sites of traumatized bone and not necessarily through direct communication with synovial fluid.[74]

SUMMARY

While cartilage loss is a central feature of OA, it is clear that that cartilage damage cannot be considered in isolation. OA is the result of local biomechanical factors acting within the context of systemic susceptibility. Progressive cartilage loss occurs when the local biomechanical forces exceed the material properties of the osteochondral unit. Conditions such as joint malalignment and loss of normal meniscal function lead to focal concentration of compressive loads in the joint, particularly in the setting of obesity. Imaging features on MR imaging such as BMLs and meniscal extrusion may serve as indicators of this condition and may serve as imaging biomarkers for excessive joint loading. Weakened material properties of cartilage produced by damage of the extracellular matrix or delamination injuries of the bone cartilage interface may indicate articular sites at risk for progressive tissue loss. These injuries are associated with altered signal intensity on clinical T2-weighted and PD-weighted MR images, and may be assessed quantitatively using cartilage T2 mapping. Placing these findings in the context of joint biomechanics will allow for further refinement of our understanding of rapid OA progression, and may lead to the development of specific imaging biomarkers to indicate patients at risk.

REFERENCES

1. Altman R, Asch E, Bloch D, et al. Development of criteria for the classification and reporting of osteoarthritis. Classification of osteoarthritis of the knee. Diagnostic and Therapeutic Criteria Committee of the American Rheumatism Association. Arthritis Rheum 1986;29(8):1039–49.

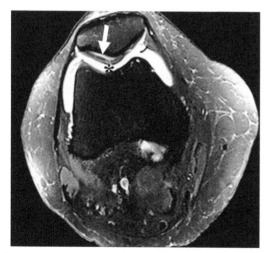

Fig. 8. PD-weighted FS MR imaging (TR/TE: 3300 ms/28 ms) demonstrates extensive chondral delamination of the lateral patellar facet (*arrow*), with communication to the articular surface through a deep fissure at the junction of the median ridge and lateral patellar facet (*asterisk*).

2. Belo JN, Berger MY, Reijman M, et al. Prognostic factors of progression of osteoarthritis of the knee: a systematic review of observational studies. Arthritis Rheum 2007;57(1):13–26.

3. Biswal S, Hastie T, Andriacchi TP, et al. Risk factors for progressive cartilage loss in the knee: a longitudinal magnetic resonance imaging study in forty-three patients. Arthritis Rheum 2002;46(11):2884–92.

4. Roemer FW, Guermazi A, Javaid MK, et al. Change in MRI-detected subchondral bone marrow lesions is associated with cartilage loss: the MOST Study. A longitudinal multicentre study of knee osteoarthritis. Ann Rheum Dis 2009;68(9):1461–5.

5. Hunter DJ, Wilson DR. Imaging the role of biomechanics in osteoarthritis. Rheum Dis Clin North Am 2009;35(3):465–83.

6. Hunter DJ, Zhang Y, Niu J, et al. Structural factors associated with malalignment in knee osteoarthritis: the Boston osteoarthritis knee study. J Rheumatol 2005;32(11):2192–9.

7. Yasuda K, Majima T, Tsuchida T, et al. A ten- to 15-year follow-up observation of high tibial osteotomy in medial compartment osteoarthrosis. Clin Orthop Relat Res 1992;282:186–95.

8. Allen PR, Denham RA, Swan AV. Late degenerative changes after meniscectomy. Factors affecting the knee after operation. J Bone Joint Surg Br 1984;66(5):666–71.

9. Schouten JS, van den Ouweland FA, Valkenburg HA. A 12 year follow up study in the general population on prognostic factors of cartilage loss in osteoarthritis of the knee. Ann Rheum Dis 1992;51(8):932–7.

10. Tetsworth K, Paley D. Malalignment and degenerative arthropathy. Orthop Clin North Am 1994;25(3):367–77.

11. Kraus VB, Vail TP, Worrell T, et al. A comparative assessment of alignment angle of the knee by radiographic and physical examination methods. Arthritis Rheum 2005;52(6):1730–5.

12. Takahashi T, Yamanaka N, Komatsu M, et al. A new computer-assisted method for measuring the tibiofemoral angle in patients with osteoarthritis of the knee. Osteoarthritis Cartilage 2004;12(3):256–9.

13. Andriacchi TP. Dynamics of knee malalignment. Orthop Clin North Am 1994;25(3):395–403.

14. Ledingham J, Regan M, Jones A, et al. Radiographic patterns and associations of osteoarthritis of the knee in patients referred to hospital. Ann Rheum Dis 1993;52(7):520–6.

15. Tanamas S, Hanna FS, Cicuttini FM, et al. Does knee malalignment increase the risk of development and progression of knee osteoarthritis? A systematic review. Arthritis Rheum 2009;61(4):459–67.

16. Brouwer GM, van Tol AW, Bergink AP, et al. Association between valgus and varus alignment and the development and progression of radiographic osteoarthritis of the knee. Arthritis Rheum 2007;56(4):1204–11.

17. McKellop HA, Llinas A, Sarmiento A. Effects of tibial malalignment on the knee and ankle. Orthop Clin North Am 1994;25(3):415–23.

18. Sharma L, Song J, Felson DT, et al. The role of knee alignment in disease progression and functional decline in knee osteoarthritis. JAMA 2001;286(2):188–95.

19. Cerejo R, Dunlop DD, Cahue S, et al. The influence of alignment on risk of knee osteoarthritis progression according to baseline stage of disease. Arthritis Rheum 2002;46(10):2632–6.

20. Sharma L, Eckstein F, Song J, et al. Relationship of meniscal damage, meniscal extrusion, malalignment, and joint laxity to subsequent cartilage loss in osteoarthritic knees. Arthritis Rheum 2008;58(6):1716–26.

21. Kellgren JH, Lawrence JS. Radiological assessment of osteo-arthrosis. Ann Rheum Dis 1957;16(4):494–502.

22. Miyazaki T, Wada M, Kawahara H, et al. Dynamic load at baseline can predict radiographic disease progression in medial compartment knee osteoarthritis. Ann Rheum Dis 2002;61(7):617–22.

23. Schipplein OD, Andriacchi TP. Interaction between active and passive knee stabilizers during level walking. J Orthop Res 1991;9(1):113–9.

24. Hurwitz DE, Ryals AB, Case JP, et al. The knee adduction moment during gait in subjects with knee osteoarthritis is more closely correlated with static alignment than radiographic disease severity, toe out angle and pain. J Orthop Res 2002;20(1):101–7.

25. Hinterwimmer S, Graichen H, Vogl TJ, et al. An MRI-based technique for assessment of lower extremity deformities-reproducibility, accuracy, and clinical application. Eur Radiol 2008;18(7):1497–505.

26. Felson DT, McLaughlin S, Goggins J, et al. Bone marrow edema and its relation to progression of knee osteoarthritis. Ann Intern Med 2003;139(5 Pt 1):330–6.

27. Yu JS, Cook PA. Magnetic resonance imaging (MRI) of the knee: a pattern approach for evaluating bone marrow edema. Crit Rev Diagn Imaging 1996;37(4):261–303.

28. Zanetti M, Bruder E, Romero J, et al. Bone marrow edema pattern in osteoarthritic knees: correlation between MR imaging and histologic findings. Radiology 2000;215(3):835–40.

29. Felson DT, Chaisson CE, Hill CL, et al. The association of bone marrow lesions with pain in knee osteoarthritis. Ann Intern Med 2001;134(7):541–9.

30. Wluka AE, Hanna F, Davies-Tuck M, et al. Bone marrow lesions predict increase in knee cartilage defects and loss of cartilage volume in middle-aged women without knee pain over 2 years. Ann Rheum Dis 2009;68(6):850–5.

31. Fairbank TJ. Knee joint changes after meniscectomy. J Bone Joint Surg Am 1948;30B(4):664–70.

32. Seedhom BB, Dowson D, Wright V. Proceedings: functions of the menisci. A preliminary study. Ann Rheum Dis 1974;33(1):111.

33. Verstraete KL, Verdonk R, Lootens T, et al. Current status and imaging of allograft meniscal transplantation. Eur J Radiol 1997;26(1):16–22.

34. Day B, Mackenzie WG, Shim SS, et al. The vascular and nerve supply of the human meniscus. Arthroscopy 1985;1(1):58–62.

35. Arnoczky SP, Warren RF. Microvasculature of the human meniscus. Am J Sports Med 1982;10(2):90–5.

36. Walker PS, Erkman MJ. The role of the menisci in force transmission across the knee. Clin Orthop Relat Res 1975;109:184–92.

37. Eyre DR, Wu JJ. Collagen of fibrocartilage: a distinctive molecular phenotype in bovine meniscus. FEBS Lett 1983;158(2):265–70.

38. Brody JM, Hulstyn MJ, Fleming BC, et al. The meniscal roots: gross anatomic correlation with 3-T MRI findings. AJR Am J Roentgenol 2007;188(5):W446–50.

39. Skaggs DL, Warden WH, Mow VC. Radial tie fibers influence the tensile properties of the bovine medial meniscus. J Orthop Res 1994;12(2):176–85.

40. Adams JG, McAlindon T, Dimasi M, et al. Contribution of meniscal extrusion and cartilage loss to joint space narrowing in osteoarthritis. Clin Radiol 1999; 54(8):502–6.

41. Allaire R, Muriuki M, Gilbertson L, et al. Biomechanical consequences of a tear of the posterior root of the medial meniscus. Similar to total meniscectomy. J Bone Joint Surg Am 2008;90(9):1922–31.

42. Fukubayashi T, Kurosawa H. The contact area and pressure distribution pattern of the knee. A study of normal and osteoarthrotic knee joints. Acta Orthop Scand 1980;51(6):871–9.

43. Hunter DJ, Zhang YQ, Niu JB, et al. The association of meniscal pathologic changes with cartilage loss in symptomatic knee osteoarthritis. Arthritis Rheum 2006;54(3):795–801.

44. Noble J. Lesions of the menisci. Autopsy incidence in adults less than fifty-five years old. J Bone Joint Surg Am 1977;59(4):480–3.

45. Poehling GG, Ruch DS, Chabon SJ. The landscape of meniscal injuries. Clin Sports Med 1990;9(3): 539–49.

46. Englund M, Guermazi A, Gale D, et al. Incidental meniscal findings on knee MRI in middle-aged and elderly persons. N Engl J Med 2008;359(11): 1108–15.

47. Peterfy CG, Guermazi A, Zaim S, et al. Whole-organ magnetic resonance imaging score (WORMS) of the knee in osteoarthritis. Osteoarthritis Cartilage 2004; 12(3):177–90.

48. Annandale T. An operation for displaced semilunar cartilage. 1885. Clin Orthop Relat Res 1990;260:3–5.

49. Noble J, Erat K. In defence of the meniscus. A prospective study of 200 meniscectomy patients. J Bone Joint Surg Br 1980;62-B(1):7–11.

50. Noble J. Clinical features of the degenerate meniscus with the results of meniscectomy. Br J Surg 1975;62(12):977–81.

51. Sonne-Holm S, Fledelius I, Ahn NC. Results after meniscectomy in 147 athletes. Acta Orthop Scand 1980;51(2):303–9.

52. Roos H, Lauren M, Adalberth T, et al. Knee osteoarthritis after meniscectomy: prevalence of radiographic changes after twenty-one years, compared with matched controls. Arthritis Rheum 1998;41(4):687–93.

53. Englund M, Guermazi A, Lohmander SL. The role of the meniscus in knee osteoarthritis: a cause or consequence? Radiol Clin North Am 2009;47(4): 703–12.

54. Northmore-Ball MD, Dandy DJ, Jackson RW. Arthroscopic, open partial, and total meniscectomy. A comparative study. J Bone Joint Surg Br 1983; 65(4):400–4.

55. Englund M, Lohmander LS. Risk factors for symptomatic knee osteoarthritis fifteen to twenty-two years after meniscectomy. Arthritis Rheum 2004; 50(9):2811–9.

56. Noyes FR, Barber-Westin SD, Rankin M. Meniscal transplantation in symptomatic patients less than fifty years old. J Bone Joint Surg Am 2005; 87(Suppl 1(Pt 2)):149–65.

57. Venn M, Maroudas A. Chemical composition and swelling of normal and osteoarthrotic femoral head cartilage. I. Chemical composition. Ann Rheum Dis 1977;36(2):121–9.

58. Shindle MK, Foo LF, Kelly BT, et al. Magnetic resonance imaging of cartilage in the athlete: current techniques and spectrum of disease. J Bone Joint Surg Am 2006;88(Suppl 4):27–46.

59. Winalski CS, Gupta KB. Magnetic resonance imaging of focal articular cartilage lesions. Top Magn Reson Imaging 2003;14(2):131–44.

60. Mandelbaum BR, Browne JE, Fu F, et al. Articular cartilage lesions of the knee. Am J Sports Med 1998;26(6):853–61.

61. Goodwin DW, Wadghiri YZ, Zhu H, et al. Macroscopic structure of articular cartilage of the tibial plateau: influence of a characteristic matrix architecture on MRI appearance. AJR Am J Roentgenol 2004;182(2):311–8.

62. Mosher TJ, Dardzinski BJ. Cartilage MRI T2 relaxation time mapping: overview and applications. Semin Musculoskelet Radiol 2004;8(4):355–68.

63. Maroudas AI. Balance between swelling pressure and collagen tension in normal and degenerate cartilage. Nature 1976;260(5554):808–9.

64. Levy AS, Lohnes J, Sculley S, et al. Chondral delamination of the knee in soccer players. Am J Sports Med 1996;24(5):634–9.

65. Wong M, Carter DR. Articular cartilage functional histomorphology and mechanobiology: a research perspective. Bone 2003;33(1):1–13.

66. Tomatsu T, Imai N, Takeuchi N, et al. Experimentally produced fractures of articular cartilage and bone. The effects of shear forces on the pig knee. J Bone Joint Surg Br 1992;74(3):457–62.

67. Redler I, Mow VC, Zimny ML, et al. The ultrastructure and biomechanical significance of the tidemark of articular cartilage. Clin Orthop Relat Res 1975;112:357–62.

68. Kendell SD, Helms CA, Rampton JW, et al. MRI appearance of chondral delamination injuries of the knee. AJR Am J Roentgenol 2005;184(5):1486–9.

69. Mosher TJ. MRI of osteochondral injuries of the knee and ankle in the athlete. Clin Sports Med 2006;25(4): 843–66.

70. Prakash D, Learmonth D. Natural progression of osteo-chondral defect in the femoral condyle. Knee 2002;9(1):7–10.

71. Pape D, Filardo G, Kon E, et al. Disease-specific clinical problems associated with the subchondral bone. Knee Surg Sports Traumatol Arthrosc 2010; 18(4):448–62.

72. Tanamas SK, Wluka AE, Pelletier JP, et al. The association between subchondral bone cysts and tibial cartilage volume and risk of joint replacement in people with knee osteoarthritis: a longitudinal study. Arthritis Res Ther 2010;12(2):R58.

73. Crema MD, Roemer FW, Marra MD, et al. MR imaging of intra- and periarticular soft tissues and subchondral bone in knee osteoarthritis. Radiol Clin North Am 2009;47(4):687–701.

74. Crema MD, Roemer FW, Zhu Y, et al. Subchondral cystlike lesions develop longitudinally in areas of bone marrow edema-like lesions in patients with or at risk for knee osteoarthritis: detection with MR Imaging—The MOST Study. Radiology 2010; 256(3):855–62.

Magnetic Resonance Imaging in Knee Osteoarthritis Research: Semiquantitative and Compositional Assessment

Michel D. Crema, MD[a,b,c,d],*, Frank W. Roemer, MD[a,b,e], Ali Guermazi, MD[a,b]

KEYWORDS

- Magnetic resonance imaging • Knee • Osteoarthritis
- Semiquantitative assessment

Over the past 2 decades magnetic resonance (MR) imaging has become established as the most important imaging modality in the assessment of joint disease in both the clinical and research environments. Regarding knee osteoarthritis (OA), MR imaging-based studies first focused on the assessment of hyaline articular cartilage as the main outcome measure in clinical and epidemiologic studies.[1–6] However, it is widely accepted now that OA is a disease of the whole joint including the subchondral bone, synovium, menisci, and ligaments. Because MR imaging is able to depict all tissues of the joint directly, the joint can be assessed as a whole organ, providing a detailed picture of the structural changes associated with OA, as well as the role of such changes in predicting pain and progression of disease. Validated MR imaging-based semiquantitative (SQ) scoring systems are available for the assessment of the whole knee joint in OA and have been applied to many OA studies. The analyses based on SQ scoring have added deeply to our understanding of the physiopathology and natural history of knee OA, as well as to the clinical implications of the structural changes.[7–17]

Several MR imaging techniques are available to evaluate composition of hyaline cartilage, and degenerative changes can be detected before morphologic changes are seen. These techniques have increased our understanding of early and potentially reversible disease, and may help to avoid the permanent morphologic changes commonly seen in knee OA. This review discusses MR imaging-based SQ scoring systems for the evaluation of knee OA, focusing on the role of different intra-articular structural pathologies in predicting pain and progression of disease. The review also discusses available MR imaging

[a] Department of Radiology, Quantitative Imaging Center, Boston University School of Medicine, 820 Harrison Avenue, FGH Building, 3rd Floor, Boston, MA 02118, USA
[b] Boston Imaging Core Lab (BICL), 601 Albany Street, Boston, MA 02118-2771, USA
[c] Institute of Diagnostic Imaging (IDI), Avenida Saudade 456, Ribeirão Preto, São Paulo 14085-000, Brazil
[d] Division of Radiology, Department of Internal Medicine, Avenida Bandeirantes 3900, Ribeirão Preto School of Medicine, University of São Paulo (USP), Ribeirão Preto, São Paulo 14048-900, Brazil
[e] Klinikum Augsburg, Stenglinstrasse 2, Augsburg 86156, Germany
* Corresponding author. Department of Radiology, Quantitative Imaging Center, Boston University School of Medicine, 820 Harrison Avenue, FGH Building, 3rd Floor, Boston, MA 02118.
E-mail address: michelcrema@gmail.com

Magn Reson Imaging Clin N Am 19 (2011) 295–321
doi:10.1016/j.mric.2011.02.003
1064-9689/11/$ – see front matter © 2011 Elsevier Inc. All rights reserved.

techniques for the assessment of hyaline cartilage composition, as well as its importance in detecting and monitoring cartilaginous degeneration.

SQ SCORING METHODS FOR MR IMAGING ASSESSMENT OF WHOLE KNEE JOINT

Assessment based on SQ scoring methods has added greatly to the understanding of the pathophysiology and natural history of knee OA as well as the clinical implications of the structural changes.[8,10,11,16–20] These techniques allow assessment of articular structures that are currently believed to be relevant to the functional integrity of the knee or that are potentially involved in the pathophysiology of OA in terms of progression and pain. These structural features include articular cartilage morphology, subchondral bone marrow abnormalities, presence of marginal and central osteophytes, meniscal morphology and position, cruciate and collateral ligament integrity, presence of synovitis and effusion, and intra-articular loose bodies, as well as periarticular cysts and bursitis.

Whole-organ assessment scoring of different joint structures on MR imaging has shown adequate reliability, specificity, and sensitivity, as well as the ability to detect lesion progression.[11,21–23] Three SQ scoring systems for whole-organ assessment of knee OA have been validated: the whole-organ magnetic resonance imaging score (WORMS),[22] the knee osteoarthritis scoring system (KOSS),[23] and the Boston-Leeds osteoarthritis knee score (BLOKS).[21] Additional scoring tools have been introduced for joint conditions that may not be adequately assessed by the current systems or that offer alternative approaches. Examples are the assessment of synovitis on contrast-enhanced MR imaging or detailed evaluation of the intercondylar tibial region.[9,24] An overview of the 3 different whole-organ scoring systems is presented in **Table 1**.

Several epidemiologic studies and clinical trials have used WORMS, introduced by Peterfy and colleagues,[22] to evaluate OA features of the knee.[7,12,17–19,25,26] WORMS uses a complex subregional division of the different knee compartments (**Fig. 1**). Features assessed by WORMS are: cartilage morphology and signal, subchondral bone marrow edemalike lesions or the synonymous bone marrow lesions (BMLs), subchondral cysts, osteophytes, subchondral bone attrition, meniscal morphology and position, and a combined effusion/synovitis score as well as collateral and cruciate ligaments status. In addition, several periarticular features are evaluated such as meniscal and popliteal cysts, periarticular bursitis, and loose bodies. BMLs and cysts are

scored depending on the percentage amount of subregion. Unlike the other systems, WORMS uses a strict subregional rather than a lesion-oriented approach especially to the scoring of cartilage, BMLs, and subchondral cysts. This strategy offers the advantage of summing several lesions per subregion and facilitates assessment and subsequent analyses.

The KOSS system, introduced by Kornaat and colleagues,[23] covers similar MR imaging-detected OA features as WORMS, but with differences: cartilage status, subchondral BMLs, and cysts are scored individually for each subregion and each score is differentiated by lesion size. Osteophytes are differentiated into marginal, intercondylar, and central. Although KOSS uses a more complex meniscal score for tear morphology than WORMS, it does not describe regional subdivisions or partial or total meniscal maceration/resection.

The BLOKS system was published by Hunter and colleagues[21] in 2008. BLOKS uses an approach similar to KOSS in the regional division of the knee joint, focusing on the weight-bearing components versus the patellofemoral joint (**Fig. 2**). BMLs and cysts are evaluated by taking into account number and size of BMLs, percentage of involved subchondral surface area of the BML and the percentage of BML that is cystic. Thus, subchondral cysts are defined as part of the BML and are not assessed separately as in WORMS and KOSS. The lesional approach for BML assessment allows for superior longitudinal analysis of individual lesions. On the other hand, defining the exact number of individual lesions is sometimes difficult because lesions may be directly adjacent to each other or merge or split in longitudinal assessments.[21,23,27] Cartilage scoring takes into account percentage of any cartilage loss in the subregion and percentage of cartilage damage that represents full-thickness loss. Signal changes in the Hoffa fat pad are scored as a surrogate for synovitis.[28–30] BLOKS uses a complex system to evaluate the meniscal status including different types of tears, intrasubstance signal changes, and meniscal extrusion.

Recent work based on Osteoarthritis Initiative (OAI) data evaluated how differences between WORMS and BLOKS in scoring cartilage, meniscus, and subchondral BMLs affected the assessment of presence, extent, and severity of structural changes of knee OA.[31–33] The investigators concluded that the ideal MR imaging reading system for OAI data should include elements from both systems. Excellent reliability data have been published for all 3 whole-organ SQ scoring systems (**Table 2**).

Table 1
Comparison of 3 different SQ scoring systems of knee OA

	BLOKS	KOSS	WORMS
Number of knees scored in original publication	10 knees (71 knees for validity exercise of BML scoring)	25 knees	19 knees
MR imaging protocol of original publication (all publications used 1.5-T systems)	For reliability exercise (10 knees): sag/cor T2w FS, sag T1 SE, axial/cor 3D FLASH. For validity of BML assessment: sag PD/T2w. Cor/axial PD/T2w FS	Cor/sag T2w and PDw, sag 3D SPGR, axial PD, and axial T2w FS	Axial T1 SE, cor T1 SE, sag T1 SE, sag T2 FS, sag 3D SPGR
Subregional division of knee	9 subregions: medial/lateral patella, medial/lateral trochlea, medial, lateral weight-bearing femur, medial/lateral weight-bearing tibia, subspinous tibia	9 subregions: medial patella, patellar crest, lateral patella, medial/ lateral trochlea, medial/lateral femoral condyle, medial/lateral tibial plateau	15 subregions: medial/lateral patella, medial/lateral femur (anterior/central/posterior), medial/lateral tibia (anterior/central/posterior), subspinous tibia
Interreader reliability	Performed on 10 knees. w-κ between 0.51 (meniscal extrusion) and 0.79 (meniscal tear)	Performed on 25 knees. w-κ between 0.57 (osteochondral defects) and 0.88 (bone marrow edema)	Performed on 19 knees. ICC between 0.74 (bone marrow abnormalities and synovitis/effusion) and 0.99 (cartilage)
Intrareader reliability	Not presented	Performed on 25 knees. w-κ between 0.56 (intrasubstance meniscal degeneration) and 0.91 (bone marrow edema and Baker cyst)	Not presented
Scored MR Features			
Cartilage	Two different scores. Score 1: subregional approach. (A) Percentage of any cartilage loss in subregion; (B) percentage of full-thickness cartilage loss in subregion. Score 2: Site-specific approach. Scoring of cartilage thickness at 11 specific locations (not subregions) from 0 (none) to 2 (full-thickness loss)	Subregional approach: focal and diffuse defects are differentiated. Depth of lesions is scored from 0 to 3. Diameter of lesion is scored from 0 to 3. Osteochondral defects are scored separately	Subregional approach: scores from 0 to 6 depending on depth and extent of cartilage loss. Intrachondral signal additionally scored as present/absent

(continued on next page)

Table 1
(continued)

	BLOKS	KOSS	WORMS
BMLs	Scoring of individual lesions Three different aspects of BMLs are scored: 1. Size of BML scored from 0 to 3 concerning percentage of subregional bone volume 2. Percentage of surface area adjacent to subchondral plate 3. Percentage of BML that is noncystic	Scoring of individual lesions from 0 to 3 concerning maximum diameter of lesion	Summed BML size/volume for subregion from 0 to 3 in regard to percentage of subregional bone volume
Subchondral cysts	Scored together with BMLs	Scoring of individual lesions from 0 to 3 concerning maximum diameter of lesion	Summed cyst size/volume for subregion from 0 to 3 in regard to percentage of subregional bone volume
Osteophytes	Scored at 12 sites from 0 to 3	Scored from 0 to 3 Marginal, intercondylar and central osteophytes are differentiated Locations/sites of osteophyte scoring not forwarded	Scored at 16 sites from 0 to 7
Bone attrition	Not scored	Not scored	Scored in 14 subregions from 0 to 3
Effusion	Scored from 0 to 3	Scored from 0 to 3	Scored from 0 to 3
Synovitis	1. Scoring of size of signal changes in Hoffa fat pad 2. Five additional sites scored as present/absent (details of scoring not described)	Synovial thickening scored as present/absent on sagittal T1w SPGR sequence (location not described)	Combined effusion/synovitis score
Meniscal status	Anterior horn, body, posterior horn scored separately in medial/lateral meniscus Presence/absence scored: intrameniscal signal vertical tear horizontal tear complex tear root tear macerated meniscal cyst	No subregional division of meniscus described Presence/absence of following tears horizontal tear vertical tear radial tear complex tear bucket-handle tear meniscal intrasubstance degeneration scored from 0 to 3	Anterior horn, body, posterior horn scored separately in medial/lateral meniscus from 0 to 4: minor radial or parrot beak tear nondisplaced tear or prior surgical repair displaced tear or partial resection complete maceration/destruction or complete resection

Feature			
Meniscal extrusion	Scored as medial and lateral extrusion on coronal image and anterior extrusion for medial/lateral meniscus on sagittal image from 0 to 3	Scored on coronal image from 0 to 3	Not scored
Ligaments	Cruciate ligaments scored as normal or complete tear. Associated insertional BMLs are scored in tibia and in femur	Not scored	Cruciate ligaments and collateral ligaments scored as intact or torn
Periarticular features	Patella tendon: no signal change and signal abnormality. The following features are scored as present or absent: Pes anserine bursitis, Iliotibial band signal, Popliteal cyst, Infrapatellar bursa, Prepatellar bursa, Ganglion cysts of the TFJ, meniscus, ACL, PCL, semimembranosus, semitendinosus, other	Only popliteal cysts scored from 0 to 3	Popliteal cysts, anserine bursitis, semimembranosus bursa meniscal cyst, infrapatellar bursitis, prepatellar bursitis, tibiofibular cyst scored from 0 to 3
Loose bodies	Scored as absent/present	Not scored	Scored from 0 to 3

Abbreviations: ACL, anterior cruciate ligament; BML, bone marrow lesion; cor, coronal; ICC, intraclass correlation coefficient; PCL, posterior cruciate ligament; PD, proton density-weighted; sag, sagittal; TFJ, tibiofemoral joint; T2w FS, T2-weighted fat-suppressed sequence; T1 SE, T1-weighted spin echo sequence; 3D FLASH, three-dimensional fast low-angle shot sequence; 3D SPGR, three-dimensional spoiled gradient echo sequence; w-κ, weighted κ.

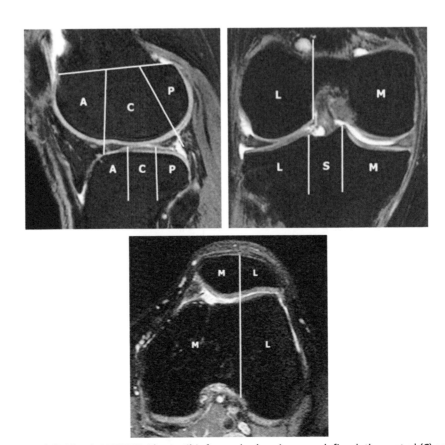

Fig. 1. Subregional division in WORMS. Eleven tibiofemoral subregions are defined: the central (C) and posterior (P) femur medially and laterally, the anterior (A), central (C), and posterior (P) tibia medially and laterally, and the subspinous (S) region. Four patellofemoral subregions are defined: the medial (M, including the patellar crest) and lateral (L) patella and the anterior (A) subregions of the femur (trochlea) medially (M) and laterally (L).

Several factors have to be considered when deciding which scoring system should be applied for the assessment of a given study. The most important are the outcome measures that are relevant to the study. Second, resources have to be taken into account because assessment using a complete whole-organ score differs from scoring only certain selected features. Last, the image data set is important because not all features are scorable on all sequences or with any given sequence protocol.

No literature is available concerning knee OA to determine whether several consecutive MR imaging examinations from the same patient should be evaluated semiquantitatively with chronologic order known to readers or if the images should be presented with readers blinded to the sequence in which they were acquired.[32] The primary rationale behind blinding to sequence is to reduce reader bias toward change in the expected direction. However, as long as readers are blinded to treatment assignment in a clinical trial it is not necessary to blind them to the chronologic sequence of the image data because bias cannot influence the trial results. If the research aim is not treatment but rather the natural history and detection of change, blinding might be of advantage.

ROLE OF MR IMAGING-DETECTED STRUCTURAL ABNORMALITIES IN PREDICTING PAIN AND PROGRESSION OF DISEASE IN KNEE OA
Subchondral BMLs

BMLs are defined on MR imaging as noncystic subchondral areas of ill-defined hyperintensity on proton density-weighted, intermediate-weighted, T2-weighted or short tau inversion recovery (STIR) sequences, displaying low signal intensity on T1-weighted spin echo images.[34–37] MR imaging assessment of BMLs should be

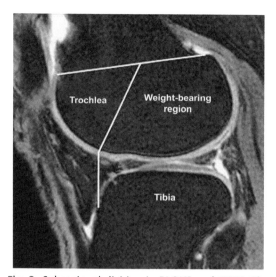

Fig. 2. Subregional division in BLOKS and KOSS. The femur is subdivided into the femoral trochlea (patello-femoral compartment) and the weight-bearing region (tibiofemoral compartment). The medial and lateral tibial plateaus are defined as 1 subregion, respectively. As in WORMS, the patella is divided in medial and lateral subregions in BLOKS (see **Fig. 1**). In KOSS, the patellar crest is a separate entity; thus, the patella has 3 subregions.

performed only on such sequences, because gradient recalled echo (GRE)-type sequences such as spoiled gradient echo at a steady state, fast low-angle shot, 3-point Dixon, double-echo steady state (DESS) and others are insensitive to marrow abnormalities because of trabecular magnetic susceptibility or T2* effects, and may lead to underestimation of BML size (**Fig. 3**).[37–39] It is important to distinguish degenerative BMLs from other marrow alterations of traumatic or non-traumatic origin,[40] because the differential diagnoses are broad. These degenerative lesions are frequently detected in conjunction with cartilage damage in the same region,[41–42] along with other OA features such as adjacent osteophytes. Knowing the specific MR imaging characteristics of such lesions is crucial for accurate detection and quantification.

BMLs play an important role in predicting structural progression and pain incidence as well as fluctuation of symptoms in patients with knee OA.[10,11,16,17,26,27,43] The term bone marrow edemalike lesion or the synonymous bone marrow lesion is now widely accepted to describe these alterations, because edema seems to be only a minor constituent of these abnormalities.[34,44]

Concerning the natural history of these lesions, BMLs represent a highly variable feature in patients with or at risk for development of knee OA, because their size may increase or decrease over time.[11,16,26,45] Mechanical limb alignment is believed to directly affect location, prevalence, and change in BMLs, because medial knee BMLs occur mainly in varus-aligned limbs, and lateral lesions occur mostly in valgus-aligned limbs.[10] Furthermore, these lesions are associated with concomitant increased local bone density, suggesting that they may be secondary to long-term excess loading.[46]

Several studies evaluating the role of BMLs in the progression of knee OA are available. In a longitudinal study assessing the association between BMLs and radiographic progression of knee OA, Felson and colleagues[10] reported that BMLs are powerful predictors of risk of local structural deterioration. Changes in BML size over time seem to have a direct effect on progression of knee OA. In a longitudinal MR imaging-based study, Roemer and colleagues[16] showed that subregions within the knee having incident and progressive BMLs had a higher risk of cartilage loss at follow-up and that absence of BMLs was associated with a lesser risk of cartilage loss in the same subregion. Hunter and colleagues[26] reported in a longitudinal study that, compared with stable BMLs, enlarging lesions were strongly associated with cartilage loss at follow-up. In the same study, presence of BMLs was strongly associated with malalignment and the effect of these lesions on cartilage loss was diluted after adjustment for limb alignment. In a recent longitudinal study, Davies-Tuck and colleagues[47] showed that development of new BMLs was associated with progressive cartilage loss after 2 years, whereas resolution of prevalent BMLs was associated with reduced progression of cartilage loss.

One could argue that the relationship between BMLs and degenerative cartilage lesions in knee OA might be seen as mutually predictive, because both features are highly related cross-sectionally. In a recent longitudinal study of patients with or at risk for knee OA, the investigators considered baseline degenerative cartilage lesions as predictors of BMLs in the same subregion.[48] They found a strong association between prevalent cartilage damage and incident BMLs in the same subregion after adjustment for potential confounders. It seems that subchondral bone and cartilage cannot be assessed and managed separately in OA, and the concept of an osteochondral unit might be fruitful in future OA research.

Another type of BML includes those in areas not covered by articular cartilage, such as the interspinous region at the tibia and the femoral notch. These lesions, known as traction or insertional

Table 2
Published interobserver and intraobserver reliability results for reading of MR imaging features using different whole-joint scoring systems

Joint Feature	WORMS Interreader Agreement (ICC)	KOSS Interreader (ICC [95% CI]/w-κ)	KOSS Intrareader (ICC [95% CI]/w-κ)	BLOKS Interreader (w-κ [95% CI])
BML size	0.74	0.91 [0.88–0.93]/ 0.88	0.93 [0.91–0.94]/ 0.91	0.72 [0.58–0.87]
BML % area (BLOKS only)	N/A	N/A	N/A	0.69 [0.55–0.82]
% of lesion BML (BLOKS only)	N/A	N/A	N/A	0.72 [0.58–0.87]
Osteophytes	0.97	0.71 [0.67–0.76]/ 0.67	0.76 [0.72–0.80]/ 0.79	0.65 [0.52–0.77]
Cartilage morphology	0.99	0.64 [0.58–0.69]/ 0.57	0.78 [0.74–0.81]/ 0.67	0.72 [0.59–0.85]
Cartilage 2 (BLOKS only)	N/A	N/A	N/A	0.73 [0.60–0.85]
Osteochondral defects (KOSS only)	N/A	0.63 [0.55–0.70]/ 0.66	0.87 [0.83–0.90]/ 0.87	N/A
Synovitis	0.74	0.74 [0.58–0.85]	0.81 [0.69–0.89]/ 0.77	0.62 [0.05–1.00]
Effusion	See synovitis; scores combined	See synovitis; scores combined	See synovitis; scores combined	0.61 [0.05–0.85]
Meniscal extrusion/ subluxation	N/A	0.67 [0.57–0.75]/ 0.65	0.82 [0.75–0.86]/ 0.82	0.51 [0.24–0.78]
Meniscal signal/ intrasubstance degeneration	N/A	0.78 [0.68–0.85]/ 0.66	0.76 [0.66–0.83]/ 0.56	0.68 [0.44–0.93]
Meniscal tear	0.87	0.70 [0.61–0.77]/ 0.70	0.78 [0.70–0.83]/ 0.78	0.79 [0.40–1.00]
Ligaments	1.0	N/A	N/A	N/A
Subchondral cysts	0.94	0.87 [0.83–0.89]/ 0.83	0.90 [0.87–0.92]/ 0.87	Part of % BML score
Baker cysts	N/A	0.89 [0.76–0.95]/ 0.80	0.96 [0.90–0.98]/ 0.91	N/A

Abbreviations: 95% CI, 95% confidence interval; ICC, intraclass correlation coefficient; N/A, not applicable; w-κ, weighted κ.

BMLs, are highly associated with cruciate ligament tears, and may be a consequence of tensile stress on these ligaments (**Fig. 4**).[9] No relationship between lesions at the interspinous region and femoral notch and cartilage loss has been shown.[9] However, lesions at the interspinous region extending to the subchondral bone of the medial tibial plateau are associated with regional cartilage loss.

The role of BMLs in predicting pain in patients with knee OA is controversial. In a cross-sectional study Felson and colleagues[27] reported that patients with radiographic knee OA and pain were more likely to have BMLs than patients without pain. Larger BMLs were found predominantly in the painful group. In a longitudinal study evaluating the relationship between fluctuation of BML size and knee pain, the same group[11] found that individuals without frequent knee pain who developed knee pain at follow-up were more likely to show an increase in BML size. In contrast, Kornaat and colleagues[45] found in a longitudinal study that changes in BMLs did not correlate with severity of pain as measured by WOMAC scores

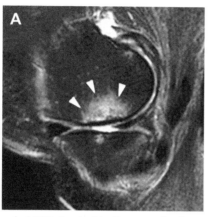
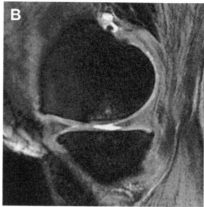

Fig. 3. Subchondral BML located in the central subregion (weight-bearing) of the medial femoral condyle. (A) Sagittal T2-weighted fat-suppressed (FS) fast spin echo (FSE) image depicts a typical BML showing high signal intensity with ill-defined margins (arrowheads). Note a tiny BML in the medial tibia. (B) Sagittal water-excitation (WE) DESS image, a GRE-type sequence, clearly underestimates the size of the medial femoral BML compared with T2-weighted FS FSE.

(Western Ontario and McMaster Universities Osteoarthritis Index). Furthermore, patients in whom BML size increased did not have a higher WOMAC score than patients with a decrease in BML size. Sowers and colleagues[49] found that frequency of BMLs was similar in both painful and painless knee OA, but larger BMLs were more frequent in patients with pain.

Subchondral Cystlike Lesions

Subchondral cystlike lesions are a common finding in patients with knee OA. These lesions have a characteristic appearance on MR imaging,

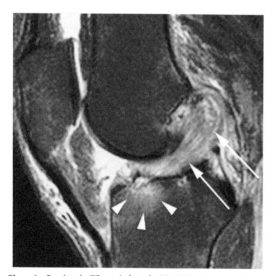

Fig. 4. Sagittal T2-weighted FS FSE image shows a typical insertional BML (arrowheads) at the tibial insertion of a partially ruptured ACL (arrows).

showing well-defined rounded areas of fluidlike signal intensity on nonenhanced imaging.[34,50] The term subchondral cystlike lesion is probably more appropriate than subchondral cyst because no evidence of epithelial lining was detected in several histologic studies.[50–53] Furthermore, in a recent cross-sectional study of patients with or at risk of knee OA, most of these lesions enhanced on MR imaging after intravenous administration of paramagnetic contrast agent, a feature not expected of pure cystic lesions.[54]

The cause of subchondral cystlike lesions is controversial. Two principal theories have been proposed, the synovial fluid intrusion and the bony contusion theories (Fig. 5). The synovial fluid intrusion theory posits that increased intra-articular pressure may lead to the intrusion of joint fluid into the subchondral bone via fissured or ulcerated cartilage,[53–55] creating the lesions. The bony contusion theory suggests that subchondral cystlike lesions are a consequence of traumatic bone necrosis after impact of 2 opposing articular surfaces.[17,52,56]

A recent cross-sectional MR imaging-based study reported that subchondral cystlike lesions were present in subregions without full-thickness cartilage defects in about half of the cases, which does not support the synovial fluid intrusion theory.[57] Subchondral cystlike lesions are strongly associated with BMLs in the same subregion, and may develop within areas of noncystic BMLs,[18,58] which favors the bony contusion theory. A recent longitudinal MR imaging-based study assessed the incidence of subchondral cystlike lesions in subregions presenting at baseline with full-thickness cartilage loss (synovial intrusion theory)

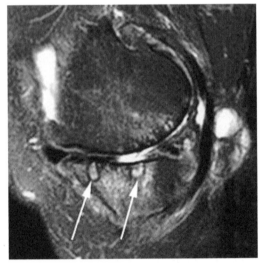

Fig. 5. Sagittal T2-weighted FS FSE image depicts typical subchondral cystlike lesions in the medial tibial plateau (*arrows*), associated with adjacent BMLs and full-thickness cartilage loss.

versus BMLs (bony contusion theory), showing an important association of incident subchondral cystlike lesions with baseline BMLs, even after adjustment for potential confounders, which strongly supports the bony contusion theory of subchondral cyst formation.[17]

Subchondral cystlike lesions do not seem to play a role in predicting knee pain. Two studies have found no association between the presence of subchondral cystlike lesions and pain in patients with knee OA.[59,60]

Subchondral Bone Attrition

Subchondral bone attrition is defined as depression or flattening of the subchondral bony surface unrelated to gross fracture. It can be assessed on radiographs or semiquantitatively on MR imaging.[22,61] Although attrition is usually observed in advanced knee OA, it may also appear in knees with mild OA that do not show joint space narrowing on radiographs.[62]

The pathogenesis of subchondral bone attrition in knee OA is unknown. Subchondral microfracturing and remodeling caused by alterations in mechanical loading, which are reflected as subchondral BMLs, may explain the presence and development of bone attrition in OA. A strong association between prevalent subchondral bone attrition and subchondral BMLs in the same subregion has been reported (**Fig. 6**), and the association increased with BML size.[18] Furthermore, the risk of incident subchondral bone attrition was increased for subregions with baseline BMLs.[18] Neogi and colleagues[20] reported that both prevalence and incidence of subchondral bone attrition are associated with knee malalignment, suggesting that attrition is a reflection of compartment-specific mechanical load, a finding that also approaches BMLs from subchondral attrition. The same group[63] found that subchondral bone attrition is a good predictor of cartilage loss longitudinally.

Subchondral bone attrition seems to play a role in predicting knee pain. In a recent cross-sectional study, Hernandez-Molina and colleagues[64] reported that bone attrition was associated with knee pain in OA, even after adjustment for other known factors linked to pain, suggesting an independent association of these features. Other studies have also suggested that subchondral bone attrition predicts knee pain.[59,61]

Meniscal Disease

The meniscus plays a critical protective role in the tibiofemoral compartments because of its

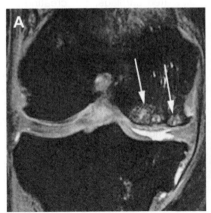
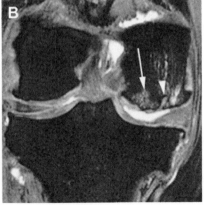

Fig. 6. Bone attrition. Coronal WE DESS images show irregularity and flattening of subchondral bone at the medial femoral condyle, in association with subchondral BMLs (*arrows, A* and *B*). Note a small subchondral cyst in B (*arrowhead*).

shock-absorbing and load-distributing properties. The menisci act on transmission of axial and torsional forces across the tibiofemoral joint and distribute mechanical loads over a wider area.[65] Meniscal disease is commonly observed in patients with and without radiographic knee OA.[13,66,67] It is rare to find normal meniscal morphology in compartments with OA; instead, the meniscus is often torn, macerated, or even totally destroyed, suggesting a strong association between tibiofemoral OA and meniscal disease.[7,13,67] Meniscal tears as well as partial or complete loss of overall normal morphology of the menisci (meniscal maceration/resection) may interfere with its functions and may lead to cartilage loss of the same compartment as well as in the subchondral bone, ultimately contributing to progression of OA.[7,8,68–72] The peak and average contact stresses in the medial compartment increase in a range of 40% to 700% when these functions are lost.[73–75]

Meniscal pathology plays a role in predicting cartilage loss in the tibiofemoral compartments (**Fig. 7**). In a recent longitudinal study, Hunter and colleagues[7] showed that displaced meniscal tears and meniscal maceration (**Fig. 8**) had a higher association with regional cartilage loss than non-displaced meniscal tears, with the most normal meniscus (without tears or maceration) used as the reference group. Another recent longitudinal study reported that not only maceration but also single horizontal tears in the medial meniscus were associated with cartilage loss in the medial compartment.[8] Horizontal meniscal tears (**Fig. 9**) are believed to be degenerative lesions, often

associated with older age and preexisting or incipient osteoarthritic disease.[76–78] Thus, horizontal (degenerative) meniscal tears could be an early sign of degeneration of the tibiofemoral compartment, including the underlying articular cartilage. After meniscal tearing and loss of its function, the underlying articular cartilage is less able to withstand the increased loading, and progression of cartilage loss is seen.

Abnormal signal within the substance of the meniscus not touching the articular surface is often detected in middle-aged and elderly patients. These signal changes, often globular or linear in shape (**Fig. 10**), are believed to represent either intrameniscal degeneration or intrasubstance tear.[79,80] The role of intrasubstance meniscal alterations in predicting knee pain is controversial,[81] and little is known about their role in progression of cartilage loss in the same compartment of the knee. A recent longitudinal study showed that abnormal intrasubstance medial meniscal signal detected at baseline was not associated with cartilage loss in the medial compartment 24 months later.[8] This finding may indicate that medial meniscal function may be preserved even when such signal alterations are present, although one could argue that follow-up in that study was short.

Meniscal extrusion is commonly seen among middle-aged and elderly patients, especially in compartments with OA.[82,83] Meniscal extrusion also predicts cartilage loss longitudinally (**Fig. 11**), because it may increase the contact stress on tibial and femoral articular cartilage, and may also contribute to increased joint space

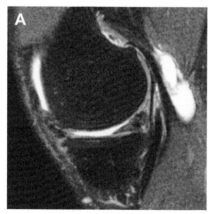 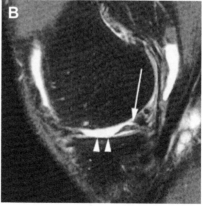

Fig. 7. Incident meniscal tear associated with tibiofemoral cartilage loss longitudinally. (*A*) Baseline sagittal T2-weighted FS FSE image depicts thinning of medial tibiofemoral cartilage, especially at the central subregion of the medial femoral condyle. Abnormal signal within the posterior horn of the medial meniscus is seen, with no evidence of tears. (*B*) 24-month follow-up sagittal T2-weighted FS FSE image shows an incident flap tear in the posterior horn of the medial meniscus (*arrow*). Cartilage loss in the medial compartment is also seen, especially at the central subregion of the medial tibia (*arrowheads*).

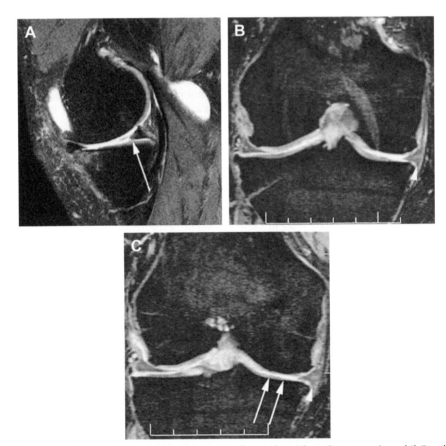

Fig. 8. Baseline meniscal maceration associated with tibiofemoral cartilage loss over time. (A) Baseline sagittal T2-weighted FS FSE image shows maceration (loss of substance and morphology) of the posterior horn of the medial meniscus (*arrow*). Areas of cartilage damage in the medial compartment are already seen at baseline. Compared with baseline coronal WE DESS image (B), follow-up coronal WE DESS image (C) shows evidence of cartilage loss in the medial tibial plateau (*arrows*). Note mild medial meniscal extrusion (*arrowheads*, B and C).

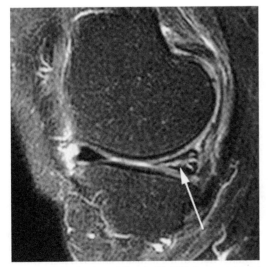

Fig. 9. Sagittal T2-weighted FS FSE image depicts a typical horizontal tear of the posterior horn of the medial meniscus (*arrow*).

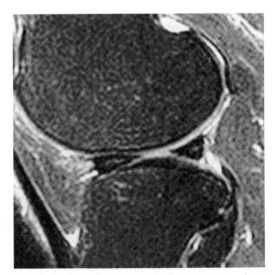

Fig. 10. Sagittal T2-weighted FS FSE image shows abnormal signal within the substance of the lateral meniscus not touching the articular surfaces.

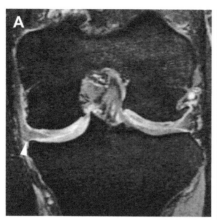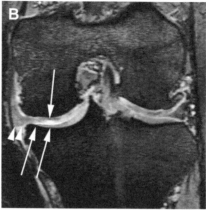

Fig. 11. Meniscal maceration associated with tibiofemoral cartilage loss over time. (*A*) Baseline coronal WE DESS image shows mild extrusion of the medial meniscus (*arrowhead*). Medial tibiofemoral cartilage is normal. (*B*) Compared with baseline, follow-up coronal WE DESS image shows evidence of cartilage loss in the medial femorotibial compartment (*arrows*). Note worsening of medial meniscal extrusion (*arrowheads*).

narrowing seen on radiographs.[7,70,84] Meniscal tears are considered the main predictor of extrusion, because tearing interrupts the circumferential hoop collagen fiber orientation. A recent cross-sectional study using a large cohort (more than 1000) with or at risk for knee OA showed a strong and significant association between meniscal tears and meniscal extrusion, with a direct relationship between degree of extrusion and severity of meniscal lesion.[85] The same study showed also that not only meniscal tears but also knee malalignment as well as cartilage damage were associated with meniscal extrusion after adjustment for the presence of concomitant meniscal tears in the same compartment. Meniscal tears in OA may be associated with symptoms, but not with most lesions.[67] Pain or discomfort might be present, especially in peripheral tears (red zone) or in dislocated tear fragments.

Synovitis

Synovitis in OA is believed to be a secondary phenomenon related to cartilage deterioration. However, its importance in the OA process is well recognized.[24,28,29,86–88] Furthermore, degenerative joints usually show signs of synovitis, even in the early phase of disease.[30,89,90]

Several nonenhanced and contrast-enhanced MR imaging techniques for detecting and quantifying synovitis are available. In a pathologic study conducted by Fernandez-Madrid and colleagues,[30] MR imaging detected signal alterations in the Hoffa fat pad correlated with mild chronic synovitis. This work led to the assumption that synovitis may be assessed on nonenhanced images, mainly on proton density-weighted or

T2-weighted sequences, using signal alterations in the Hoffa fat pad as a surrogate for whole-knee synovitis (**Fig. 12**).[28,29] However, signal alterations in the Hoffa fat pad are a common finding on MR imaging of the knee and present many possible diagnoses.[91] Roemer and colleagues[92] found that signal alterations in the Hoffa fat pad seen on noncontrast-enhanced sequences were a sensitive but not a specific sign of peripatellar synovitis, compared with contrast-enhanced sequences. Recently another scoring system for the assessment of synovitis using nonenhanced scans was introduced,[93] but it has not been tested

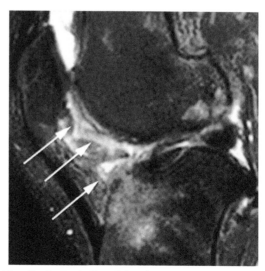

Fig. 12. Sagittal T2-weighted FS FSE image showing high signal intensity within the Hoffa fat pad (*arrows*) adjacent to the synovial lining, used as surrogate for synovitis in OA research.

against an established reference standard such as contrast-enhanced MR imaging or histology.[94] In a recent study comparing 3 scoring systems for evaluating synovitis and joint effusion on MR imaging, Loeuille and colleagues[95] found that only scoring of contrast-enhanced T1-weighted images correlated with microscopically proved synovitis. Furthermore, no correlation with microscopic synovitis was found when MR imaging was performed without contrast intravenous administration. Thus, ideally, synovitis should be assessed on contrast-enhanced T1-weighted MR imaging sequences, allowing evaluation of enhancement and thickening of the synovial membrane (**Fig. 13**).[96–98] Only contrast-enhanced images can differentiate between synovium and joint effusion. A new scoring system that uses contrast-enhanced T1-weighted sequences to assess synovitis at multiple sites in patients with knee OA was presented recently.[24] Synovial thickness was measured at the peripatellar region, around the cruciate ligaments and menisci, and around popliteal cysts and loose bodies if present, allowing assessment of synovitis in the whole joint. The reliability of the reading was good to excellent for the 11 different synovitis locations. The region around the cruciate ligaments seems to be the most commonly affected, a novel finding of possible clinical relevance in regard to the role of ligament integrity in the OA process.[99]

There is evidence that synovitis also plays a role in progression of cartilage loss in knee OA. In a longitudinal study with 422 patients, Ayral and colleagues[87] assessed the medial perimeniscal synovium and the medial tibiofemoral cartilage using arthroscopy, and found that 123 (29%) patients had a reactive aspect and 89 (21%) had an inflammatory aspect of the synovium. Only the inflammatory synovitis group showed an association with cartilage loss at follow-up. Although histologic evaluation was not performed, previous studies have shown a good correlation between arthroscopic and microscopic findings of synovitis.[100,101]

Synovial inflammation is believed to contribute to pain in patients with knee OA, even although nociceptive fibers are inconsistently present within the synovial membrane.[102] Hill and colleagues[29] showed that alterations in the Hoffa fat pad signal changes over time were modestly and directly correlated with changes in knee pain, but not with cartilage loss. The effect of these signal alterations on pain was independent of changes in joint effusion. In another cross-sectional study, the same group found that these alterations were more common in patients with knee pain and radiographic OA than those with radiographic OA and no pain.[28] However, both studies relied on noncontrast-enhanced MR imaging sequences. Recent studies assessing synovitis on contrast-enhanced MR imaging in patients with or at risk for knee OA reported that high-grade synovitis (graded semiquantitatively from 0 to 2) was associated with knee pain compared with patients with no or low-grade synovitis.[24,88]

Effusion

Joint effusion is commonly detected in patients with moderate to advanced knee OA,[28,103] and reflects synovial activation secondary to ligament injury, loose bodies, hyaline cartilage deterioration, and meniscal damage.[15] Joint effusion is ideally assessed and quantified on proton

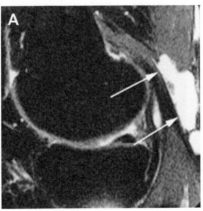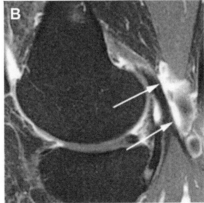

Fig. 13. (*A*) Sagittal proton density-weighted FS FSE image shows fluid signal within the medial gastrocnemius-semimembranosus bursa (popliteal cyst, *arrows*). (*B*) Sagittal T1-weighted FS FSE image after intravenous administration of gadolinium shows synovial enhancement and thickening (synovitis) around the popliteal cyst (*arrows*).

density-weighted, T2-weighted, and STIR MR imaging sequences. However, synovial thickening as seen in synovitis increases the total synovial volume in such sequences, and differentiating synovium from effusion on nonenhanced MR imaging sequences is often difficult.[99]

The prevalence of joint effusion in knee OA has a direct relationship with radiographic severity in the knee joint.[103] In a cohort of 1368 knees without radiographic knee OA, the prevalence of joint effusion was 33.7% and most effusions were small.[15] Hill and colleagues[28] reported a high prevalence of joint effusion in individuals with radiographic knee OA. Effusion was present in 91.7% of patients with radiographic OA and knee pain, and in 82.3% of those with radiographic OA and no pain. The same study reported that moderate and large effusions (graded from 0 to 3) were significantly more common among those with knee pain. A significant association between grades of effusion (graded in conjunction with synovitis on nonenhanced MR imaging) with knee pain severity was found by Torres and colleagues[59] in a cohort of 143 patients with knee OA. The joint capsule contains pain fibers, and capsule distension associated with joint effusions may contribute to knee pain in OA.

Cruciate and Collateral Ligaments

Traumatic complete anterior cruciate ligament (ACL) tears may lead to premature knee OA.[104–107] However, the role of traumatic incomplete ACL tears in predicting knee OA is controversial.[108] ACL disruption inevitably causes alterations in knee kinematics, because the ACL is the primary restraint against tibial translation.[109] Furthermore, ACL failure increases the external adduction moment and consequently medial loading, increasing the risk of medial tibiofemoral OA.[110] ACL tears are frequently associated with other traumatic lesions in the knee such as meniscal tears and chondral/osteochondral lesions, making the assessment of their role in knee degeneration more difficult.[111]

Incidental ACL tears are common among patients with knee OA, with reported prevalence ranging from 20% to 35%.[110,112,113] Patients with knee OA and incidental ACL tears are often unable to recall significant knee injury. Degeneration within the ligament fibers, alterations in notch width and depth, and the presence of notch osteophytes (**Fig. 14**) may predispose to ACL tears in patients with knee OA.[114–117] Evaluation of cruciate ligaments must include not only assessment for tears but also for insertional or traction BMLs. Hernandez-Molina and colleagues[9] showed that traction BMLs, detected on MR

imaging at the femoral and tibial insertions of the ACL, are strongly related to ACL disease.

The role of ACL tears in predicting structural progression in patients with knee OA remains unclear. In a recent longitudinal study, Amin and colleagues[118] found that the presence of an ACL tear at baseline increased the risk for cartilage loss in the medial compartment at 30-month follow-up. However, adjustment for medial meniscal damage diluted the effect. In a large cohort of 245 elderly individuals (aged 70–79 years), the prevalence of any ligament tear in the knee was 27% in men and 30% in women, and a good correlation with cartilage loss was found.[119] However, there was no longitudinal assessment.

The contribution of ACL tears to pain severity in patients with knee OA is also unclear. Hill and colleagues[110] showed that complete ACL tears were common (22.8%) in a population with symptomatic knee OA and poor recall of knee trauma, and rare (2.7%) among those without knee symptoms. Another group reported that patients with a complete ACL tear tended to have greater knee pain at baseline, but no overall differences in pain severity were found after adjustment for potential confounders.[118] In both studies, the ACL was scored as pathologic when a complete tear was detected.

The posterior cruciate ligament (PCL) plays a role in the kinematics of the knee, especially for the medial compartment, and a tear with a subsequent PCL deficiency may increase the incidence of knee OA.[120,121] In a long follow-up study of 58 patients with isolated partial or complete PCL tears treated conservatively and evaluated after 2 to 19.3 years (mean 6.9 years), Patel and colleagues[122] found that 10 (17.2%) developed medial tibiofemoral radiographic OA. Incidental complete PCL tears are rare among patients with knee OA.

Incidental collateral ligament tears are infrequent among patients with knee OA.[59] In a small cohort of 30 patients with medial compartment knee OA with no history of trauma and 30 age-matched patients with atraumatic knee pain but without OA, signal changes in or around the medial collateral ligament (MCL) (grade 1 and 2 lesions) were seen in 27 (90%) of the first group, but in only 2 (6.6%) from the control group,[123] suggesting that grade 1 and 2 MCL lesions may be related to medial knee OA in patients without history of trauma. The role of collateral ligament abnormalities in predicting structural progression and pain in patients with OA is unknown.

Periarticular Cysts and Bursae

A wide spectrum of periarticular cystic lesions may be encountered around the knee in patients with

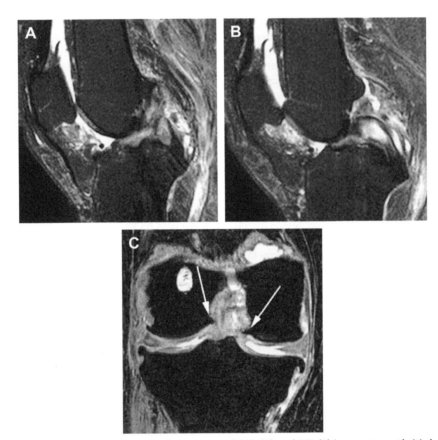

Fig. 14. Sagittal T2-weighted FS FSE images show ruptured ACL (*A*) and PCL (*B*) in an osteoarthritic knee. Coronal WE DESS (*C*) shows central osteophytes adjacent to the intercondylar notch (*arrows*).

OA.[124,125] Most cystic lesions around the knee are encapsulated fluid collections showing low signal intensity on T1-weighted images and high signal intensity on T2-weighted images.[124,125]

Popliteal (Baker) cysts are not true cysts, but fluid in the semimembranosus-medial gastrocnemius bursa, and are commonly detected in patients with knee OA.[28,103,126] Hill and colleagues[28] found that the prevalence of these lesions was 43.2% in knees with moderate or larger effusions, compared with 22.7% in those with little or no effusion. In this study, presence of popliteal cysts was not associated with pain. However, different grades of synovitis may be present around popliteal cysts,[24] and such a feature should be assessed on contrast-enhanced MR imaging (see **Fig. 13**). Moderate to large popliteal cysts are associated with incident radiographic knee OA.[127]

A wide spectrum of bursitides may occur in patients with knee OA.[124] Prepatellar bursitis may be seen in conjunction with knee OA, but its pathogenesis is believed not to be directly linked to degeneration. A less common site of bursitis is the superficial infrapatellar bursa, appearing on MR imaging as a fluid collection anterior to the tibial tubercle. A tiny amount of fluid within the deep infrapatellar bursa is frequently detected on MR imaging of the knee, including patients with OA.[128] However, this may be considered a normal finding without clinical significance, because of its high prevalence in asymptomatic patients.[128,129] Anserine bursitis may be detected in conjunction with knee OA, but its association with degeneration is controversial. Chronic anserine bursitis is believed to be most common in elderly patients with degenerative disease or rheumatoid arthritis.[130] However, a recent case-control study found no association between prevalent anserine bursitis and radiographic knee OA.[131] Furthermore, anserine bursitis shows no significant association with incident knee pain or incident radiographic OA.[127]

Parameniscal cysts are believed to be formed by fluid extravasation through a meniscal tear into the parameniscal soft tissue.[129] Most of these cysts result from horizontal tears, which are believed to be of degenerative origin and are a common finding in knee OA.[77,132,133] Lateral meniscal cysts are associated with incident knee pain longitudinally.[127]

Ganglion cysts around the knee are routinely detected on MR imaging examinations.[124] They may be seen in conjunction with OA, but accepted theories for ganglia formation are not directly related to OA.[134–136] Tibiofibular synovial cysts are more prevalent in patients with knee effusion, because in 10% of adults the proximal tibiofibular joint communicates with the knee joint. The reported prevalence in patients with knee OA is low.[128] Other cystic lesions around the osteoarthritic knee are rare.

Loose Bodies

Loose bodies are frequently detected in conjunction with knee OA on MR imaging, especially in severe cases. Loose bodies are a catchall term that may include, for example, chondral fragments, detached osteophytes, and meniscal fragments. Synovial osteochondromatosis secondary to OA should also be considered.[137] Loose bodies are related to internal knee derangement in patients with OA,[138,139] because they may trigger synovial inflammation as shown by a recent study using contrast-enhanced MR imaging,[24] and are a common indication for arthroscopic treatment.[138,139] On MR imaging, loose bodies are best visualized in joints with prevalent effusion and may be delineated as solitary or multiple low signal intensity abnormalities within the joint (Fig. 15).

Compositional Imaging of Cartilage in Knee OA

The articular cartilage is composed of a fluid-filled macromolecular network responsible for supporting mechanical loading. During joint loading, the electrolyte-containing interstitial fluid, which represents about 75% of cartilage by weight, becomes pressurized to the extent that its movement is restricted by the macromolecular network, distributing and supporting the mechanical loading. The cartilaginous macromolecular network is composed of collagen and proteoglycans. Collagen is the most abundant macromolecule, accounting for about 20% of cartilage volume by weight, whereas aggrecan, a large aggregating proteoglycan, is the second most abundant. In knees without OA, the collagen network acts as the structural framework of the tissue, providing the main source of tensile and shear strength. The proteoglycans have glycosaminoglycans (GAG) attached as side chains with abundant negatively charged carboxyl and sulfate groups, which give the cartilage considerable compressive strength.

Osteoarthritic changes are characterized by significant changes in cartilage biochemical composition. Loss of GAG and increased water content represent the earliest stage of cartilage degeneration, although the collagenous component of the extracellular matrix still remains intact. Several MR imaging techniques allow detection of biochemical changes that precede the morphologic degeneration in cartilage, attempting to selectively visualize the GAG components and/or the collagen fiber network of the extracellular matrix.[140,141]

T2 of hyaline articular cartilage reflects interactions between water molecules and between water and surrounding macromolecules, especially collagen. Increased interactions between water and collagen result in decreased T2. Therefore, T2 relaxation time mapping has been used to describe the composition of cartilage, because it is

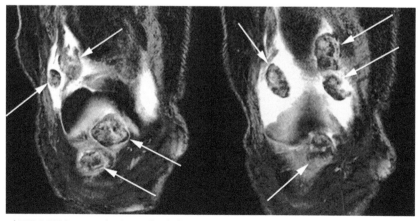

Fig. 15. Coronal WE DESS images depict multiple low signal intensity loose bodies in the suprapatellar and parapatellar articular recesses (arrows).

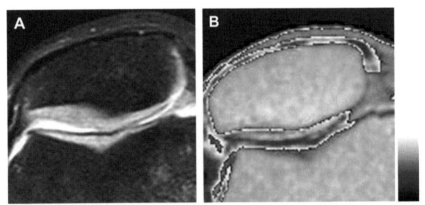

Fig. 16. 26-year-old man with type II collagenopathy (Stickler syndrome). (*A*) Axial proton density-weighted FS FSE image shows normal morphology of patellar articular cartilage. (*B*) Axial multi-echo spin-echo, MESE cartilage T2 map shows markedly increased T2 values (90 ms to 100 ms, corresponding to lighter colors in color map) with loss of normal spatial variation caused by lack of normal type II collagen network. (*Courtesy of* Timothy J. Mosher, MD, Penn State University College of Medicine.)

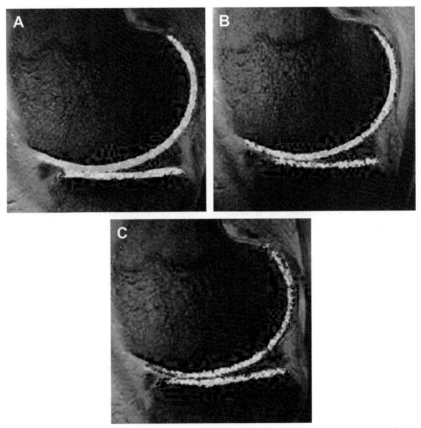

Fig. 17. Sagittal dGEMRIC images of the medial compartment of the knee before (*A*), 1 day after (*B*), and 1 week after running a marathon (*C*). The dGEMRIC index decreased over this period. However, in other case studies, the dGEMRIC index returned to baseline after 1 week. Larger studies need to determine whether these transient effects affect or predict the long-term health of articular cartilage. (*Courtesy of* Deborah Burstein, PhD, Harvard Medical School.)

highly sensitive to changes in hydration (or, nearly equivalently, collagen concentration),[142] as well as to orientation of the anisotropic arrangement of collagen fibrils within the extracellular cartilage matrix.[143] In normal cartilage, regional and zonal differences in density and organization of collagen matrix appear as variations in T2. Therefore zonal evaluation of articular cartilage is crucial. A multiecho spin echo technique is used to measure T2 values. There is good evidence that T2 mapping is useful for identifying sites of early degeneration (early disruption of the collagen matrix), which appear as early increase in cartilage T2 (**Fig. 16**).[144] Compared with T2 maps of normal hyaline cartilage, T2 maps of osteoarthritic cartilage are more heterogeneous. It is controversial whether there is a linear relationship between T2 and OA severity.[144,145] Furthermore, physical activity seems to play a role in cartilage T2 values.[146]

The delayed gadolinium MR imaging of cartilage (dGEMRIC) technique is based on the general principle that ions in the interstitial fluid are distributed in cartilage in relation to the concentration of the negatively charged GAG molecules. The contrast agent gadolinium diethylenetriamine pentaacetate anion (Gd-DTPA^{2-}), once penetrated into the cartilage, concentrates where the cartilage GAG content is relatively low. Because the concentration of Gd-DTPA^{2-} can be approximated from a T1 measurement, a T1 map of the cartilage after administration of Gd-DTPA^{2-} allows assessment of GAG content. The term delayed in dGEMRIC reflects the time needed (about 90 minutes) to allow penetration of Gd-DTPA^{2-} into the full cartilage thickness. Areas of cartilage with

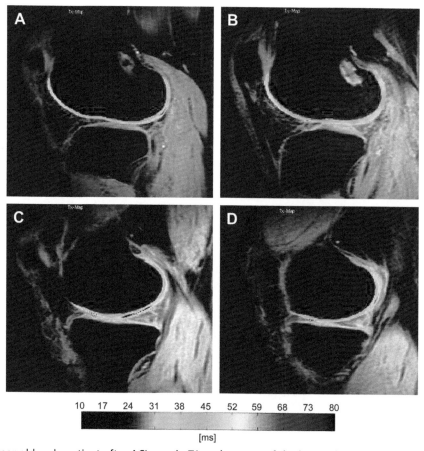

10 17 24 31 38 45 52 59 68 73 80

[ms]

Fig. 18. 51-year-old male patient after ACL repair. T1ρ color maps of the lateral femoral condyle (*A, B*) and the medial femoral condyle (*C, D*). Sagittal 3D T1ρ sequence was performed at 3 T using the following acquisition parameters: repetition time (TR)/echo time (TE) = 9.3/3.7 ms, time of recovery = 1500 ms, field of view = 14 cm, matrix = 256 × 192, slice thickness = 3 mm, bandwidth = 31.25 kHz. Higher T1ρ values indicate lower concentration of macromolecules/glycosaminoglycans. (*Courtesy of* Thomas Baum, MD, University of California at San Francisco.)

depleted GAG show lower dGEMRIC indexes (often called lesions), which are commonly observed in joints with radiographic findings of OA, as well as in compartments with overloading.[147] Variations in the dGEMRIC index in the same articular compartment may be seen even in early and potentially reversible stages of OA,[147] because such stages are characterized by reduction in tissue GAG. The dGEMRIC index has been shown to be sensitive to several physiologic factors, including exercise (**Fig. 17**)[148] and body mass index (calculated as weight in kilograms divided by the square of height in meters).[149] It may also be sensitive to acute physical stress. The dGEMRIC measurements have been validated in clinical studies, corresponding to reference standard measurements for GAG histology and biochemistry.[150] In particular, dGEMRIC has been reported to show variations in morphologically intact cartilage and to predict progression of OA.[151]

T1ρ relaxation time describes the spin-lattice relaxation in the rotating frame with an additional radiofrequency pulse applied after the magnetization is tipped into the transverse plane. The interactions between motion-restricted water molecules and their local macromolecular environment including collagen and GAG can be monitored by T1ρ measurements. Changes to the extracellular matrix, such as proteoglycan depletion, may alter T1ρ measurements.[152] In knee OA, damaged cartilage shows higher T1ρ values than normal cartilage (**Fig. 18**), and is more sensitive than T2 for differentiating healthy individuals from patients with early OA.[153] There is evidence that several factors other than proteoglycan depletion may contribute to variations in T1ρ values, such as collagen fiber orientation and concentration, as well as other macromolecules.[154] Even although T1ρ imaging cannot specify the macromolecular change in cartilage degeneration, its nonspecific sensitivity in the detection of early

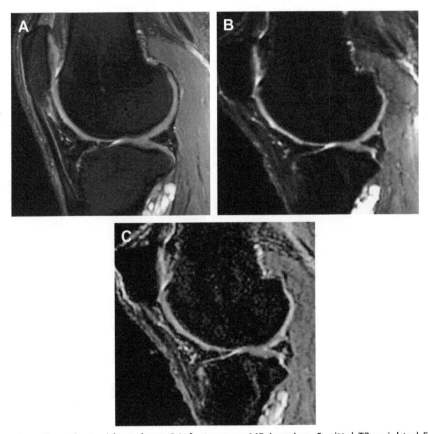

Fig. 19. Asymptomatic patient with no knee OA features on MR imaging. Sagittal T2-weighted FS FSE image (*A*) and corresponding diffusion images for b = 0 (*B*) and apparent diffusion coefficient map (*C*). All images were performed at 3 T using the following acquisition parameters: TR/TE = 2200/73 ms, b factor = 600s/mm², slice thickness = 5 mm, matrix = 192 × 192. (*Courtesy of* Thomas Baum, MD, University of California at San Francisco.)

degenerative lesions may provide valuable etiologic, diagnostic, or prognostic information regarding knee OA. To our knowledge, no large clinical studies on knee OA have been performed using T1ρ imaging.

The negatively charged GAG is responsible for higher concentrations of positively charged sodium (Na^{23}) in the cartilaginous interstitial fluid, compared with its concentration in the surrounding synovial fluid or bone. Normal (GAG-rich) cartilage has higher concentrations of sodium, and areas of cartilage with depletion of the negatively charged GAG have lower concentrations of sodium. Because sodium possesses a nuclear spin momentum, it shows MR, and therefore is MR imaging observable. The advantages of sodium imaging are that sodium occurs naturally in the cartilage matrix, its signal in cartilage is high compared with background, and it can depict regions of proteoglycan depletion, which show lower signal intensity on sodium MR imaging, compared with areas of normal cartilage.[155–157] Therefore, sodium may be useful in differentiating normal cartilage from early degenerated cartilage.[155] Because of short T2 relaxation times of sodium, this technique is commonly performed using a spectrally weighted twisted projection technique. Care should be taken when interpreting sodium MR imaging of cartilage because some spatial variation in sodium concentration (and thus in signal) may be present in normal cartilage. To our knowledge, no large clinical studies on knee OA have been performed using sodium MR imaging.

Diffusion-weighted MR imaging of cartilage is based on the molecular motion of water, which is believed to be related to the macromolecular environment. Consequently, diffusion-weighted MR imaging may provide useful information about cartilage composition by measuring the molecular movement, which reflects biochemical structure and architecture of hyaline cartilage (Fig. 19). It has been shown that disruption of the cartilage matrix results in enhanced water mobility, which increases the apparent diffusion coefficient of cartilage.[158] To our knowledge, no large clinical studies on knee OA have been performed using diffusion-weighted MR imaging.

SUMMARY

OA of the knee is considered a disease of the whole joint. MR imaging has added much to our understanding of all the joint tissues involved in the disease process such as the subchondral bone, synovium, menisci, ligaments, and periarticular soft tissues and their significance in explaining

pain and structural progression. The use of appropriate MR imaging pulse sequences is crucial, allowing accurate assessment and quantification of these alterations. Reliable MR imaging-based SQ scoring systems are available to assess the structural integrity of subchondral bone, synovium, menisci, ligaments, and periarticular alterations. Contrast-enhanced MR imaging should be considered in the assessment of whole-knee synovitis, because it enables accurate evaluation and quantification of synovial thickness. MR imaging-based compositional techniques for the assessment of hyaline cartilage have added to the understanding and detection of early degenerative changes, before morphologic changes can be seen in knees at risk of OA. MR imaging biomarkers have proved in recent years to be a powerful and applicable tool that has contributed to our understanding of the processes and natural history of OA.

REFERENCES

1. Eckstein F, Schnier M, Haubner M, et al. Accuracy of cartilage volume and thickness measurements with magnetic resonance imaging. Clin Orthop Relat Res 1998;352:137–48.
2. Burgkart R, Glaser C, Hyhlik-Dürr A, et al. Magnetic resonance imaging-based assessment of cartilage loss in severe osteoarthritis: accuracy, precision, and diagnostic value. Arthritis Rheum 2001;44(9):2072–7.
3. Cicuttini F, Forbes A, Asbeutah A, et al. Comparison and reproducibility of fast and conventional spoiled gradient-echo magnetic resonance sequences in the determination of knee cartilage volume. J Orthop Res 2000;18(4):580–4.
4. Gahunia HK, Babyn P, Lemaire C, et al. Osteoarthritis staging: comparison between magnetic resonance imaging, gross pathology and histopathology in the rhesus macaque. Osteoarthritis Cartilage 1995;3(3):169–80.
5. Broderick LS, Turner DA, Renfrew DL, et al. Severity of articular cartilage abnormality in patients with osteoarthritis: evaluation with fast spin-echo MR vs arthroscopy. AJR Am J Roentgenol 1994;162(1):99–103.
6. Blackburn WD Jr, Bernreuter WK, Rominger M, et al. Arthroscopic evaluation of knee articular cartilage: a comparison with plain radiographs and magnetic resonance imaging. J Rheumatol 1994;21(4):675–9.
7. Hunter DJ, Zhang YQ, Niu JB, et al. The association of meniscal pathologic changes with cartilage loss in symptomatic knee osteoarthritis. Arthritis Rheum 2006;54(3):795–801.
8. Crema MD, Guermazi A, Li L, et al. The association of prevalent medial meniscal pathology with

cartilage loss in the medial tibiofemoral compartment over a 2-year period. Osteoarthritis Cartilage 2010;18(3):336–43.

9. Hernández-Molina G, Guermazi A, Niu J, et al. Central bone marrow lesions in symptomatic knee osteoarthritis and their relationship to anterior cruciate ligament tears and cartilage loss. Arthritis Rheum 2008;58(1):130–6.

10. Felson DT, McLaughlin S, Goggins J, et al. Bone marrow edema and its relation to progression of knee osteoarthritis. Ann Intern Med 2003; 139(5 Pt 1):330–6.

11. Felson DT, Niu J, Guermazi A, et al. Correlation of the development of knee pain with enlarging bone marrow lesions on magnetic resonance imaging. Arthritis Rheum 2007;56(9):2986–92.

12. Englund M, Guermazi A, Roemer FW, et al. Meniscal tear in knees without surgery and the development of radiographic osteoarthritis among middle-aged and elderly persons: the Multicenter Osteoarthritis Study. Arthritis Rheum 2009;60(3):831–9.

13. Englund M, Guermazi A, Gale D, et al. Incidental meniscal findings on knee MRI in middle-aged and elderly persons. N Engl J Med 2008;359(11):1108–15.

14. Hunter DJ, Zhang YQ, Tu X, et al. Change in joint space width: hyaline articular cartilage loss or alteration in meniscus? Arthritis Rheum 2006;54(8): 2488–95.

15. Roemer FW, Guermazi A, Hunter DJ, et al. The association of meniscal damage with joint effusion in persons without radiographic osteoarthritis: the Framingham and MOST osteoarthritis studies. Osteoarthritis Cartilage 2009;17(6):748–53.

16. Roemer FW, Guermazi A, Javaid MK, et al. Change in MRI-detected subchondral bone marrow lesions is associated with cartilage loss: the MOST Study. A longitudinal multicentre study of knee osteoarthritis. Ann Rheum Dis 2009;68(9):1461–5.

17. Crema MD, Roemer FW, Zhu Y, et al. Subchondral cystlike lesions develop longitudinally in areas of bone marrow edema-like lesions in patients with or at risk for knee osteoarthritis: detection with MR imaging–the MOST study. Radiology 2010; 256(3):855–62.

18. Roemer FW, Neogi T, Nevitt MC, et al. Subchondral bone marrow lesions are highly associated with, and predict subchondral bone attrition longitudinally: the MOST study. Osteoarthritis Cartilage 2010;18(1):47–53.

19. Roemer FW, Zhang YQ, Niu J, et al. Tibiofemoral joint osteoarthritis: risk factors for MR-depicted fast cartilage loss over a 30-month period in the multicenter osteoarthritis study. Radiology 2009; 252(3):772–80.

20. Neogi T, Nevitt MC, Niu J, et al. Subchondral bone attrition may be a reflection of compartment-specific mechanical load: the MOST Study. Ann Rheum Dis 2010;69(5):841–4.

21. Hunter DJ, Lo GH, Gale D, et al. The reliability of a new scoring system for knee osteoarthritis MRI and the validity of bone marrow lesion assessment: BLOKS (Boston Leeds Osteoarthritis Knee Score). Ann Rheum Dis 2008;67(2):206–11.

22. Peterfy CG, Guermazi A, Zaim S, et al. Whole-Organ Magnetic Resonance Imaging Score (WORMS) of the knee in osteoarthritis. Osteoarthritis Cartilage 2004;12(3):177–90.

23. Kornaat PR, Ceulemans RY, Kroon HM, et al. MRI assessment of knee osteoarthritis: Knee Osteoarthritis Scoring System (KOSS)–inter-observer and intra-observer reproducibility of a compartment-based scoring system. Skeletal Radiol 2005; 34(2):95–102.

24. Guermazi A, Roemer FW, Crema MD, et al. A novel semiquantitative whole-knee scoring system for the assessment of synovitis in knee OA on contrast-enhanced MRI– the MOST study. Osteoarthritis Cartilage 2008;16(Suppl 4):S174–5.

25. Reichenbach S, Yang M, Eckstein F, et al. Does cartilage volume or thickness distinguish knees with and without mild radiographic osteoarthritis? The Framingham Study. Ann Rheum Dis 2010; 69(1):143–9.

26. Hunter DJ, Zhang Y, Niu J, et al. Increase in bone marrow lesions associated with cartilage loss: a longitudinal magnetic resonance imaging study of knee osteoarthritis. Arthritis Rheum 2006;54(5): 1529–35.

27. Felson DT, Chaisson CE, Hill CL, et al. The association of bone marrow lesions with pain in knee osteoarthritis. Ann Intern Med 2001;134(7): 541–9.

28. Hill CL, Gale DG, Chaisson CE, et al. Knee effusions, popliteal cysts, and synovial thickening: association with knee pain in osteoarthritis. J Rheumatol 2001;28(6):1330–7.

29. Hill CL, Hunter DJ, Niu J, et al. Synovitis detected on magnetic resonance imaging and its relation to pain and cartilage loss in knee osteoarthritis. Ann Rheum Dis 2007;66(12):1599–603.

30. Fernandez-Madrid F, Karvonen RL, Teitge RA, et al. Synovial thickening detected by MR imaging in osteoarthritis of the knee confirmed by biopsy as synovitis. Magn Reson Imaging 1995;13(2): 177–83.

31. Lynch JA, Roemer FW, Nevitt MC, et al. Comparison of BLOKS and WORMS scoring systems part I. Cross sectional comparison of methods to assess cartilage morphology, meniscal damage, and bone marrow lesions on knee MRI: data from the Osteoarthritis Initiative. Osteoarthritis Cartilage 2010;18(11):1393–401.

32. Felson DT, Nevitt MC. Blinding images to sequence in osteoarthritis: evidence from other diseases. Osteoarthritis Cartilage 2009;17(3):281–3.

33. Felson DT, Lynch J, Guermazi A, et al. Comparison of BLOKS and WORMS scoring systems part II. Longitudinal assessment of knee MRIs for osteoarthritis and suggested approach based on their performance: data from the Osteoarthritis Initiative. Osteoarthritis Cartilage 2010;18:1402–7.

34. Zanetti M, Bruder E, Romero J, et al. Bone marrow edema pattern in osteoarthritic knees: correlation between MR imaging and histologic findings. Radiology 2000;215(3):835–40.

35. Yu JS, Cook PA. Magnetic resonance imaging (MRI) of the knee: a pattern approach for evaluating bone marrow edema. Crit Rev Diagn Imaging 1996;37(4):261–303.

36. Bergman AG, Willén HK, Lindstrand AL, et al. Osteoarthritis of the knee: correlation of subchondral MR signal abnormalities with histopathologic and radiographic features. Skeletal Radiol 1994;23(6):445–8.

37. Roemer FW, Hunter DJ, Guermazi A. MRI-based semiquantitative assessment of subchondral bone marrow lesions in osteoarthritis research. Osteoarthritis Cartilage 2009;17(3):414–5 [author reply: 416–7].

38. Yoshioka H, Stevens K, Hargreaves BA, et al. Magnetic resonance imaging of articular cartilage of the knee: comparison between fat-suppressed three-dimensional SPGR imaging, fat-suppressed FSE imaging, and fat-suppressed three-dimensional DEFT imaging, and correlation with arthroscopy. J Magn Reson Imaging 2004;20(5):857–64.

39. Peterfy CG, Gold G, Eckstein F, et al. MRI protocols for whole-organ assessment of the knee in osteoarthritis. Osteoarthritis Cartilage 2006;14(Suppl A):A95–111.

40. Roemer FW, Frobell R, Hunter DJ, et al. MRI-detected subchondral bone marrow signal alterations of the knee joint: terminology, imaging appearance, relevance and radiological differential diagnosis. Osteoarthritis Cartilage 2009;17(9):1115–31.

41. Guymer E, Baranyay F, Wluka AE, et al. A study of the prevalence and associations of subchondral bone marrow lesions in the knees of healthy, middle-aged women. Osteoarthritis Cartilage 2007;15(12):1437–42.

42. Baranyay FJ, Wang Y, Wluka AE, et al. Association of bone marrow lesions with knee structures and risk factors for bone marrow lesions in the knees of clinically healthy, community-based adults. Semin Arthritis Rheum 2007;37(2):112–8.

43. Zhang Y, Nevitt MC, Niu J. Reversible MRI features and fluctuation of knee pain severity. Osteoarthritis Cartilage 2008;16(Suppl 4):S145.

44. Taljanovic MS, Graham AR, Benjamin JB, et al. Bone marrow edema pattern in advanced hip osteoarthritis: quantitative assessment with magnetic resonance imaging and correlation with clinical examination, radiographic findings, and histopathology. Skeletal Radiol 2008;37(5):423–31.

45. Kornaat PR, Kloppenburg M, Sharma R, et al. Bone marrow edema-like lesions change in volume in the majority of patients with osteoarthritis; associations with clinical features. Eur Radiol 2007;17(12):3073–8.

46. Lo GH, Hunter DJ, Zhang Y, et al. Bone marrow lesions in the knee are associated with increased local bone density. Arthritis Rheum 2005;52(9):2814–21.

47. Davies-Tuck ML, Wluka AE, Forbes A, et al. Development of bone marrow lesions is associated with adverse effects on knee cartilage while resolution is associated with improvement–a potential target for prevention of knee osteoarthritis: a longitudinal study. Arthritis Res Ther 2010;12(1):R10.

48. Crema MD, Roemer FW, Wang K, et al. The association of prevalent cartilage damage and cartilage loss over time with incident bone marrow edema-like lesions at the tibiofemoral compartments: the MOST study. Osteoarthritis Cartilage 2010;18(Suppl 2):S12–3.

49. Sowers MF, Hayes C, Jamadar D, et al. Magnetic resonance-detected subchondral bone marrow and cartilage defect characteristics associated with pain and X-ray-defined knee osteoarthritis. Osteoarthritis Cartilage 2003;11(6):387–93.

50. Pouders C, De Maeseneer M, Van Roy P, et al. Prevalence and MRI-anatomic correlation of bone cysts in osteoarthritic knees. AJR Am J Roentgenol 2008;190(1):17–21.

51. Resnick D, Niwayama G, Coutts RD. Subchondral cysts (geodes) in arthritic disorders: pathologic and radiographic appearance of the hip joint. AJR Am J Roentgenol 1977;128(5):799–806.

52. Rhaney K, Lamb DW. The cysts of osteoarthritis of the hip; a radiological and pathological study. J Bone Joint Surg Br 1955;37:663–75.

53. Landells JW. The bone cysts of osteoarthritis. J Bone Joint Surg Br 1953;35:643–9.

54. Crema MD, Roemer FW, Marra MD, et al. Contrast-enhanced MRI of subchondral cysts in patients with or at risk for knee osteoarthritis: the MOST study. Eur J Radiol 2010;75:e92–6.

55. Freund E. The pathological significance of intra-articular pressure. Edinb Med J 1940;47:192–203.

56. Ferguson AJ. The pathological changes in degenerative arthritis of the hip and treatment by rotational osteotomy. J Bone Joint Surg Am 1964;46:1337–52.

57. Crema MD, Roemer FW, Marra MD, et al. MRI-detected bone marrow edema-like lesions are strongly associated with subchondral cysts in

patients with or at risk for knee osteoarthritis: the MOST study. Osteoarthritis Cartilage 2008; 16(Suppl 4):S160.

58. Carrino JA, Blum J, Parellada JA, et al. MRI of bone marrow edema-like signal in the pathogenesis of subchondral cysts. Osteoarthritis Cartilage 2006; 14(10):1081–5.

59. Torres L, Dunlop DD, Peterfy C, et al. The relationship between specific tissue lesions and pain severity in persons with knee osteoarthritis. Osteoarthritis Cartilage 2006;14(10):1033–40.

60. Kornaat PR, Bloem JL, Ceulemans RY, et al. Osteoarthritis of the knee: association between clinical features and MR imaging findings. Radiology 2006;239(3):811–7.

61. Dieppe PA, Reichenbach S, Williams S, et al. Assessing bone loss on radiographs of the knee in osteoarthritis: a cross-sectional study. Arthritis Rheum 2005;52(11):3536–41.

62. Reichenbach S, Guermazi A, Niu J, et al. Prevalence of bone attrition on knee radiographs and MRI in a community-based cohort. Osteoarthritis Cartilage 2008;16(9):1005–10.

63. Neogi T, Felson DT, Niu J, et al. Cartilage loss occurs in the same subregions as subchondral bone attrition: a within-knee subregion-matched approach from the Multicenter Osteoarthritis Study. Arthritis Rheum 2009;61(11):1539–44.

64. Hernández-Molina G, Neogi T, Hunter DJ, et al. The association of bone attrition with knee pain and other MRI features of osteoarthritis. Ann Rheum Dis 2008;67(1):43–7.

65. Seedhom BB, Dowson D, Wright V. Proceedings: functions of the menisci. A preliminary study. Ann Rheum Dis 1974;33(1):111.

66. Guermazi A, Hunter DJ, Roemer FW, et al. Magnetic resonance imaging prevalence of different features of knee osteoarthritis in persons with normal knee X-Rays. Arthritis Rheum 2007;56:S128–9.

67. Bhattacharyya T, Gale D, Dewire P, et al. The clinical importance of meniscal tears demonstrated by magnetic resonance imaging in osteoarthritis of the knee. J Bone Joint Surg Am 2003;85(1):4–9.

68. Biswal S, Hastie T, Andriacchi TP, et al. Risk factors for progressive cartilage loss in the knee: a longitudinal magnetic resonance imaging study in forty-three patients. Arthritis Rheum 2002; 46(11):2884–92.

69. Lo GH, Hunter DJ, Nevitt MC, et al. Strong association of MRI meniscal derangement and bone marrow lesions in knee osteoarthritis: data from the osteoarthritis initiative. Osteoarthritis Cartilage 2009;17(6):743–7.

70. Berthiaume MJ, Raynauld JP, Martel-Pelletier J, et al. Meniscal tear and extrusion are strongly associated with progression of symptomatic knee osteoarthritis as assessed by quantitative magnetic resonance imaging. Ann Rheum Dis 2005;64(4): 556–63.

71. Lynch JA, Javaid MK, Roemer FW, et al. Associations of medial meniscal tear and extrusion with the sites of cartilage loss in the knee–results from the MOST study. Arthritis Rheum 2008;58: S235–6.

72. Sharma L, Eckstein F, Song J, et al. Relationship of meniscal damage, meniscal extrusion, malalignment, and joint laxity to subsequent cartilage loss in osteoarthritic knees. Arthritis Rheum 2008; 58(6):1716–26.

73. Baratz ME, Fu FH, Mengato R. Meniscal tears: the effect of meniscectomy and of repair on intraarticular contact areas and stress in the human knee. A preliminary report. Am J Sports Med 1986; 14(4):270–5.

74. Kurosawa H, Fukubayashi T, Nakajima H. Load-bearing mode of the knee joint: physical behavior of the knee joint with or without menisci. Clin Orthop Relat Res 1980;149:283–90.

75. Fukubayashi T, Kurosawa H. The contact area and pressure distribution pattern of the knee. A study of normal and osteoarthrotic knee joints. Acta Orthop Scand 1980;51(6):871–9.

76. Noble J. Lesions of the menisci. Autopsy incidence in adults less than fifty-five years old. J Bone Joint Surg Am 1977;59(4):480–3.

77. Noble J, Hamblen DL. The pathology of the degenerate meniscus lesion. J Bone Joint Surg Br 1975; 57(2):180–6.

78. Poehling GG, Ruch DS, Chabon SJ. The landscape of meniscal injuries. Clin Sports Med 1990;9(3): 539–49.

79. Stoller DW, Martin C, Crues JV 3rd, et al. Meniscal tears: pathologic correlation with MR imaging. Radiology 1987;163(3):731–5.

80. Kaplan PA, Nelson NL, Garvin KL, et al. MR of the knee: the significance of high signal in the meniscus that does not clearly extend to the surface. AJR Am J Roentgenol 1991;156(2):333–6.

81. Low AK, Chia MR, Carmody DJ, et al. Clinical significance of intrasubstance meniscal lesions on MRI. J Med Imaging Radiat Oncol 2008;52(3): 227–30.

82. Adams JG, McAlindon T, Dimasi M, et al. Contribution of meniscal extrusion and cartilage loss to joint space narrowing in osteoarthritis. Clin Radiol 1999; 54(8):502–6.

83. Gale DR, Chaisson CE, Totterman SM, et al. Meniscal subluxation: association with osteoarthritis and joint space narrowing. Osteoarthritis Cartilage 1999;7(6):526–32.

84. Ding C, Martel-Pelletier J, Pelletier JP, et al. Knee meniscal extrusion in a largely non-osteoarthritic cohort: association with greater loss of cartilage volume. Arthritis Res Ther 2007;9(2):R21.

85. Crema MD, Roemer FW, Englund M, et al. Factors associated with prevalent magnetic resonance imaging (MRI)-detected meniscal extrusion in persons with or at risk for knee osteoarthritis–the MOST study. Osteoarthritis Cartilage 2010; 18(Suppl 2):S175–6.

86. Pelletier JP, Martel-Pelletier J, Abramson SB. Osteoarthritis, an inflammatory disease: potential implication for the selection of new therapeutic targets. Arthritis Rheum 2001;44(6):1237–47.

87. Ayral X, Pickering EH, Woodworth TG, et al. Synovitis: a potential predictive factor of structural progression of medial tibiofemoral knee osteoarthritis–results of a 1 year longitudinal arthroscopic study in 422 patients. Osteoarthritis Cartilage 2005;13(5):361–7.

88. Marra MD, Roemer FW, Crema MD, et al. Peripatellar synovitis in osteoarthritis: comparison of non-enhanced and enhanced magnetic resonance imaging (MRI) and its association with peripatellar knee pain: the MOST study. Osteoarthritis Cartilage 2008;16(Suppl 4):S167.

89. Loeuille D, Chary-Valckenaere I, Champigneulle J, et al. Macroscopic and microscopic features of synovial membrane inflammation in the osteoarthritic knee: correlating magnetic resonance imaging findings with disease severity. Arthritis Rheum 2005;52(11):3492–501.

90. Lindblad S, Hedfors E. Arthroscopic and immunohistologic characterization of knee joint synovitis in osteoarthritis. Arthritis Rheum 1987;30(10): 1081–8.

91. Saddik D, McNally EG, Richardson M. MRI of Hoffa's fat pad. Skeletal Radiol 2004;33(8): 433–44.

92. Roemer FW, Guermazi A, Zhang Y, et al. Hoffa's fat pad: evaluation on unenhanced MR images as a measure of patellofemoral synovitis in osteoarthritis. AJR Am J Roentgenol 2009;192(6): 1696–700.

93. Pelletier JP, Raynauld JP, Abram F, et al. A new non-invasive method to assess synovitis severity in relation to symptoms and cartilage volume loss in knee osteoarthritis patients using MRI. Osteoarthritis Cartilage 2008;16(Suppl 3):S8–13.

94. Roemer FW, Hunter DJ, Guermazi A. Semiquantitative assessment of synovitis in osteoarthritis on non contrast-enhanced MRI. Osteoarthritis Cartilage 2009;17(6):820–1 [author reply: 822–4].

95. Loeuille D, Saulière N, Champigneulle J, et al. What is the most accurate MRI approach to assess synovitis and/or effusion in knee OA? Osteoarthritis Cartilage 2008;16(Suppl 4):S176.

96. Ostergaard M, Hansen M, Stoltenberg M, et al. Magnetic resonance imaging-determined synovial membrane volume as a marker of disease activity and a predictor of progressive joint destruction in the wrists of patients with rheumatoid arthritis. Arthritis Rheum 1999;42(5):918–29.

97. Rhodes LA, Grainger AJ, Keenan AM, et al. The validation of simple scoring methods for evaluating compartment-specific synovitis detected by MRI in knee osteoarthritis. Rheumatology (Oxford) 2005; 44(12):1569–73.

98. Clunie G, Hall-Craggs MA, Paley MN, et al. Measurement of synovial lining volume by magnetic resonance imaging of the knee in chronic synovitis. Ann Rheum Dis 1997;56(9):526–34.

99. Roemer FW, Kassim Javaid MK, Guermazi A, et al. Anatomical distribution of synovitis in knee osteoarthritis and its association with joint effusion assessed on non-enhanced and contrast-enhanced MRI. Osteoarthritis Cartilage 2010;18(10):1269–74.

100. Lindblad S, Hedfors E. Intraarticular variation in synovitis. Local macroscopic and microscopic signs of inflammatory activity are significantly correlated. Arthritis Rheum 1985;28(9):977–86.

101. Kurosaka M, Ohno O, Hirohata K. Arthroscopic evaluation of synovitis in the knee joints. Arthroscopy 1991;7(2):162–70.

102. Dye SF, Vaupel GL, Dye CC. Conscious neurosensory mapping of the internal structures of the human knee without intraarticular anesthesia. Am J Sports Med 1998;26(6):773–7.

103. Fernandez-Madrid F, Karvonen RL, Teitge RA, et al. MR features of osteoarthritis of the knee. Magn Reson Imaging 1994;12(5):703–9.

104. von Porat A, Roos EM, Roos H. High prevalence of osteoarthritis 14 years after an anterior cruciate ligament tear in male soccer players: a study of radiographic and patient relevant outcomes. Ann Rheum Dis 2004;63(3):269–73.

105. Maletius W, Messner K. Eighteen- to twenty-four-year follow-up after complete rupture of the anterior cruciate ligament. Am J Sports Med 1999;27(6): 711–7.

106. Kannus P, Järvinen M. Posttraumatic anterior cruciate ligament insufficiency as a cause of osteoarthritis in a knee joint. Clin Rheumatol 1989;8(2): 251–60.

107. Nebelung W, Wuschech H. Thirty-five years of follow-up of anterior cruciate ligament-deficient knees in high-level athletes. Arthroscopy 2005; 21(6):696–702.

108. Messner K, Maletius W. Eighteen- to twenty-five-year follow-up after acute partial anterior cruciate ligament rupture. Am J Sports Med 1999;27(4):455–9.

109. Dargel J, Gotter M, Mader K, et al. Biomechanics of the anterior cruciate ligament and implications for surgical reconstruction. Strategies Trauma Limb Reconstr 2007;2(1):1–12.

110. Hill CH, Seo GS, Gale D, et al. Cruciate ligament integrity in osteoarthritis of the knee. Arthritis Rheum 2005;52(3):794–9.

111. Crema MD, Marra MD, Guermazi A, et al. Relevant traumatic injury of the knee joint-MRI follow-up after 7–10 years. Eur J Radiol 2009;72(3):473–9.

112. Chan WP, Lang P, Stevens MP, et al. Osteoarthritis of the knee: comparison of radiography, CT, and MR imaging to assess extent and severity. AJR Am J Roentgenol 1991;157(4):799–806.

113. Link TM, Steinbach LS, Ghosh S, et al. Osteoarthritis: MR imaging findings in different stages of disease and correlation with clinical findings. Radiology 2003;226(2):373–81.

114. Cushner FD, La Rosa DF, Vigorita VJ, et al. A quantitative histologic comparison: ACL degeneration in the osteoarthritic knee. J Arthroplasty 2003;18(6):687–92.

115. Lee GC, Cushner FD, Vigoritta V, et al. Evaluation of the anterior cruciate ligament integrity and degenerative arthritic patterns in patients undergoing total knee arthroplasty. J Arthroplasty 2005;20(1): 59–65.

116. Wada M, Tatsuo H, Baba H, et al. Femoral intercondylar notch measurements in osteoarthritic knees. Rheumatology (Oxford) 1999;38(6):554–8.

117. Mullaji AB, Marawar SV, Simha M, et al. Cruciate ligaments in arthritic knees: a histologic study with radiologic correlation. J Arthroplasty 2008; 23(4):567–72.

118. Amin S, Guermazi A, Lavalley MP, et al. Complete anterior cruciate ligament tear and the risk for cartilage loss and progression of symptoms in men and women with knee osteoarthritis. Osteoarthritis Cartilage 2008;16(8):897–902.

119. Guermazi A, Taouli B, Lynch JA, et al. Prevalence of meniscus and ligament tears and their correlation with cartilage morphology and other MRI features in knee osteoarthritis (OA) in the elderly. The Health ABC Study. Arthritis Rheum 2002;46:S567.

120. Logan M, Williams A, Lavelle J, et al. The effect of posterior cruciate ligament deficiency on knee kinematics. Am J Sports Med 2004;32(8):1915–22.

121. Dejour H, Walch G, Peyrot J, et al. The natural history of rupture of the posterior cruciate ligament. Rev Chir Orthop Reparatrice Appar Mot 1988; 74(1):35–43 [in French].

122. Patel DV, Allen AA, Warren RF, et al. The nonoperative treatment of acute, isolated (partial or complete) posterior cruciate ligament-deficient knees: an intermediate-term follow-up study. HSS J 2007;3(2):137–46.

123. Bergin D, Keogh C, O'Connell M, et al. Atraumatic medial collateral ligament oedema in medial compartment knee osteoarthritis. Skeletal Radiol 2002;31(1):14–8.

124. Marra MD, Crema MD, Chung M, et al. MRI features of cystic lesions around the knee. Knee 2008;15(6):423–38.

125. Guermazi A, Zaim S, Taouli B, et al. MR findings in knee osteoarthritis. Eur Radiol 2003;13(6):1370–86.

126. Fam AG, Wilson SR, Holmberg S. Ultrasound evaluation of popliteal cysts on osteoarthritis of the knee. J Rheumatol 1982;9(3):428–34.

127. Guermazi A, Roemer FW, Niu L, et al. Periarticular cysts and their relation to symptoms in osteoarthritis: the MOST study. Osteoarthritis Cartilage 2007;15(Suppl 3):C170–1.

128. Hill CL, Gale DR, Chaisson CE, et al. Periarticular lesions detected on magnetic resonance imaging: prevalence in knees with and without symptoms. Arthritis Rheum 2003;48(10):2836–44.

129. Tschirch FT, Schmid MR, Pfirrmann CW, et al. Prevalence and size of meniscal cysts, ganglionic cysts, synovial cysts of the popliteal space, fluid-filled bursae, and other fluid collections in asymptomatic knees on MR imaging. AJR Am J Roentgenol 2003; 180(5):1431–6.

130. McCarthy CL, McNally EG. The MRI appearance of cystic lesions around the knee. Skeletal Radiol 2004;33(4):187–209.

131. Alvarez-Nemegyei J. Risk factors for pes anserinus tendinitis/bursitis syndrome: a case control study. J Clin Rheumatol 2007;13(2):63–5.

132. De Maeseneer M, Shahabpour M, Vanderdood K, et al. MR imaging of meniscal cysts: evaluation of location and extension using a three-layer approach. Eur J Radiol 2001;39(2):117–24.

133. Tyson LL, Daughters TC Jr, Ryu RK, et al. MRI appearance of meniscal cysts. Skeletal Radiol 1995;24(6):421–4.

134. Feldman F, Johnston A. Intraosseous ganglion. Am J Roentgenol Radium Ther Nucl Med 1973;118(2): 328–43.

135. Kim J, Jung SA, Sung MS, et al. Extra-articular soft tissue ganglion cyst around the knee: focus on the associated findings. Eur Radiol 2004;14(1): 106–11.

136. Bui-Mansfield LT, Youngberg RA. Intraarticular ganglia of the knee: prevalence, presentation, etiology, and management. AJR Am J Roentgenol 1997;168(1):123–7.

137. El Andaloussi Y, Fnini S, Hachimi K, et al. Osteochondromatosis of the popliteal bursa. Joint Bone Spine 2006;73(2):219–20.

138. Stuart MJ, Lubowitz JH. What, if any, are the indications for arthroscopic debridement of the osteoarthritic knee? Arthroscopy 2006;22(3):238–9.

139. Steadman JR, Ramappa AJ, Maxwell RB, et al. An arthroscopic treatment regimen for osteoarthritis of the knee. Arthroscopy 2007;23(9):948–55.

140. Crema MD, Roemer FW, Marra MD, et al. Articular cartilage in the knee: current MR imaging techniques and applications in clinical practice and research. Radiographics 2011;31:37–61.

141. Burstein D, Gray M, Mosher T, et al. Measures of molecular composition and structure in osteoarthritis. Radiol Clin North Am 2009;47(4):675–86.

142. Liess C, Lüsse S, Karger N, et al. Detection of changes in cartilage water content using MRI T2-mapping in vivo. Osteoarthritis Cartilage 2002; 10(12):907–13.

143. Mosher TJ, Smith H, Dardzinski BJ, et al. MR imaging and T2 mapping of femoral cartilage: in vivo determination of the magic angle effect. AJR Am J Roentgenol 2001;177(3):665–9.

144. Dunn TC, Lu Y, Jin H, et al. T2 relaxation time of cartilage at MR imaging: comparison with severity of knee osteoarthritis. Radiology 2004;232(2):592–8.

145. Koff MF, Amrami KK, Kaufman KR. Clinical evaluation of T2 values of patellar cartilage in patients with osteoarthritis. Osteoarthritis Cartilage 2007; 15(2):198–204.

146. Stehling C, Liebl H, Krug R, et al. Patellar cartilage: T2 values and morphologic abnormalities at 3.0-T MR imaging in relation to physical activity in asymptomatic subjects from the osteoarthritis initiative. Radiology 2010;254(2):509–20.

147. Williams A, Sharma L, McKenzie CA, et al. Delayed gadolinium-enhanced magnetic resonance imaging of cartilage in knee osteoarthritis: findings at different radiographic stages of disease and relationship to malalignment. Arthritis Rheum 2005;52(11):3528–35.

148. Tiderius CJ, Svensson J, Leander P, et al. dGEMRIC (delayed gadolinium-enhanced MRI of cartilage) indicates adaptive capacity of human knee cartilage. Magn Reson Med 2004;51(2):286–90.

149. Anandacoomarasamy A, Giuffre BM, Leibman S, et al. Delayed gadolinium-enhanced magnetic resonance imaging of cartilage: clinical associations in obese adults. J Rheumatol 2009;36(5):1056–62.

150. Bashir A, Gray ML, Hartke J, et al. Nondestructive imaging of human cartilage glycosaminoglycan concentration by MRI. Magn Reson Med 1999; 41(5):857–65.

151. Owman H, Tiderius CJ, Neuman P, et al. Association between findings on delayed gadolinium-enhanced magnetic resonance imaging of cartilage and future knee osteoarthritis. Arthritis Rheum 2008;58(6): 1727–30.

152. Duvvuri U, Charagundla SR, Kudchodkar SB, et al. Human knee: in vivo T1(rho)-weighted MR imaging at 1.5 T–preliminary experience. Radiology 2001; 220(3):822–6.

153. Stahl R, Luke A, Li X, et al. T1rho, T2 and focal knee cartilage abnormalities in physically active and sedentary healthy subjects versus early OA patients–a 3.0-Tesla MRI study. Eur Radiol 2009; 19(1):132–43.

154. Mlynárik V, Trattnig S, Huber M, et al. The role of relaxation times in monitoring proteoglycan depletion in articular cartilage. J Magn Reson Imaging 1999;10(4):497–502.

155. Borthakur A, Shapiro EM, Beers J, et al. Sensitivity of MRI to proteoglycan depletion in cartilage: comparison of sodium and proton MRI. Osteoarthritis Cartilage 2000;8(4):288–93.

156. Wang L, Wu Y, Chang G, et al. Rapid isotropic 3D-sodium MRI of the knee joint in vivo at 7T. J Magn Reson Imaging 2009;30(3):606–14.

157. Wheaton AJ, Borthakur A, Shapiro EM, et al. Proteoglycan loss in human knee cartilage: quantitation with sodium MR imaging–feasibility study. Radiology 2004;231(3):900–5.

158. Burstein D, Gray ML, Hartman AL, et al. Diffusion of small solutes in cartilage as measured by nuclear magnetic resonance (NMR) spectroscopy and imaging. J Orthop Res 1993;11(4):465–78.

MR Imaging Assessment of Articular Cartilage Repair Procedures

Gregory Chang, MD[a],*, Orrin Sherman, MD[b],
Guillaume Madelin, PhD[a], Michael Recht, MD[a],
Ravinder Regatte, PhD[a]

KEYWORDS

- MRI • Cartilage repair • Microfracture
- Osteochondral autograft • Osteochondral allograft
- Autologous chondrocyte implantation
- Biochemical MR imaging • 7 tesla MRI

Articular cartilage injury poses a serious problem for orthopedic surgeons. The associated pain and physical disability can have career-ending consequences in athletes and can restrict the ability to perform activities of daily living in any individual. In two separate studies, consisting of 31,156 and 1000 patients undergoing knee arthroscopy, cartilage lesions were found in greater than 60% of all patients, and approximately 5% of these lesions were classified as deep partial-thickness or full-thickness defects in patients less than 40 years of age.[1,2]

Because articular cartilage is avascular, the transport of inflammatory mediators and cells to the site of tissue injury is limited; thus, cartilage has no intrinsic capacity to heal itself.[3,4] Over the past two decades, there have been many exciting developments in the field of articular cartilage restoration. Patients who were previously offered only symptomatic relief now have a variety of treatment options, including microfracture, osteochondral autografting and allografting, restoration with resorbable synthetic scaffolds, and autologous chondrocyte implantation (ACI) (including matrix-assisted ACI [MACI]). This article reviews the different types of cartilage repair procedures and discusses their assessment using imaging.

BRIEF OVERVIEW OF MR IMAGING OF CARTILAGE

Many MR imaging sequences are currently used to evaluate cartilage morphology.[5] Typical sequences include fat-suppressed, 3-D, gradient-echo techniques[6,7] and fast spin-echo techniques with and without fat suppression.[8,9] These sequences have been extensively used to evaluate articular cartilage and have reported sensitivities and specificities for the detection of cartilage lesions close to or greater than 90% in some studies.

There has also been great interest recently in the use of MR imaging techniques to evaluate the biochemical composition of the cartilage matrix. These techniques include T2 mapping, delayed gadolinium-enhanced MR imaging of cartilage (dGEMRIC), T1rho mapping, and sodium MR imaging. T2 mapping reflects cartilage collagen content and hydration status,[10] whereas dGEMRIC, T1rho mapping, and sodium MR imaging are all markers of cartilage proteoglycan content.[5,11–13] Although these biochemical imaging techniques are less widely available, they may provide useful additional information regarding the status of the cartilage repair procedure.

The authors have no financial disclosures.
[a] Quantitative Multinuclear Musculoskeletal Imaging Group (QMMIG), Center for Biomedical Imaging, Department of Radiology, New York University Langone Medical Center, 660 First Avenue, Room 231, New York, NY 10016, USA
[b] Department of Orthopedic Surgery, New York University Langone Medical Center, 530 First Avenue, Suite 8U, New York, NY 10016, USA
* Corresponding author.
E-mail address: gregory.chang@nyumc.org

Magn Reson Imaging Clin N Am 19 (2011) 323–337
doi:10.1016/j.mric.2011.02.002
1064-9689/11/$ – see front matter © 2011 Elsevier Inc. All rights reserved.

mri.theclinics.com

Finally, with the development of ultra–high-field MR imaging scanners (7 T and above), there is the potential to improve on scanning techniques performed at standard clinical field strength (1.5 to 3 T).[14–16] Because of the greater intrinsic signal-to-noise ratio available at ultra–high field (signal-to-noise ratio scales approximately with the magnitude of the magnetic field), images can be obtained with increased spatial resolution or decreased scan time. Ultra–high field also facilitates the performance of biochemical imaging techniques, such as sodium MR imaging, which is limited by low signal-to-noise ratio at standard clinical field strength.

PARAMETERS ASSESSED IN MR IMAGING OF CARTILAGE REPAIR

Multiple parameters should be assessed in MR imaging examinations of cartilage repair. In one study of patients who underwent either microfracture or ACI, the following MR imaging parameters were evaluated: signal intensity relative to native cartilage; morphology with respect to native cartilage (flush, proud, or depressed); delamination (in the setting of ACI); nature of the interface with the adjacent surface (presence or absence and size of fissures); degree of defect filling; integrity of cartilage on the opposite articular surface; and bony hypertrophy.[17]

Another group has proposed a formal grading system for MR imaging assessment of cartilage repair, magnetic resonance observation of cartilage repair (MOCART).[18] Using fat-suppressed, 3-D, gradient-recalled echo, and fast spin-echo sequences, the investigators propose assessment of the following MR imaging parameters: degree of defect filling, integration to border zone, surface of repair tissue, structure of repair tissue, signal intensity of repair tissue, subchondral lamina, subchondral bone, adhesions, and synovitis. This scoring system was later validated in a 2-year longitudinal study of patients with matrix-assisted chondrocyte implantation,[19] with certain parameters, such as degree of defect filling, structure of repair tissue, change in subchondral bone, and signal intensity of repair tissue, correlating well with clinical scores.

TYPES OF CARTILAGE REPAIR PROCEDURES AND APPEARANCE ON MR IMAGING
Microfracture

Rationale
Microfracture was introduced by Steadman and colleagues[20] in the early 1980s and was described as a treatment for full-thickness posttraumatic cartilage defects. As opposed to other marrow stimulation techniques, such as drilling, there is essentially no risk for thermal necrosis of surrounding tissue.[20] Through micropenetration of the subchondral bone plate, the cartilage defect is populated with platelets, growth factors, and bone marrow-derived mesenchymal stem cells, which mediate a fibrocartilaginous repair process. Fibrocartilage that forms within the defect is less well organized than normal hyaline articular cartilage and has a higher proportion of type I collagen; as a result, its biomechanical properties are inferior to that of hyaline cartilage.[3,21,22]

Indications
Microfracture is a simple, single-stage procedure with relatively low patient morbidity. Microfracture is indicated as a first-line treatment for patients with small full-thickness cartilage defects in either the weight-bearing region of the femorotibial compartment or in an area of contact between the patella and trochlea. Unstable cartilage flaps are another indication for microfracture.[23–25]

Surgical technique
An arthroscopic awl is used to make multiple holes or microfractures in the exposed subchondral bone plate. When fat droplets are seen coming from the marrow cavity, the appropriate depth of 2 to 4 mm has been reached. Significant functional improvement after microfracture has been documented at a minimum follow-up period of 2 years with the best results observed with good fill grade, low body mass index, and a short duration of preoperative symptoms.[26] The success of the procedure in athletes who perform high-impact sports is associated with lesion size less than 200 mm², preoperative symptoms less than 12 months, and no prior surgical intervention.[27] Although weight bearing is detrimental in the first 8 weeks after surgery, continuous passive motion is a critical component of rehabilitation that may help stimulate chondocyte matrix production and remodel the repair cartilage surface so that it is congruent with the native hyaline cartilage.[28,29]

Imaging studies
The MR imaging appearance of reparative fibrocartilage after microfracture varies depending on the time after surgery. In general, the reparative fibrocartilage is hypertintense relative to native hyaline cartilage (**Figs. 1** and **2**). Adverse functional scores after 24 months have been correlated with poor percentage of fill by repair tissue and incomplete peripheral integration.[26] Lack of peripheral integration and thinning of the repair tissue may increase mechanical stress on the reparative fibrocartilage, leading to early cartilage degeneration and functional decline.

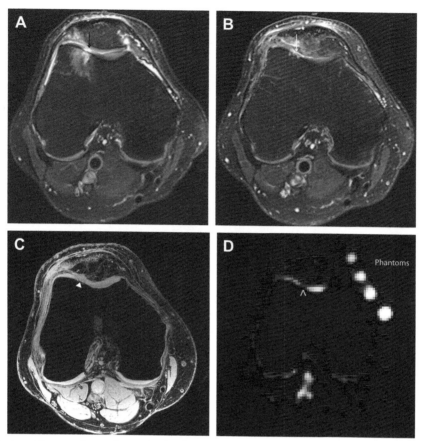

Fig. 1. A 55-year-old man who underwent microfracture repair. (*A*) Preoperative, axial, T2-weighted, fat-suppressed, 3-T MR imaging of the knee demonstrates a full-thickness cartilage defect within the lateral femoral trochlea (*arrow*) with extensive surrounding bone marrow edema. (*B*) Three-month postoperative, axial, T2-weighted, fat-suppressed, 3-T MR imaging demonstrates partial filling of the defect with fibrocartilage (*arrow*), which has an irregular surface and demonstrates fissuring. There is also decreased surrounding bone marrow edema. (*C*) Six-month postoperative, axial, 3-D, gradient-echo, T1-weighted, fat-suppressed, 7-T MR imaging (0.234 mm × 0.234 mm × 1 mm) shows slightly irregular fibrocartilage filling the defect (*arrowhead*) which has similar signal intensity characteristics to the adjacent native hyaline cartilage. (*D*) Six-month postoperative, axial, 7-T, sodium MR imaging reveals apparent decreased sodium signal (and thus proteoglycan content) within the fibrocartilage (*arrowhead*). Note the higher sodium signal within the adjacent native hyaline cartilage. Sodium chloride phantoms are seen at the medial aspect of the knee.

Two studies have used T2 mapping to evaluate the status of reparative fibrocartilage induced by microfracture. In both studies, fibrocartilage did not demonstrate the characteristic spatial variation in T2 values that is seen with native hyaline cartilage (higher T2 values near the articular surface and lower T2 values near subchondral bone).[30,31] In addition, the overall global T2 value was lower for fibrocartilage repair tissue than for native hyaline cartilage.[31]

Fibrocartilage formed after microfracture has also been evaluated using dGEMRIC. In one study, fibrocartilage demonstrated a greater difference between precontrast and postcontrast T1 relaxation time compared with repair tissue formed after

MACI[32]; this suggests a lower glycosaminoglycan content in fibrocartilage compared with other types of cartilage repair tissue.[32]

Osteochondral Autograft Transfer

Rationale

The use of osteochondral autografts was first described by Yamashita and coworkers[33] and later popularized by Bobić[34] (single plugs) and Hangody and colleagues[35,36] (multiple plugs or mosaicplasty). This technique involves repairing a cartilage defect with one or more small cylindrical osteochondral plugs harvested from a relatively non–weight-bearing portion of the

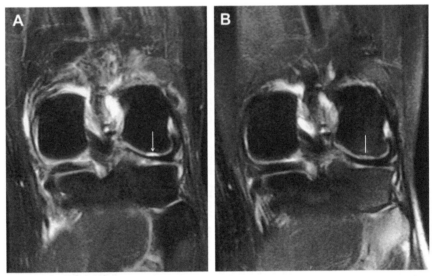

Fig. 2. A 54-year-old woman who underwent microfracture repair. (*A*) Preoperative, coronal, T2-weighted, fat-suppressed, 3-T MR imaging of the knee reveals a full-thickness cartilage defect within the posterior weight-bearing aspect of the lateral femoral condyle (*arrow*). (*B*) Six-month postoperative, coronal, T2-weighted, fat-suppressed, 3-TMR imaging shows partial filling of the defect with fibrocartilage (*line*) that is heterogeneous in signal intensity.

patellofemoral joint or from the margin of the intercondylar notch. Histologic evaluations after osteochondral autograft transfer in animal models reveal consistent survival of transplanted hyaline cartilage, deep matrix integration and formation of a composite layer with native surrounding cartilage, ingrowth of fibrocartilage at the osseous base of the defect, and osseous incorporation of the graft with recipient subchondral bone.[36–38]

Indications

The main indications for osteochondral autograft transfer are focal cartilage defects measuring 1 to 5 cm^2, typically due to trauma or osteochondritis dissecans. Under unusual circumstances, defects as large as 8 to 9 cm^2 have been repaired, but for lesions of this size, there is limited donor tissue available.[36] Fifty years is the recommended upper age limit for the procedure. Although osteochondral autografting was initially performed only on the weight-bearing surfaces of the femoral condyles and patellofemoral joints, it can also be used to treat cartilage defects of the talus, tibia, humeral capitellum, and femoral head.

Surgical technique

Osteochondral autografting can be performed arthroscopically or via an open arthrotomy. Patients are informed preoperatively of the potential need to harvest plugs from the contralateral knee, especially when treating larger cartilage defects. After gaining surgical access, the size of the cartilage

lesion is assessed, and the number, diameter, and position of graft plugs required to fill the defect are determined. Femoral condylar lesions are filled with plugs from the margins of the medial and lateral femoral condyles above the sulcus terminalis, whereas lesions in the trochlear groove are treated with plugs harvested from the intercondylar notch.[39–41]

Osteochondral autografting requires 2 weeks of non–weight-bearing during the immediate postoperative period followed by 2 weeks of partial weight bearing. Successful clinical outcomes have been reported by many groups. In a 10-year follow-up study of 831 patients, good to excellent results were reported in 92%, 87%, and 79% of femoral condylar, tibial, and patellofemoral implantations, respectively.[36] In one clinical trial comparing osteochondral autografting with ACI, osteochondral autografting was associated with faster recovery at 6, 12, and 24 months, although both procedures resulted in decreased symptoms at 24 months.[42]

Imaging studies

On MR imaging, the position of the osteochondral plug within the recipient site should be evaluated, and there should be no graft migration. Perigraft edema can be found in greater than 50% of patients at 1 year, and this gradually decreases by 3 years (**Figs. 3** and **4**).[43] The presence of subchondral cysts or persistent extensive perigraft edema at 3 years may reflect poor osseous

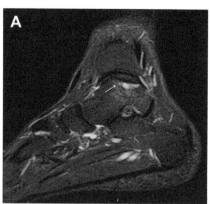 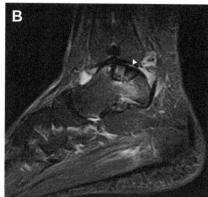

Fig. 3. A 37-year-old woman who underwent osteochondral autografting. (*A*) Preoperative, sagittal, T2-weighted, fat-suppressed, 3-T MR imaging of the ankle demonstrates an osteochondral lesion of the medial talar dome (*arrow*). There is cartilage damage, mild cortical depression, and subchondral edema/cyst formation. (*B*) Six-month postoperative, sagittal, T2-weighted, fat-suppressed, 3-T MR imaging shows restoration of the talar dome, including a thin layer of overlying cartilage (*arrowhead*) with similar signal characteristics to adjacent native hyaline cartilage and mild perigraft edema (*arrow*).

incorporation.[43,44] Rarely, osteonecrosis has been reported as a complication of osteochondral autografting.[43] The thickness and congruity of the articular surface should also be evaluated. Ideally, the thickness of the repair cartilage should be similar to that of the surrounding native hyaline cartilage with a smooth, congruent articular surface (**Fig. 5**). The deep bone-bone interface may demonstrate an incongruent surface, because the osteochondral plug may have been harvested from a location with a differing cartilage thickness.

Osteochondral Allograft

Rationale

Osteochondral allografting involves the replacement of damaged articular cartilage with mature hyaline cartilage from a suitable donor. The advantages of osteochondral allografts over autografts are (1) the avoidance of morbidity from the autograft harvesting procedure, (2) the ability to repair larger defects because more donor tissue can be harvested, and (3) the ability to harvest tissue from a site matching the exact location of a patient's cartilage defect, which allows more accurate matching of the size and contour of the graft to the defect.[45]

The rationale for this procedure is that the transplanted hyaline cartilage contains living chondrocytes that are capable of supporting the cartilage matrix within the host indefinitely.[46] The osteochondral allograft is considered immunoprivileged, because cartilage is avascular and chondrocytes are protected from host immune surveillance due to their location within the matrix.[46,47] Donor cartilage is not matched to recipient HLA type or blood type. Procurement and processing of donor tissue is, however, performed according to American Association of Tissue Banks guidelines,[48] which includes an extensive medical, social, and sexual history of the donor as well as serologic testing for HIV, hepatitis, syphilis, and other blood-borne pathogens. As a result, although fresh osteochondral allografts are necessary to ensure maximum chondrocyte survival, tissue is transplanted no sooner than 14 days and sometimes as late as 40 days after harvesting while tests for viral and bacterial contamination are conducted. Approximately 5 million fresh osteochondral allografts have been transplanted over the past decade, and few documented cases of disease transmission have been reported.[49]

Indications

In the knee, osteochondral allografting has been used for multiple indications, including traumatic or degenerative cartilage lesions, osteochondritis dissecans, osteonecrosis, or salvage of a previous cartilage repair procedure. The size of the cartilage defect can be as large as 15 cm^2.[50] Osteochondral allografting has also been performed in the ankle and hip for similar indications and when other procedures, such as osteochondral autografting, are not feasible.

Surgical technique

Osteochondral allografting is performed through a mini arthrotomy or standard arthrotomy to expose the cartilage lesion.[51] The remaining articular cartilage and damaged subchondral bone are

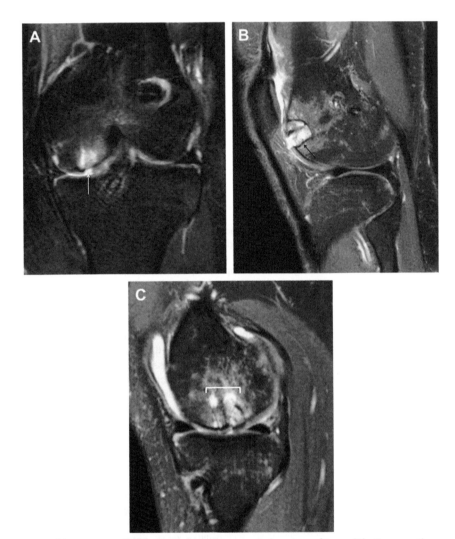

Fig. 4. A 27-year-old woman who underwent osteochondral autografting. (*A*) Preoperative, coronal, T2-weighted, fat-suppressed, 3-T MR imaging of the knee shows a full-thickness cartilage defect within the weight-bearing aspect of the medial femoral condyle (*arrow*) with surrounding subchondral bone marrow edema. (*B*) Three-month postoperative, sagittal, T2-weighted, fat-suppressed, 3-T MR imaging shows removal of two osteochondral plugs from the lateral femoral trochlea (*arrow*). (*C*) Three-month postoperative, sagittal, T2-weighted, fat-suppressed, 3-T MR imaging shows marrow hyperintensity surrounding the transplanted osteochondral autografts (*bracket*). This perigraft edema later decreased at 6-month follow-up.

removed. The allograft plug (10 to 35 mm in diameter) is then removed from the donor tissue using a coring reamer, and the graft is shaped to match the size and depth of the recipient lesion site. The graft is then gently inserted with a tamp or with joint compression during range of motion, with loose grafts fixed with bioabsorbable pins or screws. Eighty-five percent 10-year survivorship of allografts has been reported for posttraumatic defects of the femur.[52] Multiple studies have documented 80% to 84% good to excellent results at 6-year follow-up in patients treated with osteochondral allografts for a variety of conditions.[53,54]

Imaging studies

For osteochondral allografts, the same features should be evaluated on MR imaging as for osteochondral autografts (**Fig. 6**). In one animal study comparing osteochondral autografts with allografts, MR imaging revealed no statistically significant differences in the MR imaging appearance of autografts and allografts. The MR imaging features evaluated included graft cartilage signal intensity, appearance of the subchondral plate and articular surface (flush, depressed, proud, or displaced), interface with the adjacent cartilage (smooth, partial-thickness, or full-thickness offset),

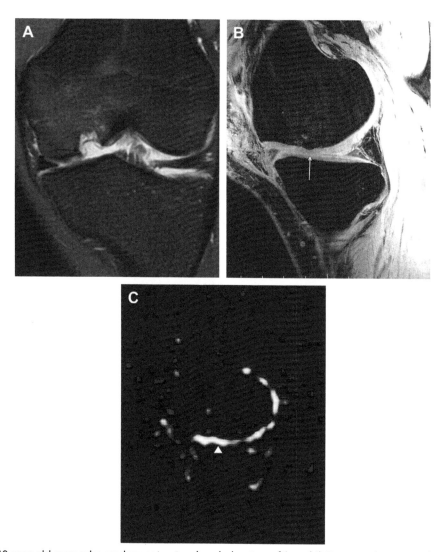

Fig. 5. A 19-year-old man who underwent osteochondral autografting. (*A*) Preoperative, coronal, T2, fat suppressed, 3-T MR image of the knee demonstrates an osteochondral lesion within the weight-bearing aspect of the medial femoral condyle (*arrow*). (*B*) Six-month postoperative, sagittal, 3-D, gradient-echo, T1-weighted, fat-suppressed, 7-T MR image (0.234 mm × 0.234 mm × 1 mm) shows an intact osteochondral autograft (*arrow*) with incorporation into surrounding subchondral bone. (*C*) Six-month postoperative, sagittal, 7-T, sodium MR image shows no detectable differences in cartilage sodium signal (and thus proteoglycan content) within the osteochondral autograft (*arrowhead*) when compared with adjacent native hyaline cartilage.

percentage fill of the defect by thirds, trabecular incorporation of the grafts (complete, partial, or poor), signal of bone graft (fat, edema, or fibrosis), and cartilage T2 relaxation times.[45] In 90% of subjects, the investigators noted a persistent cleft at the interface between the graft and host cartilage and concluded that hyaline cartilage cannot regenerate across a physical defect.

In another study involving 19 human subjects with symptomatic osteochondral lesions of the knee who were treated with hypothermically stored allografts, 2-year follow-up MR imaging examinations revealed normal graft cartilage thickness in 18 subjects, graft cartilage signal characteristics similar to native hyaline cartilage in 8 subjects, and complete or partial osseous incorporation of the allograft in 14 subjects.[50] The investigators concluded that hypothermically stored allografts are effective at short-term follow-up for treatment of symptomatic osteochondral lesions of the knee.

Finally, similar to osteochondral autografts, osteonecrosis within osteochondral allografts has been reported.[55]

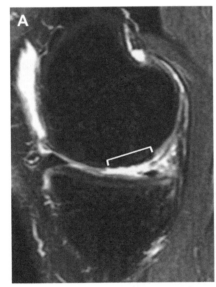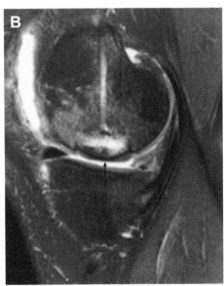

Fig. 6. A 50-year-old man who underwent osteochondral allografting. (A) Preoperative, sagittal, T2-weighted, fat-suppressed, 3-T, MR image of the knee shows a large full-thickness cartilage defect at the junction of the weight-bearing and posterior aspects of the medial femoral condyle (*bracket*). (B) Three-month postoperative, sagittal, T2-weighted, fat-suppressed, 3-T MR image shows placement of the osteochondral allograft. The cartilage surface is congruent (*arrow*), and there is extensive graft and perigraft edema.

Repair with Synthetic Resorbable Scaffolds

Rationale

In recent years, there has also been great interest in repair of cartilage lesions using synthetic resorbable scaffolds.[56–60] These scaffolds are small, cylindrical, porous plugs composed of biodegradable material (for example, a composite of polylactide-co-glycolide, calcium sulfate, and polyglycolide fibers in TruFit plugs from OsteoBiologics, San Antonio, TX, USA) that serve to facilitate the ingrowth of new healing tissue. They can be used alone or as delivery vehicles for cells and growth factors. The implants are biphasic or multiphasic in that the superficial layer has mechanical properties resembling that of hyaline cartilage and the deeper layer has mechanical properties resembling that of subchondral bone. In animal studies, the scaffolds are gradually resorbed and are replaced by hyaline cartilage and subchondral bone.[57]

Indications

The indications for the use of synthetic resorbable scaffolds for cartilage repair are similar to those for osteochondral autografts and allografts. The cartilage repair procedure is considered a potential treatment option for patients less than 50 years of age who have focal cartilage defects measuring 1 to 5 cm^2 in size. The main advantage of using synthetic resorbable scaffolds for cartilage repair is the avoidance of the limitations and potential complications associated with osteochondral autografting and allografting techniques, such as the need for an initial surgical procedure to harvest donor tissue, the lack of available donor tissue, and the risk of infection from allograft tissue.

Surgical technique

In the first step of the procedure, an osteochondral coring drill is selected such that its diameter completely covers the cartilage lesion of interest. The drill is inserted into the subchondral bone to a depth of 5 to 15 mm, and osteochondral tissue is removed. Using a delivery device with a measuring tamp, the synthetic implant is cut to the appropriate size of the surgically created osteochondral defect. The delivery device is then used to manually deliver the implant into the osteochondral defect. If further contouring is needed, the measuring tamp can be used to impact the surface of the implant such that its surface is flush with that of surrounding native hyaline cartilage. No randomized controlled trials have been performed comparing this technique with other cartilage repair techniques, although preclinical studies and isolated reports suggest promising results.[56–61]

Imaging studies

Similar to the evaluation of osteochondral autografts and allogafts, MR imaging of resorbable scaffolds should include an assessment of joint surface congruity, lesion fill, and the amount of osseous incorporation. At 3 months, the implanted scaffold has typically not integrated with the surrounding subchondral bone, and the implant can be hyperintense in signal relative to adjacent native hyaline cartilage (**Fig. 7**). By 12 months, however, the plug should be integrated with surrounding subchondral bone, such that the borders of the plug are less visible and a layer of overlying hyaline cartilage is seen (**Fig. 8**).

Autologous Chondrocyte Implantation and Matrix-Assisted Autologous Chondrocyte Implantation

Rationale
In ACI, chondrocytes are harvested from a patient and then grown in tissue culture medium. The chondrocytes are then reimplanted within the patient's cartilage defect beneath a periosteal patch and produce new cartilage repair tissue. The success of ACI in human studies was initially described by Brittberg and colleagues in 1994.[62]

Indications
ACI is indicated for near–full or full-thickness cartilage defects 2 cm^2 or greater in size. High-demand patients between the ages of 15 and 55 years with excellent treatment compliance are usually chosen. Although some surgeons believe the procedure should be reserved for patients who have failed another primary intervention, such as microfracture, others use it as a primary technique.[51] Some surgeons also treat smaller cartilage lesions less than 1 cm^2 in size with primary ACI.[51] If subchondral bone is damaged to a depth greater than 6 to 8 mm, staged or concomitant bone grafting is undertaken.

Surgical technique
ACI requires two procedures.[51] Initially, patients undergo diagnostic arthroscopy, and hyaline cartilage is harvested from a non–weight-bearing area of the knee, such as the superomedial trochlear ridge or lateral intercondylar notch. From this specimen, approximately 300,000 chondrocytes are isolated, which are grown in cell culture to produce approximately 10 million cells. In the second procedure, patients undergo arthrotomy and damaged cartilage is débrided without injuring subchondral bone. A periosteal patch is prepared (typically from the proximal medial tibial diaphysis distal to the pes anserinus insertion) and sutured over the defect, and the culture chondrocytes are injected under the periosteal patch. The patch is then sealed with additional suture and fibrin glue.

Potential complications with the use of a periosteal patch led to the development of collagen membranes to seal cartilage defects treated with ACI.[63] This led to the recognition that chondrocytes could be directly seeded onto a type I/III collagen membrane, which could then be delivered as a cell-scaffold construct for implantation. This procedure is currently referred to as matrix-assisted ACI (MACI). Other scaffolds have been developed and can be composed of carbohydrates

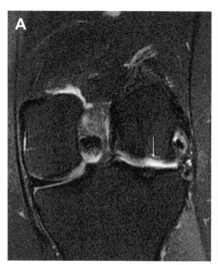
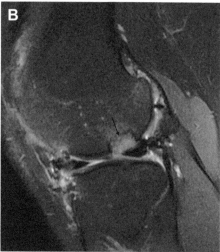

Fig. 7. A 36-year-old woman who was treated with a resorbable synthetic scaffold composed of polyglycolide-polylactide. (*A*) Preoperative, coronal, T2-weighted, fat-suppressed, 3-T, MR image of the knee shows a near full-thickness cartilage defect at the junction of the weight-bearing and posterior aspects of the lateral femoral condyle (*arrow*). (*B*) Seven-month postoperative, sagittal, T2-weighted, fat-suppressed, 3-T MR image shows that the graft is slightly hyperintense (*black arrow*) when compared with adjacent native hyaline cartilage. The graft remains congruent with the articular surface, and there is no perigraft marrow edema.

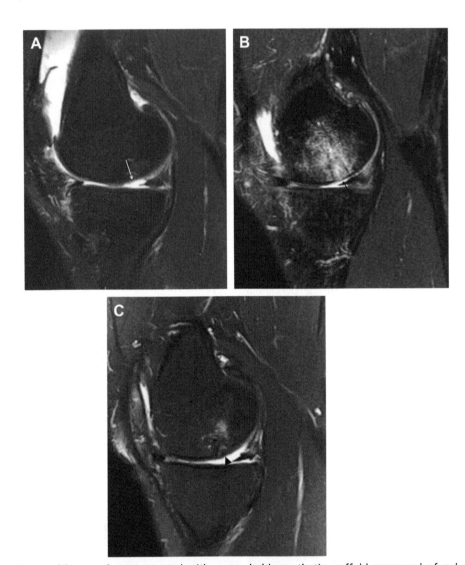

Fig. 8. A 41-year-old man who was treated with a resorbable synthetic scaffold composed of polyglycolide-polylactide. (*A*) Preoperative, sagittal, T2-weighted, fat-suppressed, 3-T MR image of the knee shows a full-thickness cartilage defect within the posterior weight-bearing aspect of the medial femoral condyle (*arrow*). (*B*) Three-month postoperative, sagittal, T2-weighted, fat-suppressed, 3-T MR image shows hyperintense signal within and surrounding the graft. The graft does not appear to be congruent with the articular surface, and no overlying hyaline articular cartilage is visible (*arrow*). (*C*) Eighteen-month, sagittal, T2-weighted, fat-suppressed, 3-T MR image shows that the degree of intragraft and perigraft edema has greatly decreased. The graft appears to be incorporated into the surrounding subchondral bone, and an overlying layer of hyaline cartilage is visible (*arrowhead*).

(polylactic/polyglycolic acid, hyaluronan, agarose, alginate), protein polymers (fibrin or gelatin), and artifical polymers (carbon fiber, hydroxyapatite, polytetrafluoroethylene, polybutyric acid). MACI obviates a periosteal patch and greatly simplifies the overall procedure. In addition, the biomatrix seeded with chondrocytes has theoretic advantages of less chondrocyte leakage, more homogeneous chondrocyte distribution, and less graft hypertrophy.[63]

In Brittberg and colleagues'[62] original *The New England Journal of Medicine* article describing ACI, 14 of 16 patients who were treated for distal femoral lesions had good to excellent clinical results. Later, the investigators published 2-year to 9-year follow-up data on their first 101 patients treated with ACI and reported 92% good to excellent results for individuals with isolated femoral condylar lesions.[64] For MACI, many studies have also shown significant improvement in clinical

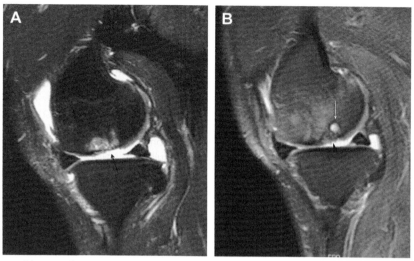

Fig. 9. A 50-year-old man who underwent ACI for a previously unsuccessful microfracture procedure. (*A*) Preoperative, sagittal, T2-weighted, fat-suppressed, 3-T, MR image of the knee shows a full-thickness cartilage defect within the weight-bearing aspect of the medial femoral condyle (*arrow*). (*B*) Six-month postoperative, sagittal, T2-weighted, fat-suppressed, 3-T MR image shows the cartilage defect partially filled in with repair tissue. At this stage, the surface of the cartilage repair tissue is slightly irregular (*arrowhead*), and a small cyst is seen within the subchondral bone marrow deep to the repair tissue (*arrow*).

outcome scores and knee function at 2-year to 7-year follow-up.[65,66]

Imaging studies

MR imaging performed shortly after ACI can demonstrate hyperintense repair cartilage, fluid signal at the interface between repair and native cartilage, and subchondral marrow edema (**Figs. 9** and **10**).[17,67,68] Over time, the signal intensity of the repair cartilage normalizes, the marrow edema decreases, and there is progressive peripheral integration of repair cartilage with

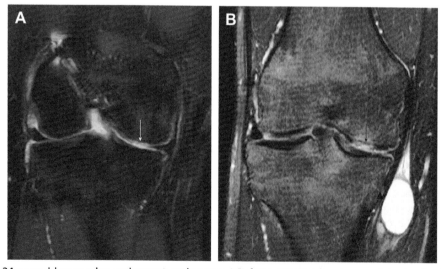

Fig. 10. A 24-year-old man who underwent underwent ACI for a previously unsuccessful microfracture procedure. (*A*) Preoperative, coronal, T2-weighted, fat-suppressed, 3-T MR image of the knee shows an anterior cruciate ligament reconstruction and irregular fibrocartilage at the weight bearing aspect of the medial femoral condyle in the region of a previous microfracture (*arrow*). (*B*) Three-month postoperative, coronal, T2-weighted, fat-suppressed, 3-T MR image shows the cartilage defect partially filled in with hyperintense cartilage repair tissue (*black arrow*) with mild underlying subchondral bone marrow edema. Incidental note is made of a postsurgical fluid collection at the medial aspect of the knee (*arrowhead*).

adjacent native hyaline cartilage as demonstrated by a lack of high T2 signal interposed between the two tissues.[68] This process can take up to 2 years to complete.

MACI has been studied using T2 mapping and, similar to native hyaline cartilage, there is spatial variation in the T2 values of repair cartilage (although the increase in mean T2 values from deep to superficial layers of cartilage is less pronounced).[30] During the first year after the procedure, global mean T2 values of MACI repair tissue can be elevated[69,70]; over time, T2 values decrease and approaches that of native hyaline cartilage.[69,71] Recently, Welsch and colleagues[72] reported that T2 mapping can distinguish between MACI performed using a collagen-based scaffold and a hyaluronan-based scaffold (higher T2 values in collagen-based scaffolds) even at 2 years after the original procedure. The investigators concluded that these differences in the MR imaging appearance of cartilage repair tissue should be taken into account when evaluating patients after MACI.

In recent years, there have also been several studies demonstrating a benefit of using dGEMRIC as a noninvasive method to monitor cartilage repair tissue formed after ACI.[32,73–77] In general, these studies have shown that in the immediate postoperative period, dGEMRIC can differentiate repair tissue from normal hyaline cartilage and suggest that dGEMRIC can be used as a means to evaluate the proteoglycan content of cartilage repair tissue. In a recent study with 9-year to 18-year follow-up of 31 patients who underwent ACI, dGEMRIC indices normalized between repair tissue and native hyaline cartilage, suggesting that proteoglycan content and perhaps the quality of the two tissues is similar.[78]

SUMMARY

As long as people remain physically active, cartilage injury will continue to represent a major clinical problem for orthopedic surgeons, rheumatologists, and other physicians who treat musculoskeletal disorders. There are currently many surgical options available to repair and restore damaged articular cartilage, including microfracture, osteochondral autografting or allografting, repair with synthetic resorbable scaffolds, and ACI (including MACI). Knowledge of the type of repair performed can be useful to interpretation of the MR imaging examination. In the current clinical realm, orthopedic surgeons rely on MR imaging to identify the number, size, and depth of cartilage lesions at the time of initial injury and to assess the status of cartilage repair tissue

from a structural standpoint (surface congruency, peripheral integration, cartilage morphology, and presence of subchondral marrow edema). These parameters are typically correlated with patient clinical outcomes to determine whether or not a procedure has been successful. In the future, imaging techniques, such as T2 mapping, dGEMRIC, and sodium MR imaging, have the potential to provide novel information regarding the biochemical composition of the repair tissue matrix, in particular, its collagen, water, and proteoglycan content. This information may help guide decision making by providing clinicians with metrics of the repair tissue quality and physiologic status in addition to its morphologic structure.

ACKNOWLEDGMENTS

The authors acknowledge grant support from the Radiological Society of North America (RSNA RR0806) and the National Institutes of Health (R01-AR053133, R01AR056260).

REFERENCES

1. Curl W, Krome J, Gordon E, et al. Cartilage injuries: a review of 31,516 knee arthroscopies. Arthroscopy 1997;13:456–60.
2. Hijelle K, Solheim E, Strand T, et al. Articular cartilage defects in 1000 knee arthroscopies. Arthroscopy 2002;18:730–4.
3. Mankin H. The response of articular cartilage to mechanical injury. J Bone Joint Surg Am 1982;64: 460–6.
4. Newman A. Articular cartilage repair. Am J Sports Med 1998;26:309–24.
5. Eckstein F, Burstein D, Link TM. Quantitative MRI of cartilage and bone:degenerative changes in osteoarthritis. NMR Biomed 2006;19:822–54.
6. Recht MP, Piraino DW, Paletta GA, et al. Accuracy of fat-suppressed three-dimensional spoiled gradient-echo FLASH MR imaging in the detection of patellofemoral articular cartilage abnormalities. Radiology 1996;198:209–12.
7. Disler DG, McCauley TR, Wirth CR, et al. Detection of knee hyaline cartilage defects using fat-suppressed three-dimensional spoiled gradient-echo MR imaging: comparison with standard MR imaging and correlation with arthroscopy. Am J Roentgenol 1995;165:377–82.
8. Potter HG, Linklater JM, Allen AA, et al. Magnetic resonance imaging of articular cartilage in the knee. An evaluation with use of fast spin echo imaging. J Bone Joint Surg Am 1998;80:1276–84.
9. Bredella MA, Tirman PFJ, Peterfy CG, et al. Accuracy of T2-weighted fast spin-echo MR imaging

with fat saturation in detecting cartilage defects in the knee: comparison with arthroscopy in 130 patients. Am J Roentgenol 1999;172:1073–80.

10. Mosher TJ, Dardzinski BJ. Cartilage MRI T2 relaxation time mapping: overview and applications. Semin Musculoskelet Radiol 2004;8:355–68.

11. Burstein D, Gray M, Mosher T, et al. Measures of molecular composition and structure in osteoarthritis. Radiol Clin North Am 2009;47:675–86.

12. Wheaton AJ, Casey FL, Gougoutas AJ, et al. Correlation of T1ρ with fixed charge density in cartilage. J Magn Reson Imaging 2004;20:519–25.

13. Shapiro EM, Borthakur A, Gougoutas A, et al. 23Na MRI accurately measures fixed charge density in articular cartilage. Magn Reson Med 2002;47: 284–91.

14. Krug R, Carballido-Gamio J, Banerjee S, et al. In vivo bone and cartilage MRI using fully-balanced steady-state free-precession at 7 Tesla. Magn Reson Med 2007;58:1294–8.

15. Banerjee S, Krug R, Carballido-Gamio J, et al. Rapid in vivo musculoskeletal MR with parallel imaging at 7T. Magn Reson Med 2008;59:655–60.

16. Regatte R, Schweitzer ME. Ultra-high-field MRI of the musculoskeletal system at 7.0 T. J Magn Reson Imaging 2007;25(2):262–9.

17. Brown WE, Potter HG, Marx RG, et al. Magnetic resonance imaging appearance of articular cartilage repair in the knee. Clin Orthop Relat Res 2004;422:214–23.

18. Marlovits S, Striessnig G, Resinger CT, et al. Definition of pertinent parameters for the evaluation of articular cartilage repair tissue with high-resolution magnetic resonance imaging. Eur J Radiol 2004; 52:310–9.

19. Marlovits S, Singer P, Zeller P, et al. Magnetic resonance observation of cartilage repair tissue (MOCART) for the evaluation of autologous chondrocyte transplantation: interobserver variability and correlation to clinical outcome after 2 years. Eur J Radiol 2006;57:16–23.

20. Steadman JR, Rodkey WG, Rodrigo JJ. Microfracture: surgical technique and rehabilitation to treat chondral defects. Clin Orthop Relat Res 2001;(391 Suppl):S362–9.

21. Robinson D, Nevo Z. Articular cartilage chondrocytes are more advantageous for generating hyaline-like cartilage than mesenchymal cells isolated from microfracture repairs. Cell Tissue Bank 2001;2:23–30.

22. Nehrer S, Spector M, Minas T. Histologic analysis of tissue after failed cartilage repair procedures. Clin Orthop Relat Res 1999;365:149–62.

23. Blevins FT, Steadman JR, Rodrigo JJ, et al. Treatment of articular cartilage defects in athletes: an analysis of functional outcome and lesion appearance. Orthopedics 1998;21:761–8.

24. Steadman JR, Rodkey WG, Singleton SB, et al. Microfracture procedure for treatment of full-thickness chondral defects: technique, clinical results and current basic science status. In: Harner CD, Vince KG, Fu FH, editors. Techniques in knee surgery. Media (PA): Williams & Wilkins; 1999. p. 23–31.

25. Steadman JR, Rodkey WG, Singleton SB, et al. Microfracture technique for full-thickness chondral defects: technique and clinical results. Oper Tech Orthop 1997;7:300–4.

26. Mithoefer K, Williams RJ 3rd, Warren RF, et al. The microfracture technique for the treatment of articular cartilage lesions in the knee. A prospective cohort study. J Bone Joint Surg Am 2005;87: 1911–20.

27. Mithoefer K, Williams RJ 3rd, Warren RF, et al. High-impact athletics after knee articular cartilage repair: a prospective evaluation of the microfracture technique. Am J Sports Med 2006;34:1413–8.

28. Salter RB. The biologic concept of continuous passive motion of synovial joints. The first 18 years of basic research and its clinical application. Clin Orthop 1989;242:12–25.

29. Rodrigo JJ, Steadman JR, Sillman J, et al. Improvement of full-thickness chondral defect healing in the human knee after debridement and microfracture using continuous passive motion. Am J Knee Surg 1994;7:109–16.

30. White LM, Sussman MS, Hurtig M, et al. Cartilage T2 assessment: differentiation of normal hyaline cartilage and reparative tissue after arthroscopic cartilage repair in equine subjects. Radiology 2006; 241:407–14.

31. Welsch GH, Mamisch TC, Domayer S, et al. Cartilage T2 assessment at 3 Tesla: in vivo differentiation of normal hyaline cartilage and reparative tissue in patients after two different cartilage repair procedures—initial experiences. Radiology 2008;247(1): 154–61.

32. Trattnig S, Mamisch TC, Pinker K, et al. Differentiating normal hyaline cartilage from post-surgical repair tissue using fast gradient echo imaging in delayed gadolinium enhanced MRI - (dGEMRIC) at 3 Tesla. Eur Radiol 2008;18(6):1251–9.

33. Yamashita F, Sacked K, Suzy F, et al. The transplantation of an autogenic osteochondral fragment for osteochondritis of the knee. Clin Orthop 1985;210: 43–50.

34. Bobić V. Arthroscopic osteochondral autograft transplantation in anterior cruciate ligament reconstruction: a preliminary clinical study. Knee Surg Sports Traumatol Arthrosc 1996;3(4):262–4.

35. Hangody L, Kish G, Karate Z, et al. Arthroscopic autogenous osteochondral mosaicplasty for the treatment of femoral condylar articular defects. A preliminary report. Knee Surg Sports Traumatol Arthrosc 1997;5:262–7.

36. Hangody L, Fule P. Autologous osteochondral mosaicplasty for the treatment of full thickness defects of weight bearing joints: ten years of experimental and clinical experience. J Bone Joint Surg Am 2003;85(Suppl 2):25–32.

37. Bodo G, Kaposi A, Hangody L, et al. The surgical technique and the age of horse both influence the outcome of mosaicplasty in a cadaver stifle model. Acta Vet Hung 2001;49:111–6.

38. Feczko P, Hangody L, Varga J, et al. Experimental results of donor site filling for autologous osteochondral mosaicplasty. Arthroscopy 2003;19:755–61.

39. Ahmed CS, Cohen ZA, Levine WN, et al. Biomechanical and topographic considerations for autologous osteochondral grafting in the knee. Am J Sports Med 2001;29:201–6.

40. Bartz RL, Kamaric E, Noble PC, et al. Topographic matching of selected donor and recipient sites for osteochondral autografting of the articular surfaces of the femoral condyles. Am J Sports Med 2001; 29:207–12.

41. Miniaci A, Evans P, Hurtig MB. Harvesting techniques for osteochondral transplantation. Proc Int Soc Arthrosc Knee Surg Orthop Sports Med 1999;86:147.

42. Horas U, Pelinkovic D, Herr G, et al. Autologous chondrocyte implantation and osteochondral cylinder transplantation in cartilage repair of the knee joint. A prospective, comparative trial. J Bone Joint Surg Am 2003;85:185–92.

43. Link TM, Mishung J, Wortler K, et al. Normal and pathological MR findings in osteochondral autografts with longitudinal follow-up. Eur Radiol 2006; 16:88–96.

44. Gudas R, Kelesinskas RJ, Kimtys V, et al. A prospective randomized clinical study of mosaic osteochondral autologous transplantation versus microfracture for the treatment of osteochondral defects in the knee joint in young athletes. Arthroscopy 2005;21:1066–75.

45. Glenn RE, McCarty EC, Potter HG, et al. Comparison of fresh osteochondral autografts and allografts. Am J Sports Med 2006;34:1084–93.

46. Gortz S, Bugbee WD. Allografts in articular cartilage repair. J Bone Joint Surg Am 2006;88(6):1374–84.

47. Langer F, Gross AE. Immunogenicity of allograft articular cartilage. J Bone Joint Surg Am 1974;56: 297–304.

48. American Association for Tissue Banks. Standards for tissue banking. 12th Edition. McLean (VA): American Association for Tissue Banking; 2008.

49. Centers for Disease Control. Allograft associated bacterial infections. MMWR Morb Mortal Wkly Rep 2002;51:207–10.

50. Williams RJ, Ranawat AS, Potter HS, et al. Fresh stored allografts for the treatment of osteochondral defects of the knee. J Bone Joint Surg Am 2007; 89:718–26.

51. Trice ME, Bugbee WD, Greenwald AS, et al. Articular cartilage restoration: a review of currently available methods for repair of articular cartilage defects. American of Academy of Orthopaedic Surgeons 76th Annual Meeting. Las Vegas (NV), February 25–28, 2009.

52. Aubin PP, Cheah HK, Davis AM, et al. Long term follow-up of fresh femoral osteochondral allografts for post traumatic defects of the knee. Clin Orthop Relat Res 2001;(391 Suppl):318–91.

53. Emmerson BC, Görtz S, Jamali AA, et al. Fresh osteochondral allografting in the treatment of osteochondritis dissecans of the femoral condyle. Am J Sports Med 2007;35(6):907–14.

54. Chu CR, Convery FR, Akeson WH, et al. Articular cartilage transplantation. Clinical results in the knee. Clin Orthop Relat Res 1999;(360):159–68.

55. Collins M, Stuart MJ. Magnetic resonance imaging osteonecrosis pattern within an osteocondral dowel allograft. J Knee Surg 2010;23:45–50.

56. Freed LE, Vunjak-Novakovic G, Biron RJ, et al. Biodegradable polymer scaffolds for tissue engineering. Biotechnology (NY) 1994;12:689–93.

57. Freed LE, Grande DA, Lingbin Z, et al. Joint resurfacing using allograft chondrocytes and synthetic biodegradable polymer scaffolds. J Biomed Mater Res 1994;28:891–9.

58. Ma PX, Schloo B, Mooney D, et al. Development of biomechanical properties and morphogenesis of in vitro tissue engineered cartilage. J Biomed Mater Res 1995;29:1587–95.

59. Cima LG, Vacanti JP, Vacanti CA, et al. Tissue engineering by cell transplantation using degradable polymer substrates. J Biomech Eng 1991;113:143–51.

60. Grande DA, Halberstadt C, Naughton G, et al. Evaluation of matrix scaffolds for tissue engineering of articular cartilage grafts. J Biomed Mater Res 1997;34:211–20.

61. Williams RJ, Niederauer GG. Articular cartilage resurfacing using synthetic resorbable scaffolds. In: Williams RJ, editor. Cartilage repair strategies. Totowa (NJ): Humana Press Inc; 2007. p. 115–35.

62. Brittberg M, Lindahl A, Nilsson A, et al. Treatment of deep cartilage defects in the knee with autologous chondrocyte transplantation. N Engl J Med 1994; 331(14):889–95.

63. Wood D, Zheng MH. Matrix-induced autologous chondrocyte implantation. In: Willliams RJ, editor. Cartilage repair strategies. Totowa (NJ): Humana Press; 2007. p. 193–206.

64. Peterson L, Minas T, Brittberg M, et al. Two- to 9-yr outcome after autologous chondrocyte transplantation of the knee. Clin Orthop Relat Res 2000;374: 212–34.

65. Ossendorf C, Kaps C, Kreuz PC, et al. Treatment of posttraumatic and focal osteoarthritic cartilage defects of the knee with autologous polymer-based

three-dimensional chondrocyte grafts: 2-year clinical results. Arthritis Res Ther 2007;9(2):640–5.

66. Marcacci M, Kon E, Delcogliano M, et al. Arthroscopic autologous osteochondral grafting for cartilage defects of the knee: prospective study results at a minimum 7-year follow-up. Am J Sports Med 2007;35(12):2014–21.

67. Alparslan L, Minas T, Winalski CS. Magnetic resonance imaging of autologous chondrocyte implantation. Semin Ultrasound CT MR 2001;22:341–51.

68. Verstraete KL, Almqvist F, Verdonk P, et al. Magnetic resonance imaging of cartilage and cartilage repair. Clin Radiol 2004;59:674–89.

69. Trattnig S, Mamisch TC, Welsch GH, et al. Quantitative T2 mapping of matrix-associated autologous chondrocyte transplantation at 3 Tesla: an in vivo cross-sectional study. Invest Radiol 2007;42:442–8.

70. Kurkijarvi JE, Mattila L, Ojala RO, et al. Evaluation of cartilage repair in the distal femur after autologous chondrocyte transplantation using T2 relaxation time and dGEMRIC. Osteoarthr Cartil 2007;15:372–8.

71. Giannini S, Battaglia M, Buda R, et al. Surgical treatment of osteochondral lesions of the talus by open-field autologous chondrocyte implantation: a 10-year follow-up clinical and magnetic resonance imaging T2-mapping evaluation. Am J Sports Med 2009;37:112S–8S.

72. Welsch GH, Mamisch TC, Zak L, et al. Matrix-associated autologous chondrocyte transplantation using a hyaluronic-based or a collagen-based scaffold with morphological MOCART scoring and biochemical T2 mapping. Am J Sports Med 2010; 38:934–42.

73. Watanabe A, Wada Y, Obata T, et al. Delayed gadolinium-enhanced MR to determine glycosaminoglycan concentration in reparative cartilage after autologous chondrocyte implantation: preliminary results. Radiology 2006;239:201–8.

74. Watanabe A, Boesch C, Anderson SE, et al. Ability of dGEMRIC and T2 mapping to evaluate cartilage repair after microfracture: a goat study. Osteoarthritis Cartilage 2009;17:1341–9.

75. Trattnig S, Burstein D, Szomolanyi P, et al. T1 (Gd) gives comparable information oas delta T1 relaxation rate in dGEMRIC evaluation of cartilage repair tissue. Invest Radiol 2009;44:598–602.

76. Domayer SE, Trattnig S, Stelzeneder D, et al. Delayed gadolinium-enhanced MRI of cartilage in the ankle at 3T: feasibility and preliminary results after matrix-asssociated autologus chondrocyte implantation. J Magn Reson Imaging 2010;31(3):732–9.

77. Welsch GH, Mamisch TC, Hughes T, et al. In vivo biochemical 7.0 Tesla magnetic resonance: preliminary results of dGEMRIC, zonal T2, and zonal T2* mapping of articular cartilage. Invest Radiol 2008;43: 619–26.

78. Vasiliadis HS, Danielson B, Ljungberg M, et al. Autologous chondrocyte implantaion in the knee: long-term evaluation with magnetic resonance imaging and delayed gadolinium-enhanced magnetic resonance imaging technique. Am J Sports Med 2010; 38:943–9.

MR Imaging Assessment of Inflammatory, Crystalline-Induced, and Infectious Arthritides

Jennifer L. Demertzis, MD*, David A. Rubin, MD

KEYWORDS

- MR imaging • Arthritis • Rheumatoid arthritis
- Spondyloarthropathies • Gout • Septic arthritis

In joints afflicted by degenerative and traumatic arthritis, magnetic resonance (MR) imaging techniques currently emphasize direct morphologic and biochemical imaging of the articular cartilage. Other arthritides primarily destroy cartilage through an inflammatory mechanism. The diagnosis of these conditions, which include primary inflammatory, crystal-induced, and septic arthritides, is typically accomplished with a combination of clinical evaluation, laboratory studies, and radiographs. Radiographs, however, are relatively insensitive to small erosions, and even combined with clinical features cannot prognosticate the disease course. Additionally in these conditions, synovitis and bone marrow changes often precede and predict later chondral disease. A major goal of MR imaging is to identify these precursor lesions before arthritis progresses to bone erosion and cartilage destruction.

For rheumatoid arthritis (RA), seronegative spondyloarthropathies, and related conditions, early diagnosis and staging has become imperative, now that targeted drugs are available to quell the inflammation before cartilage damage occurs. Gout and other crystalline diseases can also affect bone, articular cartilage, and supporting tissues over time, and these complications can be mitigated or avoided with medical and, in some cases, surgical intervention. Septic arthritis, especially bacterial, can irreversibly destroy cartilage and bone in a few days, making immediate diagnosis mandatory so that combined surgical and medical management can be instituted. This article reviews the role of MR imaging in the evaluation of patients with inflammatory, crystalline-induced, and infectious arthritides.

INFLAMMATORY ARTHRITIDES

The inflammatory arthritides, which include RA, juvenile idiopathic arthritis (JIA), and the seronegative spondyloarthropathies, are a diverse group of systemic diseases that affect the musculoskeletal systems of genetically susceptible individuals. Immune dysregulation, whether in response to an autoantigen or infectious agent, defines a common pathophysiology of activated synovium with pannus formation, resulting in cartilage and joint destruction. Inflammation of extra-articular synovium presents as bursitis and tenosynovitis. Systemic involvement of other organs such as the eye, skin, and viscera can result in significant morbidity and may be prominent features of disease.

RA affects all ethnic groups worldwide, with peak incidence in the fourth through sixth decades of life. Severity is variable, ranging from self-limited

Division of Musculoskeletal Radiology, Mallinckrodt Institute of Radiology, 510 South Kingshighway Boulevard, Campus Box 8131, St Louis, MO 63110, USA
* Corresponding author.
E-mail address: demertzisj@mir.wustl.edu

Magn Reson Imaging Clin N Am 19 (2011) 339–363
doi:10.1016/j.mric.2011.02.004
1064-9689/11/$ – see front matter © 2011 Elsevier Inc. All rights reserved.

to progressive debilitating disease. The classic presentation begins with symmetric involvement of the wrists, metacarpophalangeal joints, and proximal interphalangeal joints. The prevalence of the spondyloarthropathies parallels that of the HLA-B27 haplotype, characterized by axial inflammation of the spine and sacroiliac (SI) joints, and asymmetric peripheral arthritis of the lower extremities and small distal joints of the hands. Enthesitis (inflammation at the attachment of tendon, ligament, or joint capsule), rather than synovitis, is the primary pathologic lesion of the spondyloarthropathies that distinguishes them from RA. JIA describes a heterogeneous group of chronic arthritic conditions with features of rheumatoid and seronegative disease. By definition, JIA presents before age 16 years, but active disease often continues into adulthood. The knee is the most commonly affected joint.

Precise diagnosis of the inflammatory arthritides can be difficult. Classification criteria include a combination of clinical signs and symptoms, radiographic findings, and serologic testing. However, clinical features of the various arthritides may overlap one another, or with other conditions like connective tissue disorders. Radiographs cannot detect synovitis or other soft tissue inflammatory changes that characterize the early stages of disease, and may be relatively insensitive in detecting late findings of erosions and cartilage thinning. Serologic testing is often nonspecific and does not predict disease severity, with one notable exception. Anticyclic citrullinated peptide (anti-CCP) antibody is up to 98% specific for RA, is present in early disease in 70% of patients, and is associated with greater radiologic damage over time compared with RA patients with negative anti-CCP serology.[1]

Historically, treatment of RA and related conditions consisted of steroids and nonsteroidal anti-inflammatory drugs, which improved symptoms but did not prevent disabling and disfiguring joint damage.[2] The advent of disease-modifying antirheumatic drugs (DMARDs) has dramatically changed the management of RA. These drugs prevent joint destruction, especially when initiated early.[3] It is therefore essential to accurately assess disease activity, progression, and response to therapy. The immune cascades, resultant drug targets, and role of MR imaging have been most thoroughly investigated in adult-onset RA.

MR Imaging Technique

The MR imaging examination for inflammatory arthritis should cover critical joints, with adequate spatial resolution to demonstrate erosions and adequate contrast resolution to show bone edema and synovitis. Because rheumatoid and related arthritides commonly affect the hands and/or wrists, screening and staging studies typically image these joints as a surrogate for disease activity throughout the body. Dedicated, extremity MR imaging scanners may be used to detect erosions in hands and wrists, but the lower field strength units on the market are not as sensitive as high-field magnets for detecting bone edema, and there is high intermachine and interobserver variability for identifying synovitis and bone edema using these scanners.[4,5] In addition, the small field of view for some permanent magnet scanners limits the examination to just a few joints.[6] When using a whole-body scanner for the hands and wrists, a local coil is mandatory to achieve the necessary signal to noise ratio. Imaging can either be performed unilaterally (typically the most symptomatic or the dominant side) with a small whole-volume or surface coil, or bilaterally. The authors have found that bilateral examinations are well tolerated by patients who are positioned decubitus in the scanner, with flexion of their hips, knees, shoulders, and elbows (a modified fetal position), and with their hands in an extremity coil slightly cranial to their heads (**Fig. 1**). Bilateral imaging is useful whenever symmetry or asymmetry of the findings will affect diagnosis and management.

Short repetition time/echo time (TR/TE) spin-echo or fast spin-echo (T1-weighted) images are ideal for visualizing bone marrow, erosions, and synovial thickness. Water-sensitive sequences with fat suppression (T2-weighted fast spin-echo or short-tau inversion recovery [STIR]) demonstrate joint and tenosynovial fluid, marrow edema, soft tissue nodules, and tendons. Fat-suppressed T1-weighted images obtained after intravenous administration of gadolinium-based contrast are used to distinguish enhancing synovitis from nonenhancing effusions (unlike on T2-weighted and STIR images, where both the inflamed synovium and joint effusion demonstrate high signal intensity from increased water content) (**Figs. 2 and 3**). Contrast-enhanced images demonstrate more findings than T2-weighted images alone,[7] but more importantly, synovial enhancement represents active disease, even in patients with clinical remission.[8,9] Contrast administration also adds specificity to the examination because whereas small erosions and marrow edema may occur in some patients without inflammatory arthritis, enhancing synovitis and enhancing marrow lesions are rare or absent in healthy subjects.[10,11] Postcontrast imaging should occur within 10 minutes of injection, as contrast diffusion into the

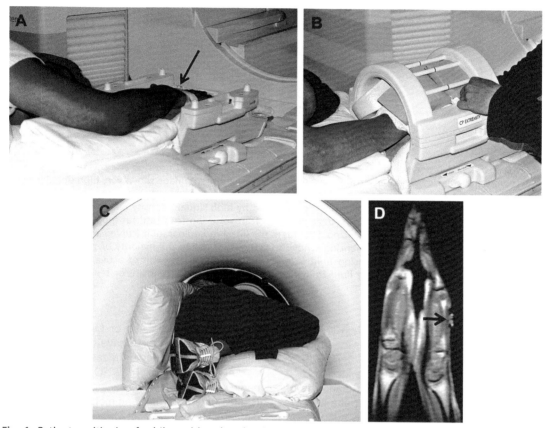

Fig. 1. Patient positioning for bilateral hand and wrist MR imaging using a whole-body, closed scanner. (*A*) A patient positioned in the lateral decubitus position, with the elbows comfortably flexed and the hands positioned slightly overhead, in a knee coil (cover removed) with the palms touching. Note the MR imaging compatible marker (*arrow*) used to designate sidedness on the final images. By convention, the authors always mark the patient's right side in their practice. (*B*) Padding is added surrounding the hands within the coil. (*C*) The patient is placed within the magnetic bore surrounded by cushioning as needed for comfort. Note the flexed attitude of the knees and hips. (*D*) Sagittal scout image, which will be used to prescribe the coronal and transverse planes. Note the marker designating the right side (*arrow*).

joint space may limit differentiation between synovium and any accompanying joint fluid.[12] Definitions of common MR imaging abnormalities in inflammatory arthritis are summarized in **Table 1**.

The anatomic coverage and imaging planes should address the target joints of the suspected arthritis. For RA, the entire wrist (including the distal radioulnar joint) and at least the metacarpophalangeal joints should be included with both coronal and transverse images (**Fig. 4**). In psoriasis and disease with more distal distributions, the coil should be positioned to include all of the finger joints and sagittal images can be substituted for coronal images (**Fig. 5**). The same imaging principles apply when performing MR imaging for other peripheral joints: the examination should use a local coil closely matched in size to the affected joints, image in at least 2 planes, and consist of a combination of short TR/TE, water-sensitive, and postcontrast sequences.

Rheumatoid Arthritis

RA, the most common inflammatory arthritis, affects approximately 25 men and 54 women per 100,000 population.[13] Although the genetic and immune abnormalities responsible for RA have not been fully elucidated, studies indicate that an antigen-specific T-cell response in the synovium initiates an immune cascade, leading to synovial proliferation and pannus formation that subsequently erode subchondral bone and to release of proteases that destroy articular cartilage.[14] Synovitis is responsible for joint pain and swelling, morning stiffness, and development of rheumatoid nodules. In the late stages, fibrosis within the joint

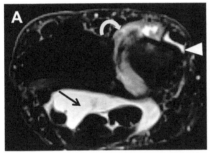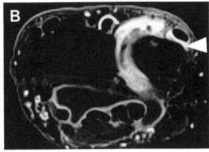

Fig. 2. Synovitis and tenosynovitis. A 32-year-old woman with rheumatoid arthritis and severe wrist swelling. (*A*) Transverse fat-suppressed water-sensitive fast spin-echo (T2-weighted) image shows very high signal intensity in the carpal tunnel involving the flexor tendon sheaths (*straight arrow*) and in the extensor carpi ulnaris tendon sheath (*arrowhead*). The distal radioulnar joint is distended by high signal intensity material that is heterogeneous and less intense than fluid (*curved arrow*). (*B*) Transverse postcontrast fat-suppressed short TR/TE (T1-weighted) image shows severe enhancing synovitis in the distal radioulnar joint (*curved arrow*). The extensor carpi ulnaris tendon sheath shows enhancing synovitis (*arrowhead*), while the majority of the enlarged flexor tendon sheaths are due to nonenhancing fluid (*straight arrow*) with a mild rim of active synovitis. Without contrast administration, distinguishing fluid from very high signal intensity synovitis or tenosynovitis may not be possible.

can lead to ankylosis (more commonly in JIA than in adult-onset RA), disuse osteoporosis, and muscle atrophy.[15]

Clinical criteria defined by the American College of Rheumatology (ACR) establish a diagnosis of RA. Radiographic findings of joint space narrowing, bony erosion, and joint deformity support the diagnosis and were incorporated into early, validated grading systems.[16,17] However, these features do not appear until after irreversible joint damage has occurred; ideally an imaging method could show soft tissue and bone findings at an earlier stage, when DMARD therapy would have the most value.[18] MR imaging is currently the ideal imaging modality fulfilling that role.[19]

Guidelines for the use of MR imaging as an outcome measure in RA have been studied and validated by the Outcome Measures in Rheumatoid Arthritis Clinical Trials (OMERACT) group, leading to an RA MR imaging scoring system (RAMRIS) for the wrists and metacarpophalangeal joints.[20] The group's scoring parameters and imaging recommendations,[21] image reference atlases,[22,23] and sample score sheets[24] are published. Quantified measurements of synovitis, bone marrow edema, and bone erosion correlate with clinical and histologic inflammatory markers, predict disease progression, and demonstrate response to therapy; these findings have also been extrapolated to describe the salient MR

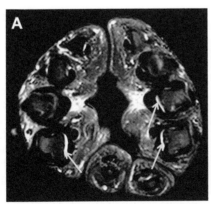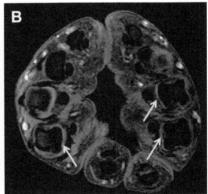

Fig. 3. Joint effusions without synovitis. A 55-year-old man with rheumatoid arthritis and joint swelling. (*A*) Transverse fat-suppressed, water-sensitive fast spin-echo (T2-weighted) image shows high signal intensity within several metacarpophalangeal joints bilaterally (*arrows*). (*B*) Transverse postcontrast fat-suppressed short TR/TE (T1-weighted) image through the same joints shows minimal if any enhancement, indicating that the findings represent simple effusions and not active synovitis (*arrows*).

Table 1
MR imaging definitions for joint and soft tissue pathology in inflammatory arthritis

Abnormality	MR Imaging Definition
Synovitis	Synovial enhancement of a thickness greater than the width of normal synovium
Bone edema	Ill-defined lesion in trabecular bone with signal characteristics consistent with increased water content (low T1-weighted and high T2-weighted signal intensity)
Bone erosion	Juxta-articular sharply marginated bone lesion with characteristic signal intensity (loss of normal cortical and trabecular T1 signal intensity, and quick postcontrast enhancement indicating pannus within the erosion) that is visible in 2 planes with a cortical break seen in at least 1 plane
Tenosynovitis	Increased water content or abnormal enhancement adjacent to a tendon in an area with a tendon sheath
Peritendonitis	Increased water content or abnormal enhancement adjacent to a tendon in an area without a tendon sheath
Tendonitis	Abnormal thickening and/or signal characteristics consistent with increased water content or abnormal enhancement within a tendon
Tendinopathy	Morphologic abnormality (thickening, attenuation or disruption) and/or signal characteristics consistent with increased water content or abnormal enhancement within a tendon
Periarticular inflammation	Increased water content or abnormal enhancement at extra-articular sites including periosteum ("periostitis") and entheses ("enthesitis"), but not the tendon sheaths ("tenosynovitis")
Bone proliferation	Abnormal periarticular (enthesophyte) or articular (ankylosis) bone formation

Adapted from Østergaard M, McQueen F, Wiell C, et al. The OMERACT psoriatic arthritis magnetic resonance imaging scoring system (PsAMRIS): definitions of key pathologies, suggested MRI sequences, and preliminary scoring system for PsA hands. J Rheumatol 2009;36:1816–24.

imaging features of RA in locations other than the hands and wrists.[25]

The earliest MR imaging finding of RA is synovitis, characterized by thickened synovial tissue and periarticular enhancement on T1-weighted images obtained after intravenous gadolinium-based contrast administration.[8,26] Symmetric synovitis typically affects the wrists, hands, and

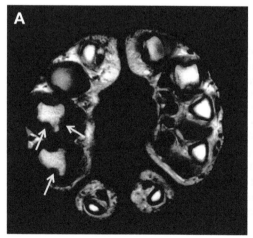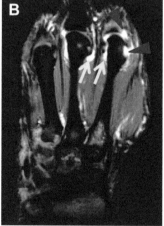

Fig. 4. Active synovitis. A 50-year-old woman with rheumatoid arthritis and polyarticular joint pain. (*A*) Transverse short TR/TE (T1-weighted) image through the metacarpophalangeal joints shows erosions in the second and third metacarpal heads (*arrows*). (*B*) Coronal postcontrast fat-suppressed short TR/TE (T1-weighted) image shows active, enhancing synovitis (*arrows*) in the metacarpophalangeal joints along with enhancement of the erosions (*arrowheads*).

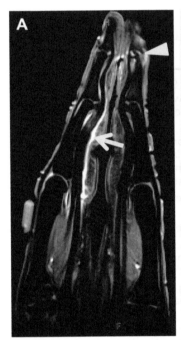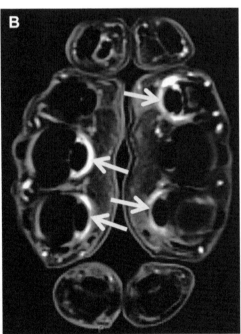

Fig. 5. MR imaging for evaluation of distal disease of the hands. A 58-year-old woman with psoriatic arthritis and distal joint pain. (*A*) Sagittal postcontrast fat-suppressed short TR/TE (T1-weighted) images of both hands are obtained with the right side marked by convention. Unlike MR imaging of RA that focuses on the wrist and meta-carpophalangeal joints, the coil has been moved distally to include the proximal and distal interphalangeal joints in this patient with spondyloarthropathy. There is tenosynovitis of the right long finger flexor digitorum sheath (*arrow*) and enhancing synovitis of the left long finger distal interphalangeal joint (*arrowhead*). (*B*) Transverse postcontrast fat-suppressed short TR/TE (T1-weighted) image demonstrates tenosynovitis of the right index and long finger and left index and ring finger flexor digitorum tendons (*arrows*). Prominent tenosynovitis, asymmetric disease, and distal joint involvement are common findings in psoriatic arthritis.

feet early in the disease,[27] often first attacking the second and third metacarpophalangeal or finger proximal interphalangeal joints (see **Fig. 4**).[28] In some patients, RA can be accurately diagnosed using MR imaging before they meet the ACR definition. Sugimoto and colleagues[29] found that MR imaging evidence of synovitis in the wrists, meta-carpophalangeal, or proximal interphalangeal joints bilaterally, combined with only one clinical finding—either a positive serum rheumatoid factor or arthritis affecting 3 or more joints—predicted development of RA with a 94% accuracy, better than the 81% to 84% accuracy with the traditional diagnostic criteria. Using MR imaging evidence of synovitis to support a diagnosis of early RA is highly sensitive even in patients with absent anti-CCP antibodies.[30] More importantly, regardless of the stage of the disease, MR imaging showing active synovitis is a strong predictor of later erosive disease[31,32] and affects the decision to begin DMARD therapy in many rheumatology practices.

Bone marrow edema, represented by poorly marginated low signal-intensity foci in the marrow compared with muscle on T1-weighted images and hyperintensity on fat-suppressed, water-sensitive, and STIR images (**Fig. 6**), is a second important imaging finding in early RA. Histologically these regions actually represent true osteitis with cellular inflammatory infiltrates,[33,34] not edema (free water) per se, although the term bone "edema" is commonly used nevertheless. There is growing evidence that these infiltrates of activated lymphocytes and osteoclasts may mediate development of erosions from the inside of the bone,[34] which would represent a second mechanism (in addition to bone invasion from the outside by pannus) of erosion formation. Bone edema usually occurs in the presence of synovitis and within the subchondral bone (**Fig. 7**), but it may occasionally be seen without accompanying synovitis [35] and deeper within bone. In the hands and wrists, the presence of bone edema is the strongest predictor of future development and progression of erosions [36–39] as well as an independent prognosticator of poor functional outcome.[34]

The third key imaging finding in RA is bone erosions,[40] characterized by circumscribed regions

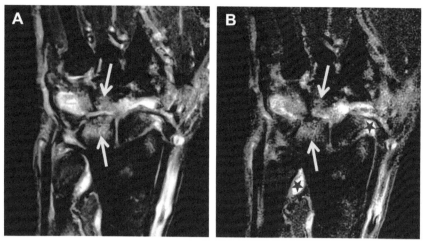

Fig. 6. Marrow edema. A 50-year-old man with rheumatoid arthritis and erosions (not shown). (*A*) Coronal STIR image though the wrist shows high signal intensity throughout several carpal bones (*arrows*). (*B*) Coronal post-contrast, fat-suppressed short TR/TE (T1-weighted) image demonstrates enhancement in the corresponding bones (*arrows*), as well as enhancing synovitis throughout all the wrist compartments (*stars*). Although the term marrow "edema" is commonly applied, the bone enhancement is due to a cellular inflammatory infiltrate and the term "osteitis" is probably more accurate.

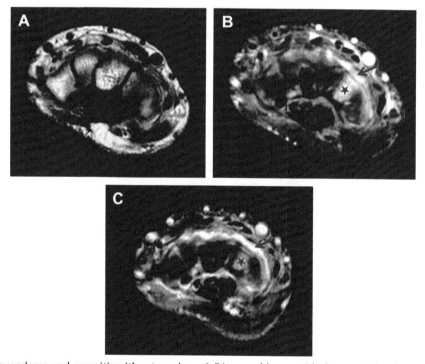

Fig. 7. Marrow edema and synovitis without erosions. A 54-year-old man with rheumatoid arthritis and morning stiffness. Transverse (*A*) short TR/TE (T1-weighted), (*B*) fat-suppressed water-sensitive fast spin-echo (T2-weighted), and (*C*) postcontrast fat-suppressed short TR/TE (T1-weighted) images of the wrist show enhancing marrow edema (*stars*) and synovitis (*arrows*) in the wrist. The patient had no erosions radiographically or on the remaining MR images. He was placed on disease modifying antirheumatoid drugs because marrow edema and synovitis are considered precursors of cartilage loss and bone erosion.

of marrow replacement along articular surfaces associated with disruption of the overlying cortex. Necessitating that erosions meet these criteria in 2 imaging planes will increase specificity and further help distinguish erosions from bone edema (**Fig. 8**). Erosions are considered a relatively late, irreversible finding in RA,[41] rarely occurring in the absence of synovitis (**Fig. 9**).[32] Nevertheless, because MR imaging is so much more sensitive than radiographs, it is common to find erosions on MR images even in cases where early disease was expected based on normal radiographs (**Fig. 10**).[42,43] Only 20% to 25% of erosions identified on MR imaging will eventually become evident radiographically, and those that do will typically undergo several years of growth before they become visible.[41] Whereas isolated erosions may occur in the normal population, increasing in incidence with age,[10] multiple erosions or erosions seen in the presence of synovitis are highly associated with RA, even in patients with negative serologic tests for anti-CCP antibodies.[30,44]

Joint space narrowing from diffuse cartilage loss and focal chondral erosions are features of RA that can be demonstrated on MR imaging,[45,46] although this is much easier to appreciate in larger articulations rather than in the hand and wrist joints (**Fig. 11**). Measurements of cartilage volume are excluded from the MR imaging scoring system because of poor reliability in the small joints of the hand and wrist.[47] Similarly, while tenosynovitis often appears in RA patients,[48] scoring of tendon and tendon sheath disease does not enter into systematic scoring systems (**Figs. 12 and 13**).[49] Rheumatoid nodules are the most common extra-articular manifestation of RA and usually form on the extensor surfaces of the elbow, hand, foot, heel, and ischial tuberosity. These nodules may present as either solid or cystic masses depending on the stage of histopathologic evolution.[50,51] Although these nodules can be identified with MR imaging, they are typically clinically evident.

In instances when MR imaging of the hands and wrists is normal but there is still strong suspicion of early RA, there may be added value to performing MR imaging examination of the dominant forefoot to assess the metatarsophalangeal joints.[52]

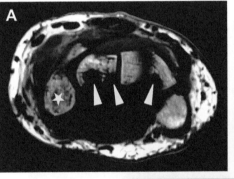
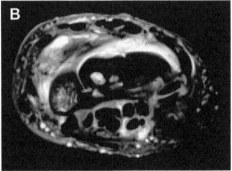
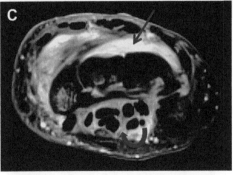

Fig. 8. Erosions and bone marrow edema. A 27-year-old woman with rheumatoid arthritis and wrist swelling. (*A*) Transverse short TR/TE (T1-weighted) images through the wrist show erosions (*arrowheads*) as relatively sharply marginated, low signal-intensity lesions in the carpal bones with focal disruption of the overlying cortex. By contrast, an area of bone marrow edema (*star*) is only slightly hypointense to the normal fatty marrow, has a reticulated, ill-defined margin, and is in a bone with intact cortex. (*B*) Transverse fat-suppressed water-sensitive fast spin-echo (T2-weighted) and (*C*) postcontrast short TR/TE (T1-weighted) images show that both the erosions (*arrowheads* in *A*) and marrow edema (*star* in *A*) are hyperintense and enhancing. Note the severe, enhancing wrist synovitis (*arrow* in *C*) and tenosynovitis of the carpal tunnel (*curved arrow* in *C*).

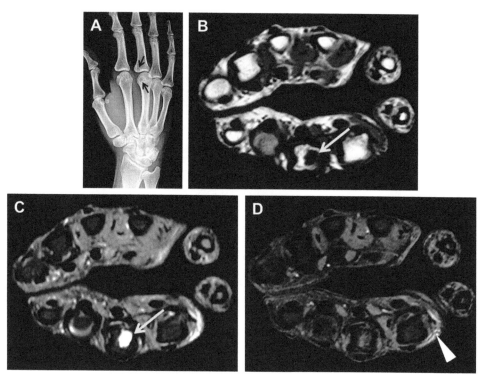

Fig. 9. Erosions without synovitis. A 41-year-old woman with rheumatoid arthritis and joint pain. (A) Oblique radiograph of the hand shows erosions in the long finger proximal phalangeal base and metacarpal head (*arrows*). (B) Transverse, short TR/TE (T1-weighted) and (C) fat-suppressed water-sensitive fast spin-echo (T2-weighted) images show the erosion in the third metacarpal head (*arrows*). (D) Transverse postcontrast short TR/TE (T1-weighted) image shows no enhancement of the erosion within the third metacarpophalangeal joint. However, there is periarticular inflammation of the right second metacarpophalangeal joint (*arrowhead*). The presence of erosions does not automatically indicate active synovitis because erosions persist even during periods of disease remission; intravenous contrast administration is necessary to demonstrate synovitis.

After the hands and feet, the cervical spine is the most common site of RA involvement. Larger joints, such as the knee, ankle, and elbow, are usually involved later in the disease (**Fig. 14**). Synovial proliferation and fluid accumulation within these joints result in expansion of the joint capsule with formation of adjacent bursae (**Fig. 15**).[53] In large joints, tendon rupture as a result of chronic tenosynovitis or adjacent bursitis is a frequent cause of morbidity in patients with long-standing RA similar to the finger tendons. Commonly involved tendons include the posterior tibialis and rotator cuff (**Fig. 16**).[54,55]

Future resexarch and clinical applications for MR imaging in the detection, monitoring, and treatment of RA will likely focus on synovitis. For clinical purposes, documenting the presence or absence of synovitis on static postcontrast images is often sufficient. However, investigators will often quantify the amount of inflammation and/or the enhancement kinetics using dynamic contrast administration. The volume of synovitis can be semiquantitatively scored as outlined by the OMERACT group or precisely measured. Quantitative synovial measurements are highly accurate but cumbersome and time-consuming without automated methods, and therefore best suited for small detailed studies. Semiquantitative scoring methods are more versatile and may be useful in both clinical settings and larger study trials.[56,57] Dynamic imaging entails rapid repetitive acquisition of images at a single slice position following bolus injection of intravenous contrast. Early enhancement, especially in the first 30 to 60 seconds after contrast administration, correlates highly with histologic evidence of active inflammation.[58] However, before it is accepted in clinical applications, automated methods of data analysis for dynamic imaging will need to be developed.

Juvenile Idiopathic Arthritis

The International League for Rheumatology (ILAR) defines JIA as a heterogeneous group of arthropathies with onset before 16 years of age and duration of at least 6 weeks; JIA affects an estimated

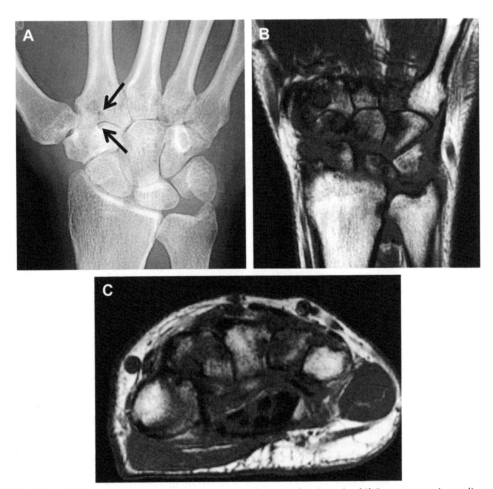

Fig. 10. Erosions. A 40-year-old man with rheumatoid arthritis and wrist pain. (A) Posteroanterior radiograph of the wrist shows mild intercarpal and carpometacarpal joint space narrowing and small erosions involving the second carpometacarpal joint (arrows), and possibly the base of the fourth metacarpal. (B) Coronal and (C) transverse short TR/TE (T1-weighted) images obtained the same day show additional erosions in virtually every carpal bone as well as the distal radius and ulna. Because of its ability to obtain thin slices in multiple planes and its high sensitivity to bone marrow changes, MR imaging is much more sensitive than radiographs for the detection of erosions.

30,000 to 50,000 patients in the United States.[59] The current JIA classification criteria replace earlier ones developed in the United States and Europe for juvenile RA and juvenile chronic arthritis. Six subtypes are recognized, 4 of which (systemic arthritis, oligoarthritis, and rheumatoid factor [RhF] positive and negative polyarthritis) share some features with adult-onset RA.[60]

The distribution of affected joints and disease course differs within each subgroup, although in general the knee is involved in up to 90% of cases (Fig. 17). Although onset is in childhood, more than half of patients will continue to have active disease as adults. The systemic arthritis subtype includes children with joint inflammation and fever who also demonstrate extensive extra-articular

manifestations, including rashes, lymphadenopathy, hepatosplenomegaly, and/or serositis. Ocular involvement is rare. The most frequently involved joints are the temporomandibular joints, wrists, knees, and ankles. Oligoarthritis, the most common subtype, classically presents in preschool-age girls with knee or ankle arthritis. This subgroup frequently demonstrates positive antinuclear antibodies (ANA) and uveitis, an asymptomatic condition that potentially threatens vision. RhF-negative polyarthritis can present at any age during childhood with marked variability in the severity of disease. Commonly affected joints are the same as those of systemic arthritis. RhF-positive polyarthritis is usually diagnosed in adolescent girls. Patients have a symmetric

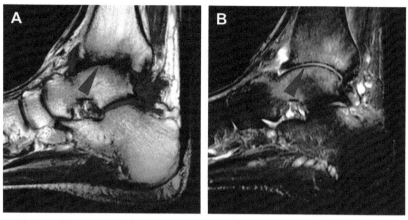

Fig. 11. Cartilage loss and marrow edema in the ankle. A 57-year-old man with ankle pain and stiffness. (A) Sagittal short TR/TE (T1-weighted) and (B) STIR images show uniform articular cartilage loss in the tibiotalar joint (arrowheads) with adjacent marrow edema. In joints larger than those of the hand and wrist, the normal articular cartilage is usually thick enough so that cartilage loss can be directly visualized on MR images. The subtalar joint shows similar, but less severe, findings.

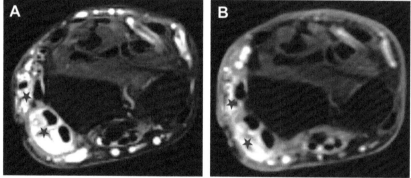

Fig. 12. Tenosynovitis without tendinitis. A 54-year-old woman with RA and wrist pain. (A) Transverse fat-suppressed water sensitive fast spin-echo (T2-weighted) and (B) postcontrast, fat-suppressed short TR/TE (T1-weighted) images through the distal forearm demonstrate tenosynovitis of the first and second extensor tendon compartments (stars), but normal morphology and signal intensity of the adjacent tendons.

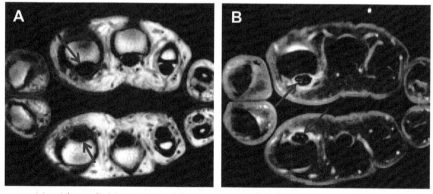

Fig. 13. Tenosynovitis with tendinitis. A 41-year-old woman with RA, hand pain, and stiffness. (A) Transverse short TR/TE (T1-weighted) image through the metacarpals shows streaks of high internal signal intensity within the flexor digitorum superficialis and profundus tendons of both index fingers (arrows). (B) Transverse postcontrast short TR/TE (T1-weighted) image shows surrounding enhancing tenosynovitis and enhancement within the tendon substance (arrows). Inflammation that involves the tendons indicates tendinitis and may be an indicator of impending tendon rupture. At the authors' institution, these changes are used as one indication for prophylactic tenosynovectomy.

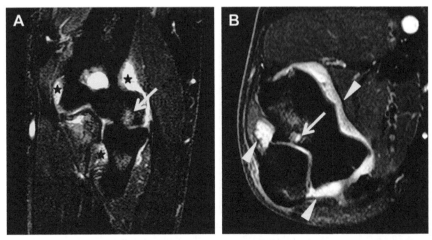

Fig. 14. Rheumatoid arthritis in the elbow. A 49-year-old man with bilateral elbow pain. (*A*) Oblique coronal fat-suppressed water-sensitive fast spin-echo (T2-weighted) image shows high signal-intensity marrow edema (*arrow*) and joint distention (*stars*). (*B*) Transverse postcontrast fat-suppressed short TR/TE (T1-weighted) image confirms that the joint distention is due to enhancing synovitis (*arrowheads*). There is also a focal erosion in the olecranon fossa (*arrow*).

polyarthritis that targets the wrist, metacarpophalangeal joints, and proximal interphalangeal joints, and commonly progresses to erosive joint destruction, a pattern typical of adult-onset RA. The temporomandibular joints, cervical spine, hips, knees, and midfeet are also commonly affected.[61]

As with RA, MR imaging is a sensitive modality for assessing disease activity, progression, and response to therapy in JIA.[62,63] However, there are unique technical, safety, and diagnostic challenges when imaging children with MR imaging that restrict its routine use.[64,65] Examination time and expense may be prohibitive, and many younger children require sedation to complete an

MR imaging study. A comprehensive examination of several involved joints is often desirable but logistically difficult, given the excessive time required when using multiple individual local coils or the limited resolution achieved with whole-body techniques. Furthermore, compared with the large body of evidence validating MR imaging as an outcome measure in RA, experience in the assessment of JIA is small. For these reasons, sonography may be a preferable method to assess articular pathology such as effusions, synovitis, cartilage thinning and erosions, and extra-articular abnormalities such as tenosynovitis and bursitis, in JIA. Sonography can also guide diagnostic joint aspirations and therapeutic joint

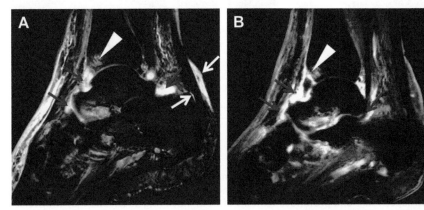

Fig. 15. RA in the hindfoot. A 70-year-old woman with ankle pain and morning stiffness. (*A*) Sagittal STIR and (*B*) postcontrast fat-suppressed short TR/TE (T1-weighted) images demonstrate enhancing osteitis (*arrowheads*) in the distal tibia and active synovitis in the ankle, subtalar, and talonavicular joints (*red arrows*). Note also the bursitis (*white arrows*) both superficial and deep to the distal Achilles tendon.

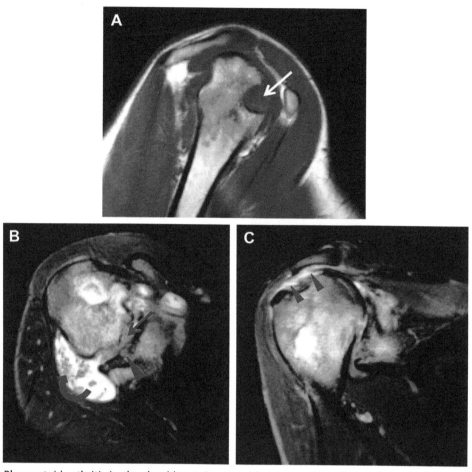

Fig. 16. Rheumatoid arthritis in the shoulder. A 24-year-old woman with polyarticular pain. (*A*) Sagittal short TR/TE (T1-weighted) image showing large erosion in the humeral head (*arrow*). (*B*) Transverse fat-suppressed water-sensitive fast spin-echo (T2-weighted) image demonstrates hypertrophic synovitis or pannus (*arrow*) ulcerating the adjacent articular cartilage (*arrowhead*) and rice bodies (*curved arrow*) in the glenohumeral joint. Contrast is not necessary to diagnose synovitis when there is nodularity of the synovium or pannus directly invading the articular cartilage. (*C*) Coronal fat-suppressed water sensitive fast spin-echo (T2-weighted) image also shows a full-thickness supraspinatus tendon tear (*arrowheads*).

injections.[66] Nonetheless, given MR imaging's superior sensitivity in detecting synovitis, unique ability to detect bone marrow edema, and access to deep structures such as spine, temporomandibular, and SI joints that cannot be examined sonographically, MR imaging remains an essential clinical and research tool in JIA.[67] Detecting joint inflammation using MR imaging is especially important to measure treatment response in children with JIA, given the side effects of systemic steroids, methotrexate, and other DMARDs used to control the disease.

Definitions of joint and soft tissue MR imaging findings, and the sequences used to detect them are the same in JIA as in RA, but the sequelae of chronic joint inflammation in the immature skeleton differ from those seen in adult patients.

Morphologic findings in the articular cartilage are rare in very young patients. However, hyperemia due to chronic inflammation directly affects the epiphyseal and growth cartilage, often leading to epiphyseal overgrowth, premature closure of the physes, growth arrest, and malalignments. Hyperemia can also cause joint ankylosis, a characteristic of JIA but not RA, most commonly affecting the tarsometatarsal joints, carpal articulations, and cervical facets (**Fig. 18**).[68]

Seronegative Spondyloarthropathies

The spondyloarthopathies are a diverse group of diseases linked by a shared genetic predisposition (association with the HLA-B27 gene), involvement of the axial skeleton, and enthesitis as a prominent

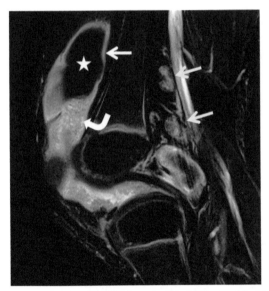

Fig. 17. MR imaging findings in JIA. A 3-year-old girl with 7 weeks of knee pain after a fall. Sagittal post-contrast fat-suppressed short TR/TE (T1-weighted) image demonstrates several classic features of JIA including enhancing synovitis (*white arrow*), nonen-hancing joint effusion (*star*), and popliteal lymphade-nopathy (*yellow arrows*). Note the frond-like pattern of synovial proliferation (*curved white arrow*). The patient was diagnosed with oligoarticular JIA, and treated with oral nonsteroidal anti-inflammatory drugs and intra-articular steroid injection.

pathologic feature in addition to synovitis (unlike RA, which lacks enthesitis). Spondyloarthopathies include ankylosing spondylitis, psoriatic arthritis (PsA), reactive arthritis, and enteropathic arthritis. The JIA psoriatic and enthesitis-related subtypes also share many features with the adult spondy-loarthropathies, with the exception that spinal involvement in enthesitis-related arthritis often does not occur until adulthood. Patients who do not meet specific diagnostic criteria are character-ized as having undifferentiated disease. Serum from patients with spondyloarthritis is often RhF negative ("seronegative"), but demonstrates elevated erythrocyte sedimentation rate and C-reactive protein.[69]

Psoriatic arthritis is the prototypic spondy-loarthropathy that affects the peripheral joints, and occurs in up to 20% of patients with psoriasis. In PsA, dermatologic disease precedes joint involvement in all but 15% to 20% of cases and may include psoriatic plaques, nail pitting, and/or onycholysis.[70] Clinical presentations vary, with most patients having either oligoarthritic or symmetric polyarthritic forms, and a minority (approximately 5% of patients) with axial disease, characterized by sacroiliitis and spondylitis. Most commonly affected locations (in descend-ing order) are the knee, proximal hand and feet interphalangeal, metatarsophalangeal, ankle,

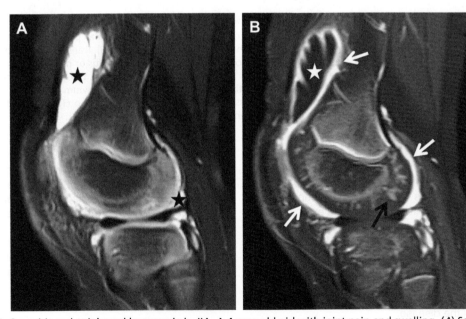

Fig. 18. Synovitis and epiphyseal hyperemia in JIA. A 4-year-old girl with joint pain and swelling. (*A*) Sagittal fat-suppressed water-sensitive fast spin-echo (T2-weighted) image of the right knee. Without contrast, it is not possible to distinguish between a joint effusion and synovitis (*black stars*). (*B*) Sagittal postcontrast fat-suppressed short TR/TE (T1-weighted) image of the knee clearly separates active enhancing synovitis (*white arrows*) from the nonenhancing joint effusion (*white star*). Also note the hyperemic epiphyseal cartilage (*black arrow*). The knee is the most commonly affected joint in JIA.

metacarpophalangeal, and distal interphalangeal joints (**Fig. 19**). Dactylitis from articular, tenosynovial, and periarticular inflammation is seen in one-third of patients, accounting for the classic "sausage digit" appearance of fingers and toes (**Fig. 20**).[71] Radiographically, reparative bone proliferation represents the healing phase of enthesitis. Periostitis and ankylosis are highly suggestive of PsA, and juxta-articular new bone formation on radiographs of the hand or foot is a diagnostic criterion of PsA according to the Classification of Psoriatic Arthritis (CASPAR) study group.[72] Reactive arthritis mimics PsA, but is typically preceded by a gastrointestinal or genitourinary infection and has a predilection for lower extremity joints.

Recently, the OMERACT group published an MR imaging scoring system for PsA in the hands (PsAMRIS-H), with characterization of key abnormalities and suggested MR imaging sequences. Definitions of synovitis, bone marrow edema, and bone erosion are the same as those for RA; additional definitions of tenosynovitis, periarticular inflammation, bone proliferation, peritendinitis, tendinitis, and tendinopathy reflect soft tissue changes throughout the digit (dactylitis) common in PsA.[73] For improved observer reproducibility, peritendinitis, tendonitis, and tendinopathy have been excluded from the scoring system even though they are recognized as important pathologic features of PsA.[74] Subsequent studies have

noted the difficulty in evaluating bone erosion, bone edema, bone proliferation, and periarticular inflammation at the proximal and distal interphalangeal joints because of their small size, which may prompt future alterations to the current scoring model.[75]

Of the spondyloarthropathies, ankylosing spondylitis (AS) is the prototype for axial disease with sacroiliitis required for diagnosis, although poor functional outcome is more closely related to spondylitis rather than sacroiliitis.[76] Patients have an insidious onset of low back pain, typically in the sacroiliac region, lasting more than 3 months that is most severe after periods of inactivity.[74] The modified New York criteria for AS diagnosis requires radiologic findings of either bilateral grade 2 sacroiliitis (small areas of erosion or reactive sclerosis without joint space narrowing) or unilateral grade 3 or 4 sacroiliitis (sclerosis, erosions, and loss of joint space in grade 3 and ankylosis in grade 4)[77] in addition to at least one clinical criteria.[78] Axial enteropathic arthritis mimics AS and runs a course independent of bowel disease. Peripheral enteropathic arthritis flares with bouts of diarrhea but tends to be nonerosive.

Patients with axial disease may be initially misclassified as having undifferentiated spondyloarthritis, because radiographic sacroiliitis may not appear until years after clinical presentation. However, more than 40% of patients with undifferentiated disease do not develop AS in long-term

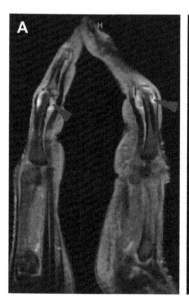
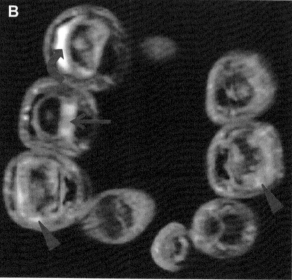

Fig. 19. Synovitis in seronegative spondyloarthropathy. A 49-year-old woman with bilateral hand stiffness. Post-contrast fat-suppressed short TR/TE (T1-weighted) images of the both hands in (*A*) sagittal and (*B*) transverse planes demonstrate synovitis of the right ring finger and left long finger proximal interphalangeal joints (*arrowheads*). Tenosynovitis of the right long finger flexor digitorum tendon (*arrow*) and synovitis of the right index finger proximal interphalangeal joint (*curved arrow*) are demonstrated on the transverse image.

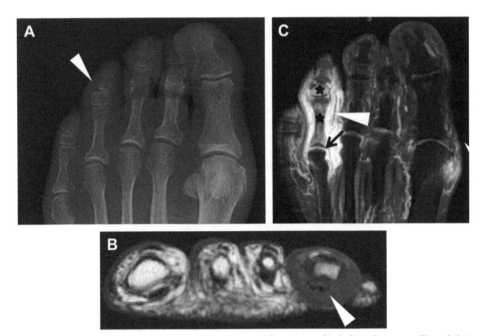

Fig. 20. Dactylitis. A 63-year-old woman, HLA B27 positive, with 2 years of left fourth toe swelling. (*A*) Dorsoplantar radiograph of the left foot shows diffuse soft tissue swelling of the symptomatic toe (*arrowhead*). (*B*) Transverse short TR/TE (T1-weighted) image of the left forefoot demonstrates circumferential swelling of the digit with edema of the subcutaneous fat (*arrowhead*). (*C*) Long-axis postcontrast fat-suppressed short TR/TE (T1-weighted) image shows diffuse enhancement of the bone (*stars*), joints (*arrow*), and soft tissues (*arrowhead*) of the digit representing dactylitis, a finding characteristic of the seronegative spondyloarthropathies. There was no soft tissue ulcer to suggest an infectious cause.

outcome studies. Therefore, MR imaging of the spine and SI joints in this population is an important tool in identifying patients who may benefit from early intervention.[79] Furthermore, in many individuals, axial disease may run a relatively benign course without treatment,[80] so that even in patients with an established diagnosis, MR imaging is useful to determine whether active inflammation is present that would require DMARD therapy.

Relevant imaging features and definitions for active sacroiliitis on MR imaging are outlined in the Assessment of SpondyloArthritis international Society (ASAS) classification criteria for axial spondyloarthritis. At a minimum, images should be obtained in a semicoronal plane parallel to the dorsal aspect of S1 and S3. Images perpendicular to this semicoronal plane may also be useful. Active inflammatory lesions are best demonstrated on STIR and postcontrast T1-weighted fat-suppressed images. Associated erosions, reactive sclerosis, and ankylosis can be seen on routine noncontrast T1-weighted images; if indeterminate on MR imaging, these findings are easily depicted by computed tomography.[81]

The ASAS criteria for active sacroiliitis on MR imaging require demonstration of typical subchondral or periarticular bone marrow edema or osteitis

(Fig. 21). In isolation—that is, without adjacent bone marrow edema or osteitis—synovitis, enthesitis, and capsulitis are insufficient for diagnosis of sacroiliitis. Similarly, structural lesions (erosions and/or ankylosis) that occur without concomitant bone marrow inflammation likely reflect prior episodes of inflammation, and therefore do not meet strict criteria for active sacroiliitis. Adjacent marrow that has undergone fatty differentiation indicates quiescent, nonactive disease. If there is only one focus of bone marrow edema for each MR imaging slice, it should be present on at least 2 consecutive 3-mm or 4-mm slices. Multiple foci of bone marrow edema in a single MR imaging slice are sufficient to suggest active inflammation.[82] Of note, the recent MORPHO study, which evaluated the diagnostic utility of MR imaging in spondyloarthritis using a simplified set of MR imaging sequences and lesions, may ultimately result in alterations to the ASAS criteria.[83] Further validation studies will be needed to resolve this issue.

CRYSTALLINE-INDUCED ARTHROPATHIES

The most common crystalline deposition diseases involve monosodium urate crystals (gout), calcium pyrophosphate dihydrate crystals (calcium

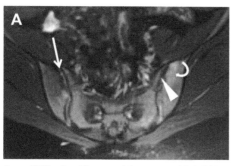
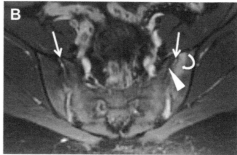

Fig. 21. Sacroiliitis. An 18-year-old woman, HLA B27 positive, with low back pain. (*A*) Transverse fat-suppressed water-sensitive fast spin-echo (T2-weighted) and (*B*) postcontrast fat-suppressed short TR/TE (T1-weighted) images of the sacroiliac joints demonstrate synovitis (*arrows*) and an erosion (*arrowheads*) of the synovial portion of the joint. Osteitis, most severe in the left iliac bone, is also present (*curved arrows*), consistent with active inflammation.

pyrophosphate deposition [CPPD] disease), and calcium hydroxyapatite (hydroxyapatite deposition disease [HADD]). Synovitis and soft tissue inflammation develop secondarily in response to crystal deposition, distinguishing these conditions from the primary inflammatory arthritides. Acute gout is usually a monoarticular disease with a predilection for the first metatarsophalangeal joint. Tophaceous gout is characterized by mass-like deposits of monosodium urate that can occur in virtually any tissue, including synovium, cartilage, tendon, ligament, bone, and bursa, and can mimic infection or neoplasm on imaging. Crystal deposition can weaken ligaments or tendons, leading to rupture. CPPD has a highly variable clinical presentation, ranging from asymptomatic to acute episodes of pseudo-gout, to a chronic destructive arthropathy. The chronic form resembles osteoarthritis, but with a predilection for

non–weight-bearing joints, such as the radiocarpal, metacarpophalangeal, elbow, and glenohumeral joints, and a bilateral, symmetric distribution. The patellofemoral joint is also commonly affected. HADD is characterized by periarticular calcifications deposited in tendons ("calcific tendinitis"), bursae, ligaments, and rarely within joints. The disease affects older patients who present with pain, swelling, erythema, and limited range of motion of the adjacent joint.

Clinical evaluation, complemented by laboratory testing and potential arthrocentesis, are frequently sufficient for disease identification. If clinically equivocal, radiographs are often diagnostic, demonstrating features such as calcified tophi in long-standing gout, chondrocalcinosis in CPPD, and soft tissue calcification in HADD. MR imaging is not used for primary diagnosis in these diseases. Rather, manifestations of these diseases may be

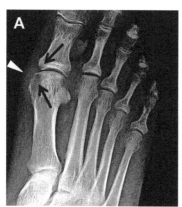
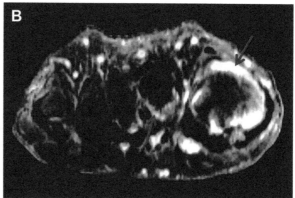

Fig. 22. Acute gout. A 63-year-old man with toe redness and pain. (*A*) Dorsoplantar radiograph of the foot shows focal soft tissue swelling medial to the first metatarsophalangeal joint (*arrowhead*) with erosions of the subjacent bones (*arrows*). Note the relative lack of joint space narrowing. (*B*) Short-axis postcontrast fat-suppressed short TR/TE (T1-weighted) image shows enhancing synovitis in the first and second metatarsophalangeal joints (*arrows*). Involvement of more than one joint as well as absence of a soft tissue ulcer and joint narrowing would be atypical for infectious arthritis.

observed on MR imaging in cases where patients are referred for undiagnosed joint pain or suspected infection or when imaged for comorbid conditions.

In acute gout, periarticular soft tissue swelling, inflammation, and a joint effusion can be detected on MR imaging (**Fig. 22**). Soft tissue tophi can erode adjacent bones, sparing the articular cartilage until late in disease. These erosions may develop an overhanging edge as reparative bone attempts to contain and encircle the tophus. On MR imaging, tophus is usually isointense to slightly hypointense to muscle on short-TE images, with near-homogeneous enhancement following intravenous contrast injection. T2-weighted signal characteristics are highly variable, presumably due to differences in internal calcium concentrations (**Fig. 23**).[84] Commonly affected areas include the foot (metatarsophalangeal joint), hand and wrist (bilateral asymmetric involvement), elbow (presenting with olecranon bursitis), and knee (marginal tibial and femoral erosions with joint space preservation and occasional prepatellar bursitis).[85] In nontophaceous disease, the imaging findings may mimic those of primary inflammatory or infectious arthritis, necessitating clinical differentiation (see **Fig. 22**).

Within the knee and wrist, CPPD affects primarily the patellofemoral and radiocarpal

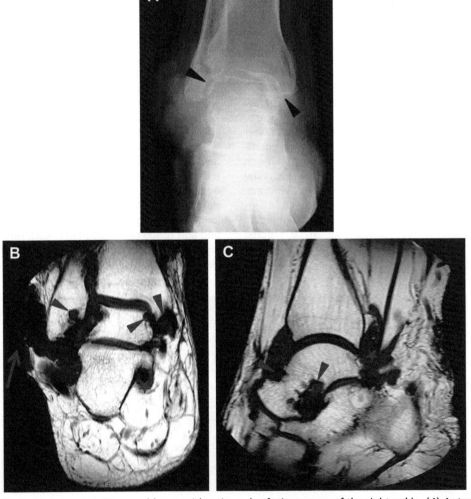

Fig. 23. Tophaceous gout. A 60-year-old man with pain and soft tissue mass of the right ankle. (*A*) Anteroposterior non–weight-bearing radiograph shows a dense mass over the lateral malleolus with erosions of the distal fibula and medial malleolus (*arrowheads*). Note the preservation of the tibiotalar joint space. (*B*) Coronal and (*C*) sagittal short TR/TE (T1-weighted) images performed in an extremity magnet show the hypointense tophus that accounts for the lateral ankle mass (*arrow*). Intra-articular tophus has resulted in bimalleolar and talar erosions (*arrowheads*) and fills the flexor hallucis longus tendon sheath (*stars*).

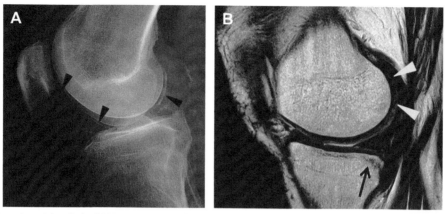

Fig. 24. Chondrocalcinosis in CPPD. A 65-year-old man with left knee pain. (*A*) Lateral radiograph of the knee clearly demonstrates chondrocalcinosis of the articular cartilage (*arrowheads*). (*B*) Sagittal high resolution water-sensitive fast spin-echo (T2-weighted) image shows speckled areas of low signal intensity in the articular cartilage of the posterior medial femoral condyle (*arrowheads*), a finding much more subtle on MR imaging than on radiograph. Also note the nondisplaced subchondral fracture of the medial tibial plateau (*arrow*).

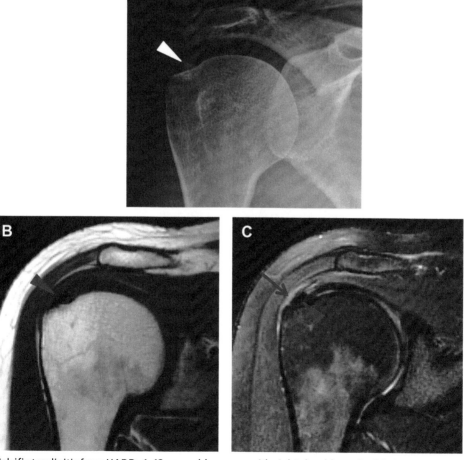

Fig. 25. Calcific tendinitis from HADD. A 42-year-old woman with right shoulder pain. (*A*) Anteroposterior radiograph of the shoulder demonstrates amorphous calcification adjacent to the greater tuberosity. Oblique coronal (*B*) short TR/TE (T1-weighted) and (*C*) fat-suppressed water-sensitive fast spin-echo (T2-weighted) images show hypointense signal in the supraspinatus tendon (*arrowhead*) with adjacent subacromial/subdeltoid bursitis (*arrow*). Findings are consistent with calcific tendinitis from HADD.

compartments. Subchondral cyst formation and chondrocalcinosis are characteristic features, though not universally present. Calcium pyrophosphate deposits in the soft tissues are typically easier to identify on radiographs rather than MR imaging (**Fig. 24**). Depending on their concentration, calcium crystals may bloom on gradient-echo recalled images, increasing their conspicuity.

Hydroxyapatite deposits may lie dormant in tissues for a long period of time without inciting an inflammatory response. Once active, however, HADD may have an aggressive appearance on MR imaging that mimics trauma, infection, or malignancy because of extensive marrow and soft tissue edema. The shoulder, and specifically the supraspinatus tendon, is the most commonly affected site (**Fig. 25**).[86]

INFECTIOUS ARTHRITIS

Joint infection results from 1 of 4 routes of contamination: (1) hematogenous seeding; (2) intra-articular extension from a contiguous source; (3) direct inoculation; and (4) postoperative infection. Regardless of cause, septic arthritis can result in catastrophic damage to the affected joint and surrounding structures.[87]

Septic arthritis is not an imaging diagnosis; when suspected clinically, arthrocentesis is indicated. MR imaging findings of septic arthritis are nonspecific and should not delay diagnostic joint aspiration. Joint effusions or synovitis are nonspecific findings caused by primary inflammatory, traumatic, and degenerative conditions as well as by infection. The value of MR imaging in septic

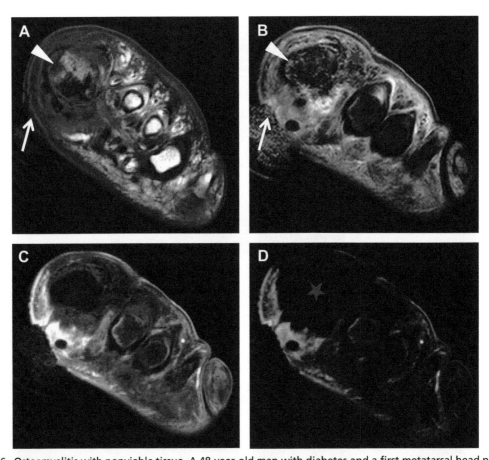

Fig. 26. Osteomyelitis with nonviable tissue. A 48-year-old man with diabetes and a first metatarsal head plantar ulcer. Short-axis (*A*) short TR/TE (T1-weighted) and (*B*) fat-suppressed water-sensitive fast spin-echo (T2-weighted) images of the forefoot demonstrate osteomyelitis of the first metatarsal head (*arrowheads*). Note the plantar soft tissue ulcer (*arrows*) and soft tissue gas (*stars*). (*C*) Contrast was given to assess for tissue viability, followed by acquisition of short-axis fat-suppressed short TR/TE (T1-weighted) images. (*D*) Subtraction of the precontrast and postcontrast T1-weighted images clearly show the nonenhancing first metatarsal and surrounding soft tissue (*star*). The presence of necrotic tissue is an indication for surgical rather than conservative management of pedal osteomyelitis.

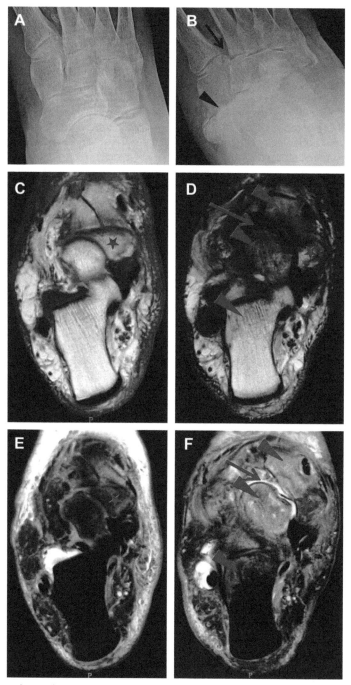

Fig. 27. Neuropathic arthropathy. A 68-year-old woman with diabetic neuropathy and right foot erythema and swelling. Sequential images of the right foot taken 1 month apart; initial presentation on the left. (*A, B*) Dorso-plantar radiographs of the right foot show mild soft tissue swelling surrounding the midfoot. There has been rapid, progressive destruction of the tarsal navicular bone (*arrowhead*), with resultant destruction of the Chopart and Lisfranc joints (*arrow*). (*C, D*) Transverse short TR/TE (T1-weighted) and (*E, F*) fat-suppressed water-sensitive fast spin-echo (T2-weighted) images of the right hindfoot show subcutaneous edema, progressive fragmentation of the navicular (*star*), development of marrow edema in the talus, calcaneus and medial cuneiform (*arrow-heads*), and destruction of the Chopart joint (*arrow*). There was no soft tissue ulcer on the MR images, and there were no systemic signs of infection. Findings are characteristic of neuropathic arthropathy.

arthritis lies in detecting associated complications such as adjacent osteomyelitis, abscesses, or retained foreign bodies, and in defining the extent of infection—findings that may alter management. Of particular importance is the use of intravenous contrast when imaging musculoskeletal infections to detect areas of nonenhancement, which are easily identified with subtraction of the precontrast and postcontrast T1-weighted images. Intravenous contrast improves conspicuity of small soft tissue abscesses and can determine the viability of adjacent infected bone and soft tissue,[88] with the assumption that nonenhancing tissue is necrotic and should be debrided (**Fig. 26**).[89]

One unique MR imaging differential diagnosis involves the distinction between septic arthritis with osteomyelitis and neuropathic arthropathy in patients with diabetic foot disease. In the acute phase, either can present with erythema and swelling. The vast majority of cases of septic arthritis with pedal osteomyelitis occur because of an adjacent skin ulcer or sinus tract. Infection tends to occur in sites at risk for developing soft tissue ulcers such as the tips and dorsum of the toes, first and fifth metatarsal heads, calcaneus, and malleoli. Infection spreads centripetally, beginning where the ulcer or sinus tract contacts bone. Deformity of the foot is uncommon, unless neuropathic arthropathy is already present.

Neuropathic arthropathy, on the other hand, is a bone-centered process with intact overlying skin. Bone findings of fragmentation, cyst formation, and marrow edema predominate; joint disease occurs secondarily, due to acquired incongruence of the articulating bone surfaces. Multiple joints within a region of the foot are usually involved, most commonly the Lisfranc and Chopart joints. With time acute inflammation may subside, associated with decreased marrow edema and enhancement. Eventual development of osteosclerosis and osteonecrosis will manifest as hypointensity of bone marrow signal on all imaging sequences (**Fig. 27**). When infection is superimposed on neuropathic arthropathy, subchondral cysts are less apparent, the bone cortices are eroded, and there is extensive marrow and soft tissue edema and enhancement with an associated ulcer or sinus tract. If imaging or clinical presentation is inconclusive, bone biopsy or joint aspiration is recommended for diagnosis.[90]

SUMMARY

Untreated inflammatory, crystalline-induced, and infectious arthritides may all lead to advanced cartilage destruction. However, when specific treatment is instituted during the early stages of the disease process, joint destruction may be avoidable. The primary role of MR imaging in these conditions is to identify key findings that occur before the articular cartilage is affected, so that timely therapy can be instituted. For rheumatic diseases, active synovitis and osteitis are the best predictors of future bone and cartilage erosions, and MR imaging has become a mainstay of both initial diagnosis and posttreatment surveillance. Crystalline-induced and infectious arthritis are typically diagnosed by means other than imaging. However, MR imaging is still useful in atypical or confusing cases to narrow the differential diagnosis and in established cases for staging the extent of disease, which ultimately affects surgical and medical treatment.

REFERENCES

1. Kroot EJ, de Jong BA, van Leeuwen MA, et al. The prognostic value of anti-cyclic citrullinated peptide antibody in patients with recent-onset rheumatoid arthritis. Arthritis Rheum 2000;43(8):1831–5.
2. Emery P. Treatment of rheumatoid arthritis. BMJ 2006;332:152–5.
3. Smolen JS, Landewe R, Breedveld FC. EULAR recommendations for the management of rheumatoid arthritis with synthetic and biological disease-modifying antirheumatic drugs. Ann Rheum Dis 2010;69:964–75.
4. Conaghan PG, Ejbjerg B, Lassere M, et al. A multicenter reliability study of extremity-magnetic resonance imaging in the longitudinal evaluation of rheumatoid arthritis. J Rheumatol 2007;34:857–8.
5. Bird P, Ejbjerg B, Lassere M, et al. A multireader reliability study comparing conventional high-field magnetic resonance imaging with extremity low-field MRI in rheumatoid arthritis. J Rheumatol 2007;34:854–6.
6. Duer-Jensen A, Ejbjerg B, Albrecht-Beste E, et al. Does low-field dedicated extremity MRI (E-MRI) reliably detect bone erosions in rheumatoid arthritis? A comparison of two different E-MRI units and conventional radiography with high-resolution CT scanning. Ann Rheum Dis 2009;68:1296–302.
7. Yao L, Magalnick M, Wilson M, et al. Periarticular bone findings in rheumatoid arthritis: T2-weighted versus contrast-enhanced T1-weighted MRI. AJR 2006;187:358–63.
8. McQueen FM. The MRI view of synovitis and tenosynovitis in inflammatory arthritis: implications for diagnosis and management. Ann N Y Acad Sci 2009;1154:21–34.
9. McQueen FM, Stewart N, Crabbe J, et al. Magnetic resonance imaging of the wrist in early rheumatoid arthritis reveals progression of erosions despite clinical improvement. Ann Rheum Dis 1999;58:156–63.

10. Olech E, Crues JV 3rd, Yocum DE, et al. Bone marrow edema is the most specific finding for rheumatoid arthritis (RA) on noncontrast magnetic resonance imaging of the hands and wrists: a comparison of patients with RA and healthy controls. J Rheumatol 2010;37:265–74.

11. Ejbjerg B, Narvestad E, Rostrup E, et al. Magnetic resonance imaging of wrist and finger joints in healthy subjects occasionally shows changes resembling erosions and synovitis as seen in rheumatoid arthritis. Arthritis Rheum 2004;50:1097–106.

12. Drapé JL, Thelen P, Gay-Depassier P, et al. Intraarticular diffusion of Gd-DOTA after intravenous injection in the knee: MR imaging evaluation. Radiology 1993;188:227–34.

13. Majithia V, Geraci SA. Rheumatoid arthritis: diagnosis and management. Am J Med 2007;120:936–9.

14. Klippel JH, Crofford LJ, Weyand CM, et al, editors. Rheumatoid arthritis: a. epidemiology, pathology and pathogenesis. In: Primer on the rheumatic diseases. 12th edition. Atlanta (GA): Arthritis Foundation; 2001. p. 209–17.

15. Imhof H, Nöbauer-Huhmann IM, Gahleitner A, et al. Pathophysiology and imaging in inflammatory and blastomatous synovial diseases. Skeletal Radiol 2002;31:313–33.

16. Arnett FC, Edworthy SM, Bloch DA, et al. The American Rheumatism Association 1987 revised criteria for the classification of rheumatoid arthritis. Arthritis Rheum 1988;31(3):315–24.

17. Sharp JT. Radiologic assessment as an outcome measure in rheumatoid arthritis. Arthritis Rheum 1989;32(2):221–9.

18. Sommer OJ, Kladosek A, Volkmar W, et al. Rheumatoid arthritis: a practical guide to state-of-the-art imaging, image interpretation, and clinical implications. Radiographics 2005;25:381–98.

19. Østergaard M, Pedersen SJ, Døhn UM. Imaging in rheumatoid arthritis—status and recent advances for magnetic resonance imaging, ultrasonography, computed tomography and conventional radiography. Best Pract Res Clin Rheumatol 2008;22(6):1019–44.

20. Peterfy C, Edmonds J, Lassere M, et al. OMERACT rheumatoid arthritis MRI studies module. J Rheumatol 2003;30:1364–5.

21. Østergaard M, Peterfy C, Conaghan P, et al. OMERACT rheumatoid arthritis magnetic resonance imaging studies. Core set of MRI acquisitions, joint pathology definitions, and the OMERACT RA-MRI scoring system. J Rheumatol 2003;30:1385–6.

22. Ejbjerg B, McQueen F, Lassere M, et al. The EULAR-OMERACT rheumatoid arthritis MRI reference image atlas: the wrist joint. Ann Rheum Dis 2005;64:i23–47.

23. Conaghan P, Bird P, Ejbjerg B, et al. The EULAR-OMERACT rheumatoid arthritis MRI reference image atlas: the metacarpophalangeal joints. Ann Rheum Dis 2005;64:i11–21.

24. Østergaard M, Edmonds J, McQueen F, et al. An introduction to the EULAR-OMERACT rheumatoid arthritis MRI reference image atlas. Ann Rheum Dis 2005;64:i3–7.

25. Hodgson RJ, O'Connor P, Moots R. MRI of rheumatoid arthritis—image quantitation for the assessment of disease activity, progression and response to therapy. Rheumatology 2008;47:13–21.

26. Sugimoto H, Takeda A, Masuyama J, et al. Early-stage rheumatoid arthritis: diagnostic accuracy of MR imaging. Radiology 1996;198:185–92.

27. Bolster MB, Monu JUV. Rheumatoid arthritis. In: Pope TL, Bloem HL, Beltran J, et al, editors. Imaging of the musculoskeletal system, vol. II. Philadelphia: Saunders Elsevier; 2008. p. 1100–12.

28. Resnick D, Kransdorf MJ. Rheumatoid arthritis. In: Resnick D, Kransdorf MJ, editors. Bone and joint imaging. 3rd edition. Philadelphia: Saunders Elsevier; 2005. p. 226–54.

29. Sugimoto H, Takeda A, Hyodoh K. Early-stage rheumatoid arthritis: prospective study of the effectiveness of MR imaging for diagnosis. Radiology 2000;216:569–75.

30. Narváez J, Sirvent E, Narváez JA, et al. Usefulness of magnetic resonance imaging of the hand versus anticyclic citrullinated peptide antibody testing to confirm the diagnosis of clinically suspected early rheumatoid arthritis in the absence of rheumatoid factor and radiographic erosions. Semin Arthritis Rheum 2008;38:101–9.

31. Huang J, Stewart N, Crabbe J, et al. A 1-year follow-up study of dynamic magnetic resonance imaging in early rheumatoid arthritis reveals synovitis to be increased in shared epitope-positive patients and predictive of erosions at 1 year. Rheumatology (Oxford) 2000;39:407–16.

32. Conaghan PG, O'Connor P, McGonagle D, et al. Elucidation of the relationship between synovitis and bone damage: a randomized magnetic resonance imaging study of individual joints in patients with early rheumatoid arthritis. Arthritis Rheum 2003;48:64–71.

33. Jimenez-Boj E, Nöbauer-Huhmann I, Hanslik-Schnabel B, et al. Bone erosions and bone marrow edema as defined by magnetic resonance imaging reflect true bone marrow inflammation in rheumatoid arthritis. Arthritis Rheum 2007;56:1118–24.

34. McQueen FM, Ostendorf B. What is MRI bone oedema in rheumatoid arthritis and why does it matter? Arthritis Res Ther 2006;8:222.

35. McGonagle D, Conaghan PG, O'Connor P, et al. The relationship between synovitis and bone changes in early untreated rheumatoid arthritis: a controlled magnetic resonance imaging study. Arthritis Rheum 1999;42:1706–11.

36. Palosaari K, Vuotila J, Takalo R, et al. Bone oedema predicts erosive progression on wrist MRI in early

RA—a 2-yr observational MRI and NC scintigraphy study. Rheumatology (Oxford) 2006;45:1542–8.

37. McQueen FM, Benton N, Perry D, et al. Bone edema scored on magnetic resonance imaging scans of the dominant carpus at presentation predicts radiographic joint damage of the hands and feet six years later in patients with rheumatoid arthritis. Arthritis Rheum 2003;48:1814–27.

38. Haavardsholm EA, Bøyesen P, Østergaard M, et al. Magnetic resonance imaging findings in 84 patients with early rheumatoid arthritis: bone marrow oedema predicts erosive progression. Rheum Dis 2008;67: 794–800.

39. Hetland ML, Ejbjerg B, Hørslev-Petersen K, et al. MRI bone oedema is the strongest predictor of subsequent radiographic progression in early rheumatoid arthritis. Results from a 2-year randomized controlled trial (CIMESTRA). Ann Rheum Dis 2009; 68:384–90.

40. McQueen F. Magnetic resonance imaging in early inflammatory arthritis: what is its role? Rheumatology 2000;39:700–6.

41. McQueen FM, Benton N, Crabbe J, et al. What is the fate of erosions in early rheumatoid arthritis? tracking individual lesions using x rays and magnetic resonance imaging over the first two years of disease. Ann Rheum Dis 2001;60:859–68.

42. Døhn UM, Ejbjerg BJ, Hasselquist M, et al. Detection of bone erosions in rheumatoid arthritis wrist joints with magnetic resonance imaging, computed tomography and radiography. Arthritis Res Ther 2008;10:R25.

43. Østergaard M, Hansen M, Stoltenberg M, et al. New radiographic bone erosions in the wrists of patients with rheumatoid arthritis are detectable with magnetic resonance imaging a median of two years earlier. Arthritis Rheum 2003;48:2128–31.

44. Solau-Gervais E, Legrand JL, Cortet B, et al. Magnetic resonance imaging of the hand for the diagnosis of rheumatoid arthritis in the absence of anti-cyclic citrullinated peptide antibodies: a prospective study. J Rheumatol 2006;33:1760–5.

45. Forslind K, Larsson EM, Johansson A, et al. Detection of joint pathology by magnetic resonance imaging in patients with early rheumatoid arthritis. Br J Rheumatol 1997;36:683–8.

46. Uhl M, Allmann KH, Ihling C, et al. Cartilage destruction in small joints by rheumatoid arthritis: assessment of fat-suppressed three-dimensional gradient-echo MR pulse sequences in vitro. Skeletal Radiol 1998;27:677–82.

47. Østergaard M, Szkudlarek M. Magnetic resonance imaging of soft tissue changes in rheumatoid arthritis wrist joints. Semin Musculoskeletal Radiol 2001;5:257–74.

48. Eshed I, Feist E, Althoff CE, et al. Tenosynovitis of the flexor tendons of the hand detected by MRI:

an early indicator or rheumatoid arthritis. Rheumatology 2009;48:887–91.

49. McQueen F, Lassere M, Edmonds J, et al. OMERACT rheumatoid arthritis magnetic resonance imaging studies. Summary of OMERACT 6 MR imaging module. J Rheumatol 2003;30:1387–92.

50. García-Patos V. Rheumatoid nodule. Semin Cutan Med Surg 2007;26(2):100–7.

51. El-Noueam KI, Giuliano V, Schweitzer ME, et al. Rheumatoid nodules: MR/pathological correlation. J Comput Assist Tomogr 1997;21(5):796–9.

52. Ostendorf B, Scherer A, Mödder U, et al. Diagnostic value of magnetic resonance imaging of the forefeet in early rheumatoid arthritis when findings on imaging of the metacarpophalangeal joints of the hands remain normal. Arthritis Rheum 2004;50:2094–102.

53. Chen AL, Joseph TN, Zuckerman JD. Rheumatoid arthritis of the shoulder. J Am Acad Orthop Surg 2003;11:12–24.

54. Soini I, Belt EA, Niemitukia L, et al. Magnetic resonance imaging of the rotator cuff in destroyed rheumatoid shoulder: comparison with findings during shoulder replacement. Acta Radiol 2004;45:434–9.

55. Bouysset M, Tebib J, Tavernier T, et al. Posterior tibial tendon and subtalar joint complex in rheumatoid arthritis: magnetic resonance imaging study. J Rheumatol 2003;30:1951–4.

56. Østergaard M, Ejbjerg B. Magnetic resonance imaging of the synovium in rheumatoid arthritis. Semin Musculoskelet Radiol 2004;8:287–99.

57. Tehranzadeh J, Ashikyan O, Dascalos J. Advanced imaging of early rheumatoid arthritis. Radiol Clin N Am 2004;42:89–107.

58. Østergaard M, Stoltenberg M, Løvgreen-Nielsen P, et al. Quantification of synovitis by MRI: correlation between dynamic and static gadolinium-enhanced magnetic resonance imaging and microscopic and macroscopic signs of synovial inflammation. Magn Reson Imaging 1998;16:743–54.

59. Lawrence RC, Helmick CG, Arnett FC, et al. Estimates of the prevalence of arthritis and selected musculoskeletal disorders in the United States. Arthritis Rheum 1998;41(5):778–99.

60. Petty RE, Southwood TR, Manners P, et al. International League of Associations for Rheumatology Classification of juvenile idiopathic arthritis: second revision, Edmonton, 2001. J Rheumatol 2004;31:390–2.

61. Davidson J. Juvenile idiopathic arthritis: a clinical overview. Eur J Radiol 2000;33:128–34.

62. Malattia C, Damasia MB, Basso C, et al. Dynamic contrast-enhanced magnetic resonance imaging in the assessment of disease activity in patients with juvenile idiopathic arthritis. Rheumatology 2010;49: 178–85.

63. Miller E, Uleryk E, Doria AS. Evidence-based outcomes of studies addressing diagnostic accuracy of MRI in juvenile idiopathic arthritis. AJR 2009;192:1209–18.

64. Frush DP, Emery K, Pitts S, et al. Practice guidelines for the performance and interpretation of pediatric magnetic resonance imaging (MRI). 2006. Available at: http://www.acr.org/SecondaryMainMenuCategories/quality_safety/guidelines/dx/mri_pediatric.aspx. Accessed August 1, 2010.

65. Kanal E, Barkovich AJ, Bell C, et al. ACR guidance document for safe MR practices: 2007. AJR Am J Roentgenol 2007;188:1447–74.

66. Doria AS, Babyn PS, Feldman B. A critical appraisal of radiographic scoring systems for assessment of juvenile idiopathic arthritis. Pediatr Radiol 2006;36: 759–72.

67. Damasio MB, Malattia C, Martini A, et al. Synovial and inflammatory diseases in childhood: role of new imaging modalities in the assessment of patients with juvenile idiopathic arthritis. Pediatr Radiol 2010;40:985–98.

68. Daldrup-Link HE, Steinbach L. MR imaging of pediatric arthritis. Magn Reson Imaging Clin N Am 2009; 17:451–67.

69. Joseph A, Brasington R, Kahl L. Immunologic rheumatic disorders. J Allergy Clin Immunol 2010;125(2): S204–15.

70. Kataria RK, Brent LH. Spondyloarthropathies. Am Fam Physician 2004;69(12):2853–60.

71. Bennet DL, Kenjirou O, El-Khoury G. Spondyloarthropathies: ankylosing spondylitis and psoriatic arthritis. Radiol Clin N Am 2004;42:121–34.

72. Taylor W, Gladman D, Helliwell P, et al. Classification criteria for psoriatic arthritis. Development of new criteria from a large international study. Arthritis Rheum 2006;54(8):2665–73.

73. Østergaard M, McQueen F, Wiell C, et al. The OMERACT psoriatic arthritis magnetic resonance imaging scoring system (PsAMRIS): definitions of key pathologies, suggested MRI sequences, and preliminary scoring system for PsA hands. J Rheumatol 2009;36:1816–24.

74. McQueen F, Lassere M, Bird P. Developing a magnetic resonance imaging scoring system for peripheral psoriatic arthritis. J Rheumatol 2007;34: 859–61.

75. McQueen F, Lassere M, Duer-Jensen A. Testing an OMERACT MRI scoring system for peripheral psoriatic arthritis in cross-sectional and longitudinal settings. J Rheumatol 2009;36:1811–5.

76. Marzo-Ortega H, McGonagle D, Bennett AN. Magnetic resonance imaging in spondyloarthritis. Curr Opin Rheumatol 2010;22:381–7.

77. Jacobson JA, Girish G, Jiang Y. Radiographic evaluation of arthritis: inflammatory conditions. Radiology 2008;248(2):378–89.

78. Mease PJ. Spondyloarthritis update. New insights regarding classification, pathophysiology, and management. Bull NYU Hosp Jt Dis 2008;66(3):203–9.

79. Colbert RA. Early axial spondyloarthritis. Curr Opin Rheumatol 2010;22:603–7.

80. Carette S, Graham D, Little H, et al. The natural disease course of ankylosing spondylitis. Arthritis Rheum 1983;26:186–90.

81. Lacout A, Rousselin B, Pelage JP. CT and MRI of spine and sacroiliac involvement in spondyloarthropathy. AJR 2008;191:1016–23.

82. Rudwaleit M, Jurik AG, Hermann KG, et al. Defining active sacroiliitis on magnetic resonance imaging (MRI) for classification of axial spondyloarthritis: a consensual approach by the ASA/OMERACT MRI group. Ann Rheum Dis 2009;68:1520–7.

83. Weber U, Lambert RGW, Ostergaard M, et al. The diagnostic utility of MRI in spondyloarthritis: an international multicentre evaluation of 187 subjects (The MORPHO study). Arthritis Rheum 2010; 62(10):3048–58.

84. Yu JS, Chung C, Recht M, et al. MR Imaging of tophaceous gout. AJR Am J Roentgenol 1997;168: 523–7.

85. Monu JUV, Pope TL. Gout: a clinical and radiologic review. Radiol Clin N Am 2004;42:169–84.

86. Steinbach LS. Calcium pyrophosphate dehydrate and calcium hydroxyapatite crystal deposition diseases: imaging perspectives. Radiol Clin N Am 2004;42:185–205.

87. Resnick D, Kransdorf MJ. Osteomyelitis, septic arthritis, and soft tissue infection: mechanisms and situations. In: Resnick D, Kransdorf MJ, editors. Bone and joint imaging. 3rd edition. Philadelphia: Saunders Elsevier; 2005. p. 713–42.

88. Kan JH, Young RS, Yu C, et al. Clinical impact of gadolinium in the MRI diagnosis of musculoskeletal infection in children. Pediatr Radiol 2010;40:1197–205.

89. Ledermann HP, Schweitzer ME, Morrison WB. Non-enhancing tissue on MR imaging of pedal infection: characterization of necrotic tissue and associated limitations for diagnosis of osteomyelitis and abscess. AJR Am J Roentgenol 2002;178:215–22.

90. Ledermann HP, Morrison WB. Differential diagnosis of pedal osteomyelitis and diabetic neuroarthropathy: MR Imaging. Semin Musculoskelet Radiol 2005;9(3):272–83.

MR Imaging of Early Hip Joint Degeneration

Donna G. Blankenbaker, MD*, Michael J. Tuite, MD

KEYWORDS

- Hip • MR imaging • MR arthrography • Articular cartilage
- Osteoarthritis

Hip pain is a common complaint seen in clinical practice and can be caused by intra-articular and extra-articular causes. The intra-articular causes of hip pain include acetabular labral tears, loose bodies, synovitis, ligamentum teres injuries, osteoarthritis, and osteochondral lesions. More recently, many of these intra-articular abnormalities have been shown to be related to underlying femoroacetabular impingement.[1–4] Magnetic resonance imaging (MR imaging) is one of the most commonly used imaging methods to evaluate patients with hip pain. Intra-articular abnormalities of the hip joint are better assessed with recent advances in MR imaging technology, such as high-field strength scanners, improved coils, and more signal-to-noise ratio (SNR)-efficient sequences. The volume of hip arthroscopy has exploded over the past decade allowing correlation between hip findings seen at arthroscopy and MR imaging.

The hip joint is one of the most common sites of debilitating osteoarthritis.[5] Osteoarthritis of the hip joint is not limited to the elderly population but may also occur in middle-aged adults and even in young individuals. Surgical treatment of osteoarthritis includes cartilage debridement and correction of deformities of the femoral head or acetabulum in patients with early joint degeneration[6,7] and total hip replacement in patients with advanced disease. Early detection of cartilage damage is paramount for proper patient selection to help identify individuals who may benefit from early medical and surgical intervention. This article discusses the causes of early hip joint degeneration and the current use of morphologic and physiologic MR imaging techniques for evaluating the articular cartilage of the hip joint. The article also discusses the role of MR arthrography in clinical cartilage imaging.

FACTORS INFLUENCING THE DETECTION OF CARTILAGE LESIONS ON MR IMAGING

Accurate measurements of articular cartilage thickness have become increasingly important in clinical practice. Osteoarthritis and hip joint injuries can result in changes in cartilage morphology. There is increasing interest in measuring and monitoring changes of articular cartilage thickness in the management of patients with prior injury or findings of femoroacetabular impingement.[8]

MR imaging evaluation of articular cartilage within the acetabulum and femoral head can be difficult. The hip joint is located off isocenter in the MR imaging scanner, which can decrease image quality. The femoral head and acetabulum are closely apposed in the normal hip, making the separate articular surfaces difficult to discriminate from each other. Additionally, the articular cartilage is thin, which also poses difficulty in the detection of cartilage lesions. Leg traction technique during MR imaging and MR arthrography has been used to allow separation of the acetabular and femoral articular surfaces.[9,10] However, in many cases, the joint space between the femoral and acetabular articular cartilage is narrow despite traction.

Department of Radiology, University of Wisconsin School of Medicine and Public Health, E3/366 Clinical Science Center, 600 Highland Avenue, Madison, WI 53792-3252, USA
* Corresponding author.
E-mail address: dblankenbaker@uwhealth.org

Magn Reson Imaging Clin N Am 19 (2011) 365–378
doi:10.1016/j.mric.2011.02.001
1064-9689/11/$ – see front matter © 2011 Elsevier Inc. All rights reserved.

Recently, hip cartilage thickness and volumes measurement have been described in cadaver hip joint,[8,11–14] within the living human hip joint,[15] and before and after periacetabular osteotomy[16] using MR imaging, MR arthrography, and computed tomography (CT) arthrography. In the study performed by Wyler and colleagues,[13] MR arthrography and CT arthrography had similar accuracy for measuring hip cartilage thickness in the coronal plane. Cartilage thickness could also be measured in the sagittal and axial planes using CT arthrography but not MR arthrography. These imaging techniques have been shown to be reproducible and sensitive to submillimeter changes in cartilage thickness and may be useful in monitoring morphologic changes caused by disease progression in patients with osteoarthritis of the hip joint.[17]

CAUSES OF EARLY HIP OSTEOARTHRITIS

The etiology of osteoarthritis of the hip joint may be primary (some underlying abnormality of articular cartilage) or secondary (congenital or developmental abnormality). Recently, primary osteoarthritis of the hip joint is thought to also be secondary to subtle developmental abnormalities that have been described as femoroacetabular impingement.[4] Femoroacetabular impingement is a cause of premature osteoarthritis in the hip

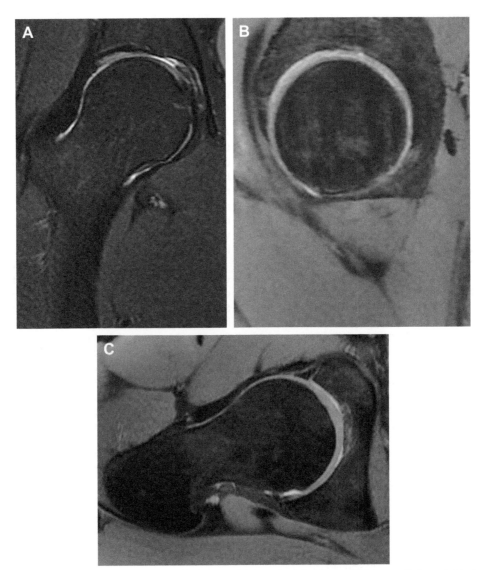

Fig. 1. Coronal T2-weighted, fat-suppressed (A), sagittal (B), and axial oblique (C) intermediate-weighted fat-suppressed conventional MR images of the hip depict normal articular cartilage as intermediate signal intensity.

joint.[18] The most frequent location for femoroacetabular impingement is the anterosuperior rim region.

Two types of femoroacetabular impingement have been described. Cam-type femoroacetabular impingement is more prevalent in young men. It is caused by a nonspherical shape of the femoral head at the femoral head-neck junction and decreased depth of the femoral waist leading to contact of the femoral head-neck junction against the acetabular rim.[19] Pincer-type femoroacetabular impingement is more prevalent in middle-aged women and is secondary to acetabular overcoverage, which limits the range of motion of the hip and leads to a contact between the acetabulum and femur.[3] Most individuals have a combination of these two mechanisms and are classified as mixed cam-pincer impingement.[1]

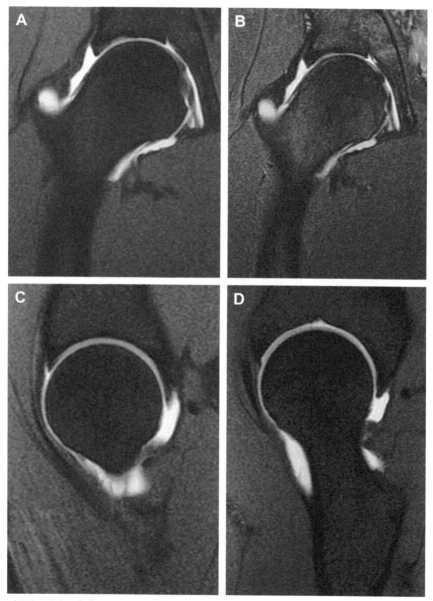

Fig. 2. Coronal T1-weighted, fat-suppressed (*A*) and T2-weighted, fat-suppressed (*B*) MR arthrogram images of the hip show the normal appearance of the articular cartilage within the acetabulum and femoral head. Sagittal T1-weighted, fat-suppressed image (*C*) depicts the normal appearance of the articular cartilage within the anterosuperior and posterosuperior acetabulum and femoral head. Axial oblique T1-weighted, fat-suppressed image (*D*) is best for visualization of articular cartilage within the anterior and posterior walls of the acetabulum.

The pattern of damage to the articular cartilage depends upon the shape of the hip joint.[1] With cam femoroacetabular impingement, the articular cartilage is commonly damaged within the anterosuperior aspect of the acetabulum. With pincer impingement, damage to the articular cartilage occurs more circumferentially, typically with only a narrow strip of involved cartilage within the posteroinferior acetabulum.[1,2] Following cartilage injury in cam impingement, tears or detachment of the anterosuperior labrum can occur.[1] Pincer impingement initially results in a labral tear or degeneration, which is the first structure to fail, followed by cartilage injury.[20] The femoral head articular cartilage remains uninvolved over a long period in pincer impingement and only late in the process will the cartilage damage occur within the posterior inferior femoral head or acetabulum called the "contrecoup lesion."[1]

It is important to recognize the type of femoroacetabular impingement because the surgical treatment differs for each type. In cam femoroacetabular impingement, the surgical technique performed is geared toward reshaping the femoral waist and restoring the spherical shape of the femoral head; whereas, in pincer impingement, the surgical technique is aimed at reducing the acetabular overcoverage by trimming the acetabular rim.[6,21–28] Surgical interventions for femoroacetabular impingement include labral repair or debridement[21,29,30] along with femoral and acetabular osteochondroplasty,[29,30] and acetabular osteotomy.[21,31] Performing these procedures before the development of advanced joint degeneration is essential for their long-term success.[7,32] The goals for surgical intervention are to relieve pain, enhance activity and function, and preserve the natural hip joint over time.[1] Recent review of the literature of hip impingement surgery has shown early relief of pain and improved function following treatment.[7] The most important role of MR imaging in evaluating patients with femoroacetabular impingement is to assess the exact extent of joint degradation.. Thus, early detection of cartilage degeneration with MR imaging can help identify patients with hip pain who may benefit from early surgical intervention.

Femoroacetabular impingement is well recognized after total hip arthroplasty. It is known to also occur in individuals with abnormal hip anatomy, such as Legg-Calve-Perthes disease, slipped capital femoral epiphysis, developmental dysplasia, or posttraumatic deformity where there is a mismatch between the femoral head-neck junction and the acetabulum.[21,33–37] Other causes of early osteoarthritis of the hip include inflammatory diseases (such as rheumatoid arthritis, ankylosing spondylitis, reactive arthritis, or lupus), as well as crystalline arthropathies, diffuse skeletal hyperostosis, and hemochromatosis. Damage to cartilage from infection, pigmented villonodular synovitis, synovial chondromatosis, and osteonecrosis can also lead to early osteoarthritis. Other congenital causes of early osteoarthritis of the hip joint include multiple epiphyseal dysplasia and spondyloepiphyseal dysplasia.

IMAGING TECHNIQUE AND DIAGNOSTIC PERFORMANCE OF CARTILAGE IMAGING SEQUENCES

Both conventional MR imaging (**Fig. 1**) and MR arthrography (**Fig. 2**) are commonly used to diagnose internal derangements of the hip joint.[38–40] MR imaging of the hip joint is best performed on 1.5-T or 3.0-T scanners because higher-field strength provides improved SNR, which is critical for high-resolution imaging. The need for a large field of view and the absence of specialized coils for evaluating the hip joint results in images with low spatial resolution. Contrary to many investigations reporting excellent results when imaging the articular cartilage of the knee joint,[41–45] evaluation of the articular cartilage of the hip joint is more difficult.[46–48] Hip imaging should be performed with either a surface-phased array coil or a multichannel cardiac coil. Intermediate echo time fast spin-echo sequences with an effective echo time

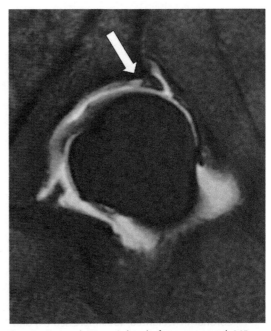

Fig. 3. Coronal T1-weighted, fat-suppressed MR arthrogram image of the hip shows a focal cartilage defect within the superior acetabulum (*arrow*) in this 25-year-old woman with mild acetabular dysplasia.

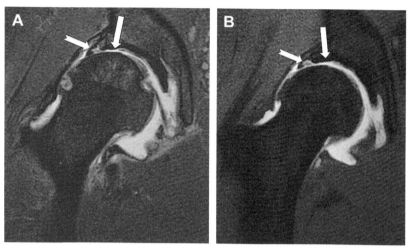

Fig. 4. Coronal T1-weighted, fat-suppressed (*A*) and T2-weighted, fat-suppressed (*B*) MR arthrogram images of the hip shows full-thickness cartilage loss within the superior acetabulum and adjacent femoral head (*arrows*) in this 49-year-old man with femoroacetabular impingement. Notched arrow depicts the anterosuperior labral tear.

of approximately 34 milliseconds at 1.5 T and 28 milliseconds at 3.0 T are recommended. The inherent magnetization transfer contrast of fast spin-echo techniques will yield differential contrast between the low signal intensity fibrocartilaginous labrum, intermediate signal intensity articular cartilage, and high signal intensity synovial fluid.[49] Coronal images best demonstrate the femoral head articular cartilage within the suprafoveal region. Sagittal images best assess the articular cartilage within the anterosuperior and posterosuperior acetabulum and femoral head; whereas, axial oblique images best depict the articular

cartilage of the anterior and posterior walls of the acetabulum (see **Fig. 2**).

CONVENTIONAL MR IMAGING AND MR ARTHROGRAPHY

Two-dimensional fast spin-echo[50] and 3-dimensional spoiled gradient-echo (SPGR) sequences[10,51] have been used to evaluate the articular cartilage of the hip joint in clinical practice. Mintz and colleagues[50] consider conventional MR imaging as having similar accuracy to MR arthrography in the detection of cartilage lesions of

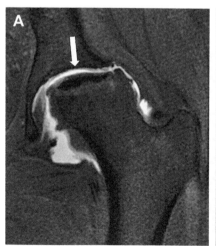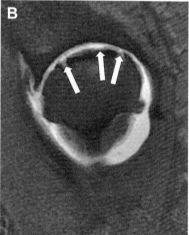

Fig. 5. Coronal (*A*) and sagittal (*B*) T1-weighted, fat-suppressed MR arthrogram images of the hip in this 19-year-old woman with old Perthes disease show diffuse cartilage loss within the acetabulum with more focal defects within the femoral head (*arrows*). Also note the collapse of the femoral head and shallow acetabulum.

the hip joint. In their study using multi-planar, 2-dimensional fast spin-echo sequences with 0.6-mm x 1.2-mm in-plane resolution and 5.0-mm slice thickness, they reported sensitivity between 86% and 93% and specificity between 72% and 85% for detecting surgically confirmed cartilage lesions in 92 subjects. Nishii and colleagues[51] evaluated 3-dimensional fat-suppressed SPGR images of the hip joint with 0.6-mm x 0.6-mm in-plane spatial resolution and 1.5-mm slice thickness and reported sensitivity between 49% and 67% and specificity between 76% and 89% for detecting surgically confirmed cartilage lesions. Possible explanations for the difference in diagnostic performance of MR imaging for evaluating the hip joint in these two studies include differences in image quality, subject population, or perhaps reader experience.

The use of sequences with higher in-plane resolution and decreased slice thickness may potentially improve the detection of cartilage lesions within the hip joint,[52] although further study is needed.

MR arthrography is considered superior to conventional MR imaging performed without intra-articular contrast material for evaluating the hip joint (**Figs. 3–5**).[39,53] The main sequences that are used in MR arthrography are fat-suppressed T1-weighted fast spin-echo sequences in the coronal, sagittal, and axial oblique planes (see **Fig. 2**). A fluid sensitive sequence and a nonfat-suppressed T1-weighted fast spin-echo sequence should also be included as part of the MR arthrogram protocol. MR arthrography has higher diagnostic performance than conventional MR imaging in the detection of labral tears.[53–55] However, MR arthrography has low

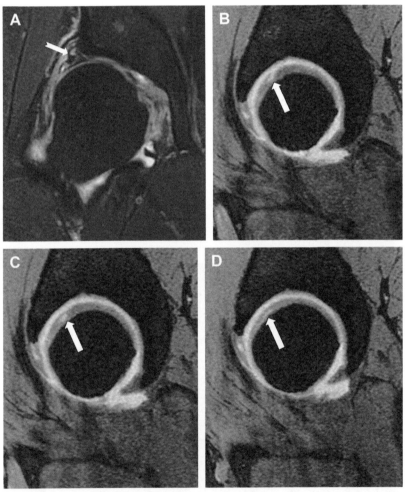

Fig. 6. Coronal T2-weighted, fat-suppressed (*A*) MR arthrogram image of the hip depicts a complex anterosuperior labral tear (*notched arrow*) in this active 35-year-old man. Sagittal (*B–D*) IDEAL-SPGR 1-mm thick MR arthrogram images demonstrate a delaminating femoral head articular cartilage lesion (*arrows*) not seen on the 2-dimensional MR arthrogram images.

diagnostic performance for evaluating the articular cartilage of the hip joint. In the study by Hodler and colleagues,[48] they correlated the anatomic and MR arthrogram measurements of femoral and acetabular cartilage thickness using a T1-weighted fast spin-echo sequence with frequency-selective fat suppression. The investigators found a significant correlation between the anatomic and MR arthrogram measurements of cartilage thickness. However, they concluded that the imaging technique was not sufficiently accurate with regard to the diagnosis for a specific patient because of the relevant scattering of data. The study by Nakanishi and colleagues[40] found

that the joint space remained narrow during MR arthrography with traction in subjects with severe osteoarthritis but not in subjects with osteonecrosis, hip dysplasia, or normal hips. Schmid and colleagues[47] evaluated the diagnostic performance of MR arthrography for detecting cartilage lesions in subjects with suspected femoroacetabular impingement or labral abnormalities. Sensitivity and specificity for detecting surgically confirmed cartilage lesions within the anterosuperior acetabulum was 65% to 100% and 40% to 80%, posterior superior acetabulum was 30% to 70% and 63% to 89%, anterior inferior acetabulum was 58% to 83% and 63% to 80%, and

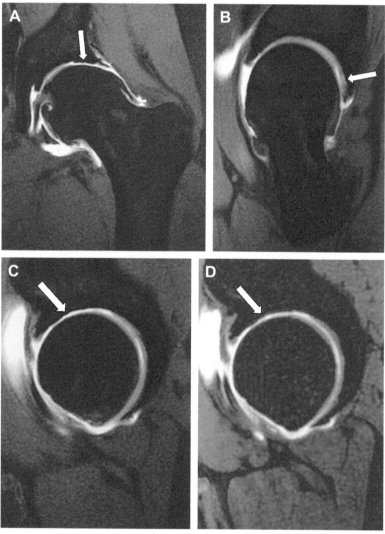

Fig. 7. Coronal (*A*), axial oblique (*B*), and sagittal (*C*) T1-weighted, fat-suppressed MR arthrogram images of the hip show diffuse cartilage loss within the acetabulum and femoral head (*arrows*) in this 49-year-old man with femoroacetabular impingement. The axial oblique image (*B*) best identifies a posterior inferior acetabular cartilage lesion (*arrow*). Sagittal (*D*) IDEAL-SPGR 1-mm thick MR arthrogram image shows the diffuse cartilage loss within the femoral head and acetabulum (*arrow*).

posteroinferior acetabulum was 20% to 60% and 91% to 94%. The sensitivity and specificity for detecting cartilage lesions of the femoral head was 40% to 60% and 88% to 91%. The study by Byrd and colleagues[54] compared conventional MR imaging and MR arthrography for evaluating the articular cartilage of the hip joint. The sensitivity and specificity for detecting surgically confirmed cartilage lesions was 41% and 100% for MR arthrography and 18% and 100% for conventional MR imaging. Furthermore, the sensitivity for detecting acetabular cartilage delamination in subjects with femoroacetabular impingement was as low as 22% for both imaging techniques.

Three-dimensional sequences may potentially improve the evaluation of the articular cartilage of the hip joint during MR arthrography (**Figs. 6–9**).[56] Two studies have directly compared 2-dimensional and 3-dimensional sequences for cartilage assessment. The study by Knuesel and colleagues[46] compared a sagittal water-excitation 3-dimensional double-echo steady-state (DESS) sequence and a sagittal fat-suppressed 2-dimensional T1-weighted fast spin-echo sequence for detecting surgically confirmed cartilage lesions within the hip joint in 21 subjects. Both sequences had similar sensitivity and specificity for detecting cartilage lesions, but cartilage lesion conspicuity was significantly (P<.05) superior for the water

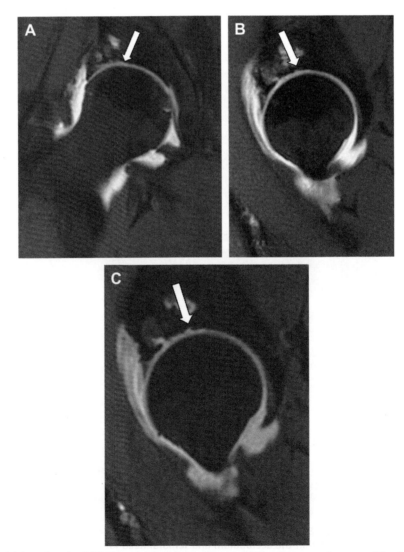

Fig. 8. Coronal (A) and sagittal (B) T1-weighted, fat-suppressed MR arthrogram images of the hip demonstrate cartilage loss within the acetabulum (arrows) in this 45-year-old woman. Sagittal (C) IDEAL-SPGR 1-mm thick MR arthrogram image also show the acetabular cartilage lesions (arrow).

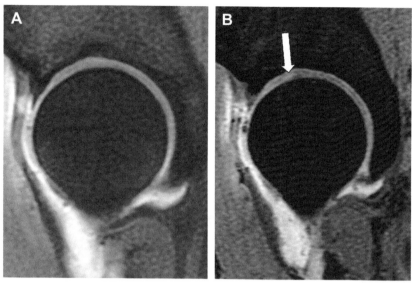

Fig. 9. Sagittal (*A*) T1-weighted, fat-suppressed MR arthrogram images of the hip demonstrate normal articular cartilage in this 38-year-old woman. Sagittal (*B*) IDEAL-SPGR 1-mm thick MR arthrogram image shows an arthroscopically proven superficial partial-thickness cartilage lesion on the anterosuperior femoral head (*arrow*).

excitation DESS sequence. In a larger study, Ullrick and colleagues[57] compared a 3-dimensional SPGR sequence with iterative decomposition of water and fat with echo asymmetry and lease squares estimation (IDEAL) fat-water separation and multi-planar fat-suppressed 2-dimensional T1-weighted fast spin-echo sequences for detecting surgically confirmed cartilage lesions within the hip joint in 67 subjects (see **Fig. 6**). IDEAL-SPGR with multi-planar reformats had significantly higher ($P<.05$) sensitivity but significantly lower ($P<.05$) specificity and accuracy than the T1-weighted fast spin-echo sequence for the detection of cartilage lesions. The sensitivity for detecting superficial cartilage lesions was extremely low with only 22% and 32% of grade 2A lesions identified using the 2-dimensional and 3-dimensional sequences.

INDIRECT MR ARTHROGRAPHY

Indirect MR arthrography has been touted as less invasive than the direct technique, does not require fluoroscopy or a physician to perform the injection, is easy to schedule, and gives improved contrast compared with conventional MR imaging. Zlatkin and colleagues[58] found indirect MR arthrography of the hip joint to be an effective means for detecting acetabular labral tears, but the imaging modality did not provide better detection of cartilage lesions when compared with conventional MR imaging. Another issue with indirect MR arthrography for hip joint evaluation is the overall long imaging time required to perform the study.

MR PHYSIOLOGIC CARTILAGE IMAGING

Newer physiologic cartilage imaging sequences are being developed and studied for clinical use in patients with hip pain. These sequences include delayed gadolinium-enhanced imaging (**Fig. 10**),[59–62] T1-rho imaging (**Fig. 11**),[52] and T2-mapping,[63–65] which may allow for improved detection of early cartilage degeneration within the hip joint.

Delayed gadolinium-enhanced MR imaging of cartilage (dGEMRIC) is a means of assessing the earliest stages of cartilage degeneration. This technique has been applied to the articular cartilage of the knee and more recently to the hip.[66,67] dGEMRIC acts under the premise that loss of glycosaminoglycan (GAG) is a prelude to early osteoarthritis.[68] This technique estimates GAG distribution in articular cartilage by measuring T1 relaxation time in the presence of gadopentetate dimeglumine (Gd-DPTA).[69] The delay refers to the time necessary for the contrast to diffuse into the articular cartilage after intravenous injection. A color-coded mapping of the cartilage displays regions of early GAG degradation. The study by Tiderus and colleagues[61] used dGEMRIC to evaluate the articular cartilage of the hip joint in asymptomatic volunteers and subjects with early osteoarthritis to determine the optimal timing after contrast injection when imaging should be performed. Bittersohl and colleagues[65] found dGEMRIC to be a reliable tool in the assessment of the articular cartilage of

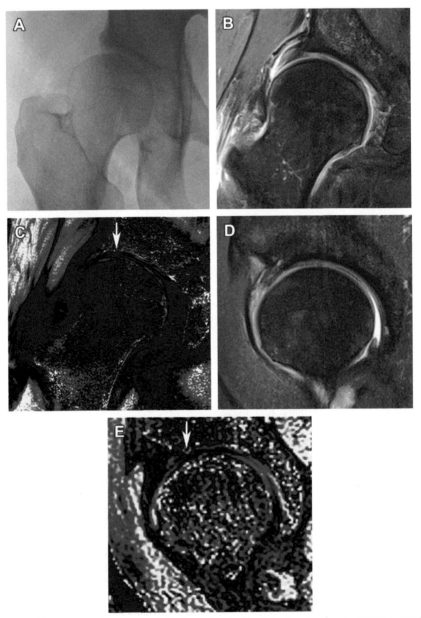

Fig. 10. A 47-year-old woman with severe right hip pain and acetabular dysplasia. Anteroposterior (A) radiograph of the hip show no evidence of osteoarthritis. MR imaging at 3.0 T was performed after intravenous injection of gadolinium. Coronal (B) and sagittal (D) intermediate-weighted, fat-suppressed fast spin-echo images of the hip demonstrate normal articular cartilage. Coronal (C) and sagittal (E) dGEMRIC images show advanced GAG loss in the anterosuperior acetabulum and femoral head (arrows), which is depicted as dark signal intensity on the color scale. (Courtesy of Young-Jo Kim, MD, PhD, Boston, MA.)

the hip joint in subjects with femoroacetabular impingement. Jessel and colleagues[59] also evaluated 30 subjects with femoroacetabular impingement using dGEMRIC. They found a significant correlation (P<.05) between dGEMRIC index, clinical symptoms, and alpha angle. Cunningham and colleagues[60] performed dGEMRIC on 47 subjects undergoing a Bernese periacetabular osteotomy

for treatment of hip dysplasia to evaluate the preoperative grade of osteoarthritis. They found the dGEMRIC index useful for assessing the degree of cartilage degeneration before surgery and for identifying subjects who had a poor outcome after pelvic osteotomy.

T2 mapping is an MR imaging technique that can evaluate the cartilage matrix status, such as

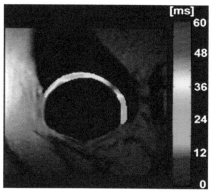

Fig. 11. $T_{1\rho}$ relaxation time map of the articular cartilage of the hip joint in an asymptomatic volunteer overlaid on the first image. (*Courtesy of* Sharmila Majumdar, PhD, San Francisco, CA.)

hydration and collagen fiber integrity.[70,71] T2 mapping uses the T2 relaxation time as an indirect indicator of structural change within articular cartilage caused by alteration in interaction between water molecules and the collagen fiber network with progressive cartilage degeneration.[72,73] A recent study by Watanabe and colleagues[64] found topographic variation in the T2 relaxation time of the articular cartilage of the hip joint in young, healthy volunteers. Nishii and colleagues[63] used T2 mapping of the hip joint to detect early cartilage degeneration in subjects with acetabular dysplasia.

THREE-DIMENSIONAL VIRTUAL CARTILAGE MODELS

MR imaging techniques have been used to assess the 3-dimensional structure of the hip joint in patients with Legg-Calve-Perthes disease. In the study be Pienkowski and colleagues,[74] 3 sets of MR images of both hip joints were obtained at different time periods. Three-dimensional virtual models of the articular cartilage were created from the MR imaging datasets, and mathematical spheres were fit to the articulating surfaces to quantify cartilage surface geometry. This technique may provide accurate and reliable assessment of the 3-dimensional deformity of the articular surface of the femoral head and acetabulum in patients with Legg-Calve-Perthes disease and other types of hip disorders.

SUMMARY

MR imaging and MR arthrography are the most commonly used imaging modalities for evaluating the articular cartilage of the hip joint in clinical practice. However, these techniques are currently suboptimal for detecting early cartilage

degeneration in patients with hip pain. Future use of high-field strength scanners, multichannel coils, and more SNR-efficient sequences may allow images of articular cartilage with higher spatial resolution and greater tissue contrast to be obtained in clinically feasible scan times, which may improve cartilage assessment. Future use of physiologic techniques, such as dGEMRIC and T2 mapping, may further improve clinical cartilage imaging and may allow for better identification of patients with early cartilage degeneration.

REFERENCES

1. Beck M, Kalhor M, Leunig M, et al. Hip morphology influences the pattern of damage to the acetabular cartilage: femoroacetabular impingement as a cause of early osteoarthritis of the Hip. J Bone Joint Surg Br 2005;87-B(7):1012–8.
2. Pfirrmann CWA, Mengiardi B, Dora C, et al. Cam and pincer femoroacetabular impingement: characteristic MR arthrographic findings in 50 Patients. Radiology 2006;240(3):778–85.
3. Ganz R, Parvizi J, Beck M, et al. Femoroacetabular impingement: a cause for osteoarthritis of the hip. Clin Orthop Relat Res 2003;(417):112–20.
4. Ganz R, Leunig M, Leunig-Ganz K, et al. The etiology of osteoarthritis of the hip an integrated mechanical concept. Clin Orthop Relat Res 2008;(466):264–72.
5. Felson DT. An update on the pathogenesis and epidemiology of osteoarthritis. Radiol Clin North Am 2004;42(1):1–9.
6. Laude F, Sariali E, Nogier A, et al. Femoroacetabular impingement treatment using arthroscopy. Clin Orthop Relat Res 2009;467:747–52.
7. Clohisy J, John LS, Schutz A. Surgical treatment of femoroacetabular impingement: a systematic review of the literature. Clin Orthop Relat Res 2010;468:555–64.
8. Cheng Y, Wang S, Yamazaki T, et al. Hip cartilage thickness measurement accuracy improvement. Comput Med Imaging Graph 2007;31(8):643–55.
9. Llopis E, Cerezal L, Kassarjian A, et al. Direct MR arthrography of the hip with leg traction: feasibility for assessing articular cartilage. AJR Am J Roentgenol 2008;190(4):1124–8.
10. Nishii T, Nakanishi K, Sugano N, et al. Articular cartilage evaluation in osteoarthritis of the hip with MR imaging under continuous leg traction. Magn Reson Imaging 1998;16(8):871–5.
11. Wyler A, Bousson V, Bergot C, et al. Hyaline cartilage thickness in radiographically normal cadaveric hips: comparison of spiral CT arthrographic and macroscopic measurements. Radiology 2007; 242(2):441–9.
12. Allen BC, Peters CL, Brown NAT, et al. Acetabular cartilage thickness: accuracy of three-dimensional

reconstructions from multidetector CT arthrograms in a cadaver study. Radiology 2010;255(2):544–52.

13. Wyler A, Bousson V, Bergot C, et al. Comparison of MR-arthrography and CT-arthrography in hyaline cartilage-thickness measurement in radiographically normal cadaver hips with anatomy as gold standard. Osteoarthritis Cartilage 2009;17(1):19–25.

14. Akiyama K, Sakai T, Koyanagi J, et al. Three-dimensional distribution of articular cartilage thickness in the elderly cadaveric acetabulum: a new method using three-dimensional digitizer and CT. Osteoarthritis Cartilage 2010;18(6):795–802.

15. Li W, Abram F, Beaudoin G, et al. Human hip joint cartilage: MRI quantitative thickness and volume measurements discriminating acetabulum and femoral head. IEEE Trans Biomed Eng 2008; 55(12):2731–40.

16. Mechlenburg I, Nyengaard J, Gelineck J, et al. Cartilage thickness in the hip measured by MRI and stereology before and after periacetabular osteotomy. Clin Orthop Relat Res 2010;468(7):1884–90.

17. Naish JH, Xanthopoulos E, Hutchinson CE, et al. MR measurement of articular cartilage thickness distribution in the hip. Osteoarthritis Cartilage 2006; 14(10):967–73.

18. Wagner S, Hofstetter W, Chiquet M, et al. Early osteoarthritic changes of human femoral head cartilage subsequent to femoro-acetabular impingement. Osteoarthritis Cartilage 2003;11(7):508–18.

19. Ito K, Minka- M-A II, Leunig M, et al. Femoroacetabular impingement and the cam-effect: a MRI-based quantitative anatomical study of the femoral head-neck offset. J Bone Joint Surg Br 2001;83-B(2): 171–6.

20. Kassarjian A, Yoon LS, Belzile E, et al. Triad of MR arthrographic findings in patients with cam-type femoroacetabular impingement. Radiology 2005; 236(2):588–92.

21. Beck M, Leunig M, Clarke E, et al. Femoroacetabular impingement as a factor in the development of nonunion of the femoral neck: a report of three cases. J Orthop Trauma 2004;18(7):425–30.

22. Mardones R, Lara J, Donndorff A, et al. Surgical correction of "cam-type" femoroacetabular impingement: a cadaveric comparison of open versus arthroscopic debridement. Arthroscopy 2009;25(2): 175–82.

23. Siebenrock KA, Schoeniger R, Ganz R. Anterior femoro-acetabular impingement due to acetabular retroversion: treatment with periacetabular osteotomy. J Bone Joint Surg Am 2003;85(2):278–86.

24. Byrd J, Jones K. Arthroscopic femoroplasty in the management of cam-type femoroacetabular impingement. Clin Orthop Relat Res 2009;467: 739–46.

25. Beaule PE, Le Duff MJ, Zaragoza E. Quality of life following femoral head-neck osteochondroplasty

for femoroacetabular impingement. J Bone Joint Surg Am 2007;89(4):773–9.

26. Beck M, Leunig M, Parvizi J, et al. Anterior femoroacetabular impingement: part II. Midterm results of surgical treatment. Clin Orthop Relat Res 2004;(418):67–73.

27. Murphy S, Tannast M, Kim Y, et al. Debridement of the adult hip for femoroacetabular impingement: indications and preliminary clinical results. Clin Orthop Relat Res 2004;(429):178–81.

28. Philippon MJ, Stubbs AJ, Schenker ML, et al. Arthroscopic management of femoroacetabular impingement. Am J Sports Med 2007;35(9):1571–80.

29. Philippon MJ, Briggs KK, Yen Y-M, et al. Outcomes following hip arthroscopy for femoroacetabular impingement with associated chondrolabral dysfunction: minimum two year follow up. J Bone Joint Surg Br 2009;91-B(1):16–23.

30. Brunner A, Horisberger M, Herzog RF. Sports and recreation activity of patients with femoroacetabular impingement before and after arthroscopic osteoplasty. Am J Sports Med 2009;37(5):917–22.

31. Sanchez-Sotelo J, Berry DJ, Trousdale RT, et al. Surgical treatment of developmental dysplasia of the hip in adults: II. Arthroplasty options. J Am Acad Orthop Surg 2002;10(5):334–44.

32. Sambandam S, Hull J, Jiranek W. Factors predicting the failure of Bernese periacetabular osteotomy: a meta-regression analysis. Int Orthop 2009;33(6): 1483–8.

33. Leunig M, Beck M, Woo A, et al. Acetabular rim degeneration: a constant finding in the aged hip. Clin Orthop Relat Res 2003;(413):201–7.

34. Eijer H, Myers SR, Ganz R. Anterior femoroacetabular impingement after femoral neck fractures. J Orthop Trauma 2001;15(7):475–81.

35. Klaue K, Durnin C, Ganz R. The acetabular rim syndrome. A clinical presentation of dysplasia of the hip. J Bone Joint Surg Br 1991;73-B(3):423–9.

36. Leunig M, Casillas MM, Hamlet M, et al. Slipped capital femoral epiphysis. Acta Orthop Scand 2000;71(4):370–5.

37. Lievense AM, Bierma-Zeinstra SMA, Verhagen AP, et al. Influence of hip dysplasia on the development of osteoarthritis of the hip. Ann Rheum Dis 2004;63: 621–6.

38. Petersilge CA, Petersilge WJ, Lewin JS, et al. Acetabular labral tears: evaluation with MR arthrography. Radiology 1996;200(1):231–5.

39. Hodler J, Yu J, Goodwin D, et al. MR arthrography of the hip: improved imaging of the acetabular labrum with histologic correlation in cadavers. Am J Roentgenol 1995;165(4):887–91 [published erratum appears in AJR Am J Roentgenol 1996; 167(1):282].

40. Nakanishi K, Tanaka H, Nishi T, et al. Evaluation of the articular cartilage of the femoral head during

traction. Correlation with resected femoral head. Acta Radiol 1999;40(1):60.

41. Bredella M, Tirman P, Peterfy C, et al. Accuracy of T2-weighted fast spin-echo MR imaging with fat saturation in detecting cartilage defects in the knee: comparison with arthroscopy in 130 patients. Am J Roentgenol 1999;172(4):1073–80.

42. Disler D, McCauley T, Kelman C, et al. Fat-suppressed three-dimensional spoiled gradient-echo MR imaging of hyaline cartilage defects in the knee: comparison with standard MR imaging and arthroscopy. Am J Roentgenol 1996;167(1):127–32.

43. Recht MP, Piraino DW, Paletta GA, et al. Accuracy of fat-suppressed three-dimensional spoiled gradient-echo FLASH MR imaging in the detection of patellofemoral articular cartilage abnormalities. Radiology 1996;198(1):209–12.

44. Broderick L, Turner D, Renfrew D, et al. Severity of articular cartilage abnormality in patients with osteoarthritis: evaluation with fast spin-echo MR vs arthroscopy. Am J Roentgenol 1994;162(1):99–103.

45. Murphy B. Evaluation of grades 3 and 4 chondromalacia of the knee using T2* weighted 3D gradient-echo articular cartilage imaging. Skeletal Radiol 2001;30(6):305–11.

46. Knuesel PR, Pfirrmann CW, Noetzli HP, et al. MR arthrography of the hip: diagnostic performance of a dedicated water-excitation 3D double-echo steady-state sequence to detect cartilage lesions. Am J Roentgenol 2004;183(6):1729–35.

47. Schmid MR, Nötzli HP, Zanetti M, et al. Cartilage lesions in the hip: diagnostic effectiveness of MR arthrography. Radiology 2003;226(2):382–6.

48. Hodler J, Trudell D, Pathria M, et al. Width of the articular cartilage of the hip: quantification by using fat-suppression spin-echo MR imaging in cadavers. Am J Roentgenol 1992;159(2):351–5.

49. Potter HG, Schachar J. High resolution noncontrast MRI of the hip. J Magn Reson Imaging 2010;31(2): 268–78.

50. Mintz DN, Hooper T, Connell D, et al. Magnetic resonance imaging of the hip: detection of labral and chondral abnormalities using noncontrast imaging. Arthroscopy 2005;21(4):385–93.

51. Nishii T, Tanaka H, Nakanishi K, et al. Fat-suppressed 3D spoiled gradient-echo MRI and MDCT arthrography of articular cartilage in patients with hip dysplasia. Am J Roentgenol 2005;185(2):379–85.

52. Carballido-Gamio J, Link TM, Li X, et al. Feasibility and reproducibility of relaxometry, morphometric, and geometrical measurements of the hip joint with magnetic resonance imaging at 3T. J Magn Reson Imaging 2008;28(1):227–35.

53. Czerny C, Neuhold A, Tschauner C, et al. Lesions of the acetabular labrum: accuracy of MR imaging and MR arthrography in detection and staging. Radiology 1996;200:225–30.

54. Byrd JW, Jones KS. Diagnostic accuracy of clinical assessment, magnetic resonance imaging, magnetic resonance arthrography, and intra-articular injection in hip arthroscopy patients. Am J Sports Med 2004;32(7):1668–74.

55. Toomayan GA, Holman WR, Major NM, et al. Sensitivity of MR arthrography in the evaluation of acetabular labral tears. Am J Roentgenol 2006;186(2): 449–53.

56. Pfirrmann CW, Duc SR, Zanetti M, et al. MR arthrography of acetabular cartilage delamination in femoroacetabular cam impingement. Radiology 2008; 249(1):236–41.

57. Ullrick S, Blankenbaker DG, Davis K, et al. Evaluation of the articular cartilage of the hip joint using IDEAL-SPGR. Presented at the Annual Meeting of the American Roentengen Ray Society. Boston (MA), April 30, 2009.

58. Zlatkin MB, Pevsner D, Sanders TG, et al. Acetabular labral tears and cartilage and lesions of the hip: indirect MR arthrographic correlation with arthroscopy–a preliminary study. Am J Roentgenol 2010;194(3):709–14.

59. Jessel RH, Zilkens C, Tiderius C, et al. Assessment of osteoarthritis in hips with femoroacetabular impingement using delayed gadolinium enhanced MRI of cartilage. J Magn Reson Imaging 2009; 30(5):1110–5.

60. Cunningham T, Jessel R, Zurakowski D, et al. Delayed gadolinium-enhanced magnetic resonance imaging of cartilage to predict early failure of Bernese periacetabular osteotomy for hip dysplasia. J Bone Joint Surg Am 2006;88(7):1540–8.

61. Tiderius CJ, Jessel R, Kim Y-J, et al. Hip dGEMRIC in asymptomatic volunteers and patients with early osteoarthritis: the influence of timing after contrast injection. Magn Reson Med 2007;57(4):803–5.

62. Bittersohl B, Steppacher S, Haamberg T, et al. Cartilage damage in femoroacetabular impingement (FAI): preliminary results on comparison of standard diagnostic vs delayed gadolinium-enhanced magnetic resonance imaging of cartilage (dGEMRIC). Osteoarthritis Cartilage 2009;17(10):1297–306.

63. Nishii T, Tanaka H, Sugano N, et al. Evaluation of cartilage matrix disorders by T2 relaxation time in patients with hip dysplasia. OsteoarthritisCartilage 2008;16(2):227–33.

64. Watanabe A, Boesch C, Siebenrock K, et al. T2 mapping of hip articular cartilage in healthy volunteers at 3T: A study of topographic variation. J Magn Reson Imaging 2007;26(1):165–71.

65. Bittersohl B, Hosalkar HS, Kim Y-J, et al. Delayed gadolinium-enhanced magnetic resonance imaging (dGEMRIC) of hip joint cartilage in femoroacetabular impingement (FAI): are pre- and postcontrast imaging both necessary? Magn Reson Med 2009; 62(6):1362–7.

66. Kim Y-J, Jaramillo D, Millis MB, et al. Assessment of early osteoarthritis in hip dysplasia with delayed gadolinium-enhanced magnetic resonance imaging of cartilage. J Bone Joint Surg Am 2003;85(10):1987–92.

67. Bashir A, Gray ML, Boutin RD, et al. Glycosaminoglycan in articular cartilage: in vivo assessment with delayed Gd(DTPA)(2-)-enhanced MR imaging. Radiology 1997;205(2):551–8.

68. Maroudas A, Venn M. Chemical composition and swelling of normal and osteoarthrotic femoral head cartilage. Ann Rheum Dis 1977;36(5):399–406.

69. Bashir A, Gray M, Burstein D. Gd-DTPA2- as a measure of cartilage degradation. Magn Reson Med 1996;36(5):665–73.

70. Nieminen MT, Rieppo J, Töyräs J, et al. T2 relaxation reveals spatial collagen architecture in articular cartilage: a comparative quantitative MRI and polarized light microscopic study. Magn Reson Med 2001;46(3):487–93.

71. Xia Y, Moody JB, Alhadlaq H. Orientational dependence of relaxation in articular cartilage: A microscopic MRI (muMRI) study. Magn Reson Med 2002;48(3):460–9.

72. White LM, Sussman MS, Hurtig M, et al. Cartilage T2 assessment: differentiation of normal hyaline cartilage and reparative tissue after arthroscopic cartilage repair in equine subjects. Radiology 2006; 241(2):407–14.

73. Welsch GH, Mamisch TC, Domayer SE, et al. Cartilage T2 assessment at 3-T MR imaging: in vivo differentiation of normal hyaline cartilage from reparative tissue after two cartilage repair procedures—initial experience. Radiology 2008;247(1): 154–61.

74. Pienkowski D, Resig J, Talwalkar V, et al. Novel three-dimensional MRI technique for study of cartilaginous hip surfaces in Legg-Calvé-Perthes disease. J Orthop Res 2009;27(8):981–8.

MR Imaging of the Articular Cartilage of the Knee and Ankle

Michael Forney, MD[a],*, Naveen Subhas, MD[a], Brian Donley, MD[b], Carl S. Winalski, MD[a]

KEYWORDS

- Cartilage • MR imaging • Knee • Ankle
- Osteochondral lesion • Cartilage lesion

INTRODUCTION TO CARTILAGE LESIONS
Clinical Background

Cartilage lesions of the knee and ankle are common problems that are not easily detected by routine physical examination.[1] In addition, cartilage lesions may be overlooked as the source of many joint symptoms, especially in the setting of a joint comorbidity. It is important for clinicians to diagnose cartilage disease correctly, as these abnormalities can be the cause of significant short and long-term morbidity. Cartilage has minimal repair capability, and untreated lesions can lead to persistent joint pain and dysfunction.[2] Moreover, alterations in joint forces related to cartilage lesions are thought to accelerate osteoarthritis of both the knee and the ankle.[1,3] Fortunately, there are new techniques for both the diagnosis and surgical treatment of cartilage lesions that have demonstrated good outcomes in recent years.[4]

Diagnosing cartilage lesions with the "gold standard," invasive technique of arthroscopy, is not practical for all patients. Magnetic resonance (MR) imaging of articular cartilage is an alternative that has been found to be a valuable tool not only for lesion detection but also for preoperative planning and postoperative assessment.[5] Accurate characterization of cartilage lesions with state-of-the-art MR imaging techniques allows clinicians to choose optimal treatments for their patients.[6] Therefore, understanding the appearance of normal articular cartilage, the spectrum of cartilage lesions, and the treatment options for these lesions in the knee and ankle will allow radiologists to more effectively guide treatment decisions.

Knee Cartilage Versus Ankle Cartilage

There are many differences between the articular cartilage of the knee and ankle. Having some understanding of these differences may help the radiologist to better appreciate the differences in the types of lesions seen clinically, as well as their imaging appearance.

Biomechanical studies suggest that variations between the articular cartilage of the knee and ankle cannot be explained by anatomic and biomechanical differences alone; rather, there are many intrinsic differences between knee and ankle cartilage.[7] Ankle cartilage is significantly thinner than knee cartilage, with a mean thickness of approximately 1.1 mm (range, 0.4–2.1 mm), whereas knee cartilage can be up to 5 mm thick.[4,8–11] It has been suggested that more congruent joints such as the hip and ankle support compressive loads with a thinner cartilage because the load is spread over a greater area.[12] The collagenous organization of knee and ankle articular cartilage is similar; however, the chondrocyte distribution is different. In the superficial zone of ankle cartilage, chondrocytes are arranged in clusters, whereas they are distributed as single chondrocytes in the superficial zone of the

No relevant disclosures for Dr Forney, Dr Subhas, or Dr Winalski.

[a] Imaging Institute, Cleveland Clinic, 9500 Euclid Avenue, Cleveland, OH 44195, USA
[b] Orthopaedic and Rheumatologic Institute, Cleveland Clinic, 9500 Euclid Avenue, Cleveland OH 44195, USA
* Corresponding author.
E-mail address: mcforney@gmail.com

Magn Reson Imaging Clin N Am 19 (2011) 379–405
doi:10.1016/j.mric.2011.02.005
1064-9689/11/$ – see front matter © 2011 Elsevier Inc. All rights reserved.

knee.[13] Ankle cartilage has been shown to have significantly higher glycosaminoglycan (GAG) content than knee cartilage.[14,15] Most important, the stiffness of ankle cartilage allows for better resistance to damage than that of knee cartilage.[16]

Although cartilage has limited repair potential, ankle cartilage has a more favorable biochemical response to injury than knee cartilage. In multiple studies, chondrocytes of the ankle were found to be more metabolically active than those of the knee after controlled mechanical stress was applied.[17–22] Specifically, ankle chondrocytes produced larger amounts of proteoglycans and collagen,[17–21] an overall anabolic response, whereas the knee chondrocytes produced an overall catabolic response.[22] Thus, although thinner, ankle cartilage has many features that make it more resistant and resilient to trauma and wear. These properties may explain why the types of cartilage lesions seen in the knee and ankle differ. Idiopathic osteoarthritis is commonly seen in the knee, whereas osteochondral lesions are more commonly seen in the ankle.

MR IMAGING APPEARANCE OF NORMAL KNEE AND ANKLE CARTILAGE

Articular cartilage has a layered appearance on MR imaging composed of a low-signal deep layer, a thicker intermediate to bright middle layer, and a thin low-signal surface layer. This trilaminate appearance is best seen with high-resolution, high–field-strength imaging (**Fig. 1**). With lower resolution imaging techniques or very short echo time (TE) acquisitions, normal cartilage may appear homogeneously intermediate to bright, as the deep and superficial layers may not be distinctly seen; this is especially true for the thin cartilage of the ankle (**Fig. 2**). Fat suppression can further decrease the conspicuity of the deep short T2 layer of cartilage because the subjacent subchondral bone and suppressed marrow fat may have similar signal intensity (**Fig. 3**). Cartilage normally demonstrates regional variations in signal intensity, largely due to variations in T2 caused by the orientation of the collagen fibrils relative to the magnetic field.[23] Normal variation in cartilage signal is smooth, whereas true cartilage abnormalities usually demonstrate abrupt signal change. Linear regions of fluid signal intensity within cartilage usually represent fissures whereas larger regions indicate cartilage loss. Focal regions of low T2 signal may also represent cartilage damage, often fissures, as shown in a recent small case series.[24] Knowledge of the normal variations of signal within the articular cartilage of the knee and ankle can help radiologists to differentiate normal regions of low and high signal from true cartilage abnormalities.

Volume-averaging artifacts can be problematic when evaluating articular cartilage. Because of the thinness of articular cartilage and the curved articular surfaces of joints, volume averaging with adjacent soft tissues such as synovial fat and fluid can give rise to falsely positive findings (**Fig. 4**). This anomaly can be minimized by obtaining thin,

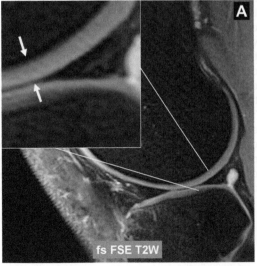
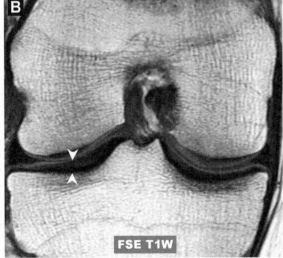

Fig. 1. Normal knee cartilage. (*A*) Cartilage in the knee is predominately intermediate in signal with thin, low signal, deep, and superficial layers (*arrows*). The calcified cartilage and subchondral bone cannot be differentiated. (*B*) Cartilage within the central tibial plateau typically has taller regions of deep low signal (*arrowheads*) due to the thicker radial zone in this region and its orientation relative to the magnetic field.

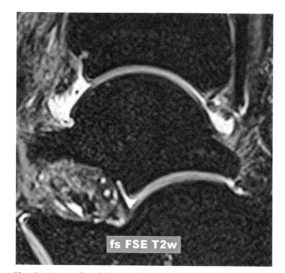

Fig. 2. Normal ankle cartilage. Ankle cartilage is much thinner than knee cartilage as seen in this sagittal fat-suppressed T2-weighted image. The trilaminate configuration that can be seen in the knee is not usually visible in the ankle. The tibial and talar chondral surfaces are often difficult to distinguish.

Normal Knee Cartilage

Knee cartilage generally displays the normal trila-minar appearance on MR imaging, with some regional variations. The central tibial plateau carti-lage typically displays a taller region of deep low signal as seen on **Fig. 1**, likely related to the greater degree of columnar organization (ie, radial zone) of collagen that is oriented parallel to the main magnetic field in this region.[5] Regions of prominent low signal are also seen in the deep central patellar cartilage and in the deep weight-bearing femoral condylar cartilage. These regions of low signal represent normal variation and should not be misinterpreted as cartilage lesions. Artifacts related to volume averaging can be particularly prominent in the trochlear cartilage because of its curved surface. Therefore, it is important to evaluate the trochlea in multiple planes, especially the sagittal plane. Cross-referencing any abnormal cartilage areas in an additional plane orthogonal to the articular surface to confirm a true abnormality can help avoid misdiagnosis of artifacts related to volume averaging (see **Fig. 4**).

Normal Ankle Cartilage

Multiple aspects of ankle cartilage make MR imaging evaluation more difficult than evaluation of knee cartilage. Ankle cartilage is very thin, making it fundamentally more susceptible to volume-averaging artifacts. Whereas in the knee the presence of the menisci provides separation of the articular surfaces, there is often little, if any, visible separation between the cartilage surfaces of the tibial plafond and talar dome. In addition, the ankle is composed of curved articular

high-resolution slices when using 2-dimensional sequences or by using high isotropic resolution 3-dimensional sequences for cartilage assess-ment. Obtaining direct obliquely oriented acquisi-tions through regions such as the inferior trochlea of the knee can help detect cartilage lesions that may be difficult to visualize on axial images. Because the dome of the talus approxi-mates a cylinder, partial volume artifacts can make detection of some cartilage lesions particu-larly difficult.

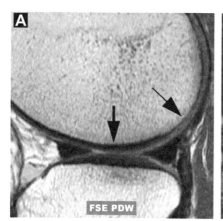

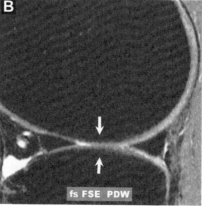

Fig. 3. The effect of fat suppression on deep cartilage. (A) Deep articular cartilage and the subchondral bone plate are most distinct on non–fat-suppressed images (*black arrows*). (B) Fat suppression may obscure the inter-face between deep cartilage and subchondral bone (*arrows*) and cause difficulty in determining cartilage thick-ness. (*From* Winalski CS, Gupta KB. Magnetic resonance imaging of focal articular cartilage lesions. Top Magn Reson Imaging 2003;14(2):131–44; with permission.)

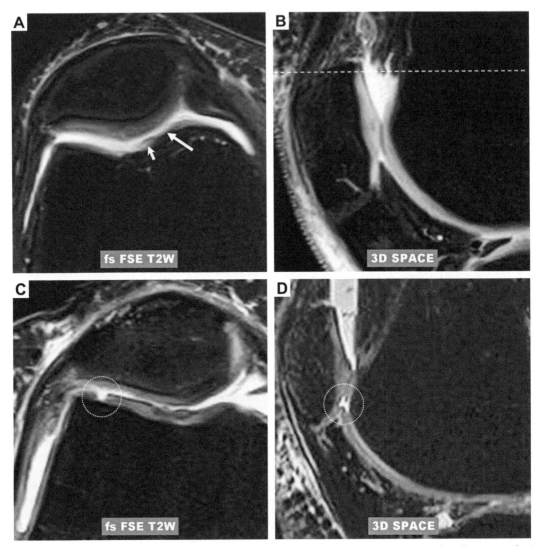

Fig. 4. Trochlear "pseudo-lesion." On the axial image (*A*), there is an apparent cartilage defect (*long arrow*) with adjacent cartilage flap (*short arrow*) in the medial trochlea. However, cross-reference to the sagittal plane (*B*, *dashed line*) shows that the apparent "cartilage lesion" on the axial image actually represents volume averaging of joint fluid and synovium. By comparison in a different patient, a cartilage true lesion (*circles*) can be clearly seen in both the axial (*C*) and sagittal planes (*D*). It is important to verify cartilage lesions in 2 planes.

surfaces, particularly the peripheral joint, resulting in volume-averaging artifacts. For these reasons, evaluation of the ankle for suspected cartilage abnormalities are best performed on the highest field-strength MR imaging unit available, preferably a 3-T MR system, with thin (≤3 mm thickness) 2-dimensional slices. When possible, a high isotropic resolution 3-dimensional volume acquisition, which can be reformatted in any desired plane, is helpful for cartilage assessment (**Fig. 5**). Even with optimized techniques, identification of partial-thickness cartilage defects and fissures in the ankle can be difficult. Fortunately, partial-thickness cartilage lesions tend to be treated conservatively. In addition to close inspection of

chondral surfaces in all imaging planes, evaluation of the subchondral bone for signal changes and irregularities is particularly helpful in identifying cartilage abnormalities. Focal, abrupt changes in signal should raise the possibility of an overlying cartilage lesion. In both the knee and the ankle, identification of subchondral edema-like marrow signal may indicate that an occult or subtle deep cartilage lesion is present.

HOW TO REPORT CARTILAGE LESIONS OF THE KNEE AND ANKLE

The description of a cartilage lesion in the radiology report should be relevant to the clinical

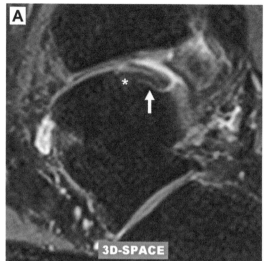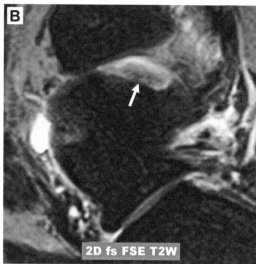

Fig. 5. High isotropic resolution 3-dimensional cartilage imaging. The osteochondral lesion of the talus (*arrows*) is more easily seen on the 3-dimensional SPACE sequence (*A*) than the 2-dimensional T2-weighted sequence (*B*). Specifically, the thin, low T2 signal, osseous attachment of the lesion (*asterisk*), is visible only on the 3-dimensional SPACE image.

situation and anticipated treatment options. To tailor the radiology report to the clinical situation and potential treatment options, it is helpful to first consider the patient's age, along with disease stage and activity level. For example, an elderly, inactive patient with diffuse osteoarthritis is more likely to undergo a joint arthroplasty than a cartilage repair surgery. Therefore, a time-consuming, detailed description of each of the individual cartilage lesions is not needed. On the other hand, a young, high-level athlete with one or two focal cartilage defects with otherwise intact cartilage may be a candidate for a cartilage repair procedure. In such cases, a detailed description of each cartilage lesion in the radiology report is required.

For the ankle, the clinical factors of age, activity level, and ankle stability play the greatest role in the clinician's determination of the treatment options for a given cartilage lesion. Cartilage repair is typically not undertaken in patients older than 50 years unless they are highly active and require optimal joint function (eg, for recreation or their profession).[2–4,25–27] A high-performance athlete is more likely to require operative repair to restore near-optimal joint function in the ankle, whereas a patient of the same age who is minimally active may not require surgery to achieve symptom relief and an adequate level of joint function. Clinical joint stability is another important factor to consider in the ankle. Postoperative rehabilitation algorithms for cartilage lesions and chronic ankle instability are in opposition: after cartilage repair

continuous passive motion is required, whereas following ankle ligamentous repair immobilization is required.[25,27,28] Therefore, in a patient with both chronic ankle instability and a cartilage lesion, cartilage repair may not be undertaken unless a staged procedure is performed. If pain is the primary complaint, debridement of the cartilage lesion is more likely to be performed in this situation. If instability is the chief complaint, debridement of the cartilage lesion may or may not be performed at the time of surgical reconstruction to correct the instability. Therefore, a detailed description of a cartilage lesion in the ankle in the radiology report is not critical unless the patient is young or highly active and chondral repair is likely to be performed.

For the knee, the overall joint status should be considered in addition to patient demographics as the radiologist tailors the radiology report. Knee joint status can be considered as 1 of 3 categories: multicompartmental lesions, unicompartmental lesions, and one or two solitary lesions. Patients with multicompartmental lesions of the knee may initially be treated nonoperatively with anti-inflammatory medications and viscosupplementation for symptom relief. Alternatively or additionally, these patients may undergo lavage and debridement. However, many will ultimately undergo total knee arthroplasty. In the case of multicompartmental disease of the knee, only a general description of cartilage lesion depth and distribution is required because surgical repair of any one of the lesions is not likely to be performed (**Fig. 6**).

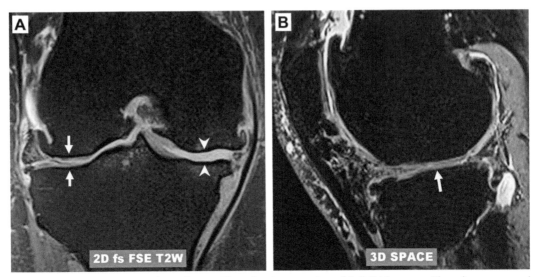

Fig. 6. Multicompartmental cartilage disease. There is a large region of full-thickness cartilage loss on opposing surfaces in the medial compartment (*A, arrowheads*). In addition, there are thinning and regions of full-thickness fissuring (*A and B, arrows*) involving the lateral compartment. The patellofemoral compartment also shows chondral thinning and fissuring. In the case of multicompartmental disease, description of individual cartilage lesions is not needed. Instead, a general description of lesion distribution and depth should be provided.

There is a different group of therapeutic options for patients with unicompartmental disease of the knee that exceeds one or two solitary lesions, including realignment osteotomy, osteochondral allograft, unicompartmental arthroplasty, and resurfacing implants. For these patients, a general description of lesion depth and distribution can be made for the involved compartment (**Fig. 7**). However, a more detailed description of any lesion found in the uninvolved compartments should be

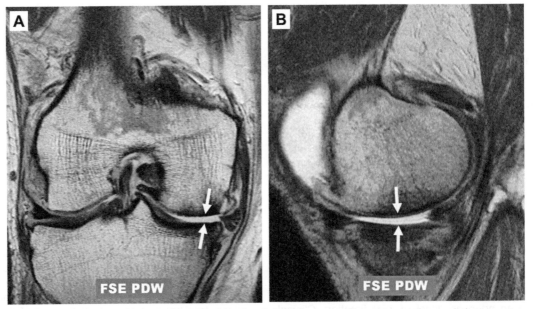

Fig. 7. Unicompartmental disease. There is extensive full-thickness cartilage loss in the medial compartment (*A and B, arrows*). Cartilage in the lateral and patellofemoral (not shown) compartments appears intact. Therefore, this patient may be a good candidate for unicompartmental therapy. When patients have severe unicompartmental disease, the radiology report should also provide a detailed description of the cartilage in the other compartments.

made, as significant lesions in multiple compartments may preclude these unicompartmental therapies. Even seemingly innocent cartilage lesions may change the joint status from what appeared to be unicompartmental arthritis by radiographs to multicompartmental disease (**Fig. 8**). In the authors' experience, MR imaging studies are more commonly being ordered on patients with severe single compartment osteoarthritis to determine whether a unicompartmental prosthesis is a more viable therapeutic option than in the past.

The solitary cartilage lesion currently presents the greatest challenge for radiologists and surgeons to evaluate and treat. The radiologist is most helpful by providing an accurate, detailed description of the solitary lesion.[6] There are many treatment options for solitary cartilage lesions, but the optimal treatment depends on the characteristics of the lesion.

How to Report a Solitary Cartilage Lesion

When a solitary cartilage lesion is observed in the knee or ankle, numerous features warrant specific comment in the radiology report to help guide therapy. The report should include a description of the lesion location, size, depth, containment, associated bone marrow edema or subchondral cysts, and any supporting structure pathology.

Lesion location

Describing the anatomic location of the cartilage lesion is important. Specific note should be made as to whether the lesion is in a weight-bearing or non–weight-bearing region of the knee. The report should also note if there are any opposing or "kissing" cartilage lesions in the knee or ankle.

Standardized intraoperative methods for defining the location of a cartilage lesion have been established for both the knee and the ankle; these methods can be adapted to MR imaging examinations as clinically appropriate. Simply put, each cartilaginous surface of the ankle or knee is divided into a 3 × 3 matrix. The International Cartilage Repair Society (ICRS) has developed cartilage mapping system for the knee in which each femoral condyle and tibial plateau are divided into anterior, central, and posterior segments and medial, central, and lateral segments. The patellar cartilage surface is divided into proximal, central, and distal segments and medial, central, and lateral segments. The trochlea is divided into only medial, central, and lateral segments.[29] For knee MR imaging, the ICRS localization grid has not been mapped onto the MR images, and the system, while useful for research, is perhaps more detailed than necessary for a radiology report. Nonetheless, basic regional descriptors provide some guidelines for terminology.

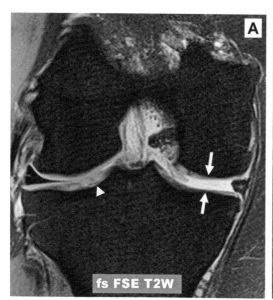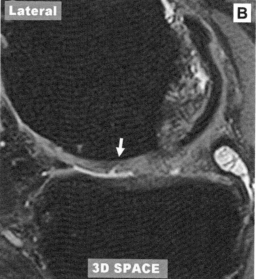

Fig. 8. Unicompartmental disease. Similar to Fig. 7, there is a large region of full-thickness loss within the medial compartment (*A, arrows*). In this case, however, there are multiple cartilage fissures of varying depths in the lateral compartment (*A and B, arrowhead and arrow*). The radiology report should detail the cartilage lesions (if any) in the uninvolved compartments as these less severe lesions may preclude a unicompartmental treatment options and require total joint arthroplasty.

In the ankle, Raikin and colleagues[9,30] have proposed a similar system for both the talar dome and tibial plafond, dividing the talar dome and tibial plafond surfaces into anterior, central, and posterior segments and medial, central, and lateral segments, thereby creating a 3 × 3 matrix for lesion localization with each location, or "cell," being assigned a zone number (1 through 9). However, for the purposes of a radiology report, anatomic descriptors with regard to the grid systems are adequate (eg, anterior medial talar dome). In the ankle, where operative exposure is more difficult, preoperative lesion localization is particularly important, as the surgeon must perform an anterior approach to address lesions within the anterior two-thirds of the joint and a posterior approach to address lesions in the posterior one-third of the joint.

Lesion size

The size of the cartilage lesion should be described as the 2 largest dimensions so that lesion area may be estimated. The area of the cartilage lesion determines the possible treatment options more so than any one dimension. Using sequences that improve intrinsic contrast between cartilage and adjacent joint structures and have higher spatial resolutions should improve lesion clarity and measurement accuracy (**Fig. 9**).[4] It is important to keep in mind that MR imaging

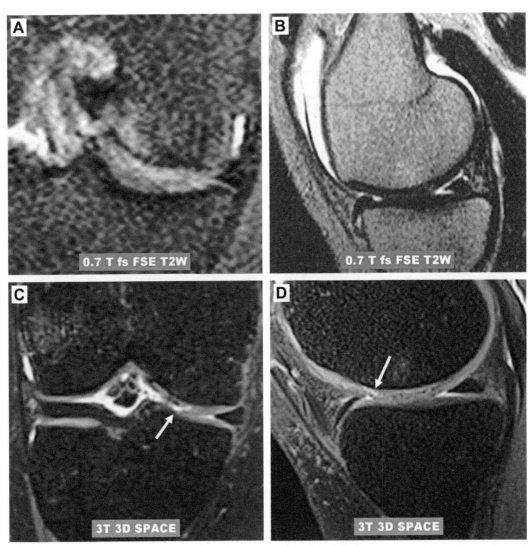

Fig. 9. Improved cartilage lesion detection and characterization with higher field strength. A patient who underwent a 0.7-T MR imaging (*A* and *B*) had a repeat examination at 3 T (*C* and *D*) just weeks later because of persistent symptoms. A small cartilage flap in the medial femoral condyle (*C* and *D*, *arrows*) was only visible on the 3-T examination.

generally underestimates cartilage lesion size when compared with direct arthroscopic evaluation for several reasons; perhaps most commonly, damaged tissue remaining within the defect cannot be readily differentiated from healthy cartilage. Partial volume-averaging artifacts and the fact that the orientation of the MR image may not be along the maximum diameters of the defect also contribute to the differences in measurements. However, MR imaging does allow for the evaluation of deep cartilage delaminations and subchondral lesions that may not be detected arthroscopically if the overlying articular cartilage is intact.[4,5]

Lesion depth

Arthroscopic grading systems have provided the basis for evaluating cartilage lesion depth. The Outerbridge classification system is a simple, commonly used method for intraoperative grading of articular cartilage lesions (**Table 1**).[31] The Outerbridge grading system has been applied in the MR imaging evaluation of cartilage lesions. However, Outerbridge grade I lesions are not reliably identified with MR imaging.[4] Although MR imaging can identify Outerbridge grade II, III, and IV lesions, accurate differentiation between these grades is not entirely reliable. Treatment options for the solitary cartilage lesion require an accurate measurement of lesion depth, and alternative grading systems have been developed for this purpose.[32] The ICRS has established an arthroscopic grading system that further stratifies lesion depth (**Table 2**).

The ICRS grading system can be adapted for quantifying cartilage lesion depth on MR imaging

Table 2
ICRS arthroscopic grading system and adapted MR imaging grading system for cartilage lesions

ICRS Arthroscopic Grade	MR Imaging Grade
1a: Mild softening or surface fibrillation	1: Abnormal signal
1b: Superficial fissures	
2: Lesion depth <50%	2: Lesion depth <50%
3a: Depth >50%, but superficial to the calcified layer	3: Lesion depth >50%
3b: Depth >50%, and reaching the calcified layer	
3c: Depth >50%, and reaching subchondral bone	
3d: Depth >50% with blistering	
4: Extension into subchondral bone	4: Osteochondral lesions (see Table 4)

Abbreviation: ICRS, International Cartilage Repair Society.
   Data from Brittberg M, Winalski CS. Evaluation of cartilage injuries and repair. J Bone Joint Surg Am 2003; 85(Suppl 2):58–69.

with some modifications. Focal low T2 signal has been shown to correlate with arthroscopically identified ICRS grade 1a lesions; therefore, these lesions can be classified as grade 1 (**Fig. 10**).[33] Discriminating between a superficial defect, that

Table 1
Outerbridge classification system for cartilage lesions

Grade	Description
0	Normal cartilage
I	Cartilage softening and or swelling
II	Partial-thickness defect with fissures on the surface that do not reach subchondral bone in an area <1.5 cm in diameter
III	Fissuring to the level of the subchondral bone in an area with a diameter >1.5 cm
IV	Cartilage lesion with exposed subchondral bone

Data from Outerbridge RE. The etiology of chondromalacia patellae. J Bone Joint Surg Br 1961;43:752–67.

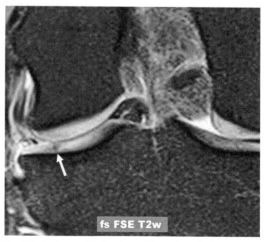

Fig. 10. Lesion with focal cartilage signal abnormality (MR imaging grade 1 lesion). There is a small, focal region of low T2 signal within the posterior lateral tibial plateau (*arrow*).

is, an ICRS grade 1b lesion, and a slightly deeper ICRS grade 2 lesion may be difficult or technically impossible, especially within the ankle where the cartilage is thin. Therefore, most radiologists categorize cartilage lesions on MR imaging as superficial when the lesion is less than 50% the expected thickness of cartilage, or deep when the lesion is greater than 50% the expected thickness (**Fig. 11**). Lesions that are less than 50% in depth are associated with a better prognosis and can have good outcomes following lavage and debridement.[28,32] MR imaging is unlikely to reliably demonstrate differences among grades 3a, 3b, and 3c at its current spatial resolution.[4] Therefore, a deep MR imaging grade 3 lesion is greater than 50% in depth but does not reach subchondral bone (**Fig. 12**). A cartilage lesion is full thickness, or grade 4, on MR imaging if it reaches or involves the subchondral bone (**Fig. 13**). When the cartilage lesion itself does not clearly extend to the subchondral bone, full-thickness extent is suggested by subchondral cysts or bone marrow edema (**Fig. 14**).

Although this grading system can be applied to both the knee and the ankle, the thinness of the articular cartilage in the ankle may not allow for detection of superficial or partial-thickness lesions (grades 1–3), especially at low field strengths. Furthermore, cartilage lesions of the ankle are commonly considered to be under the umbrella

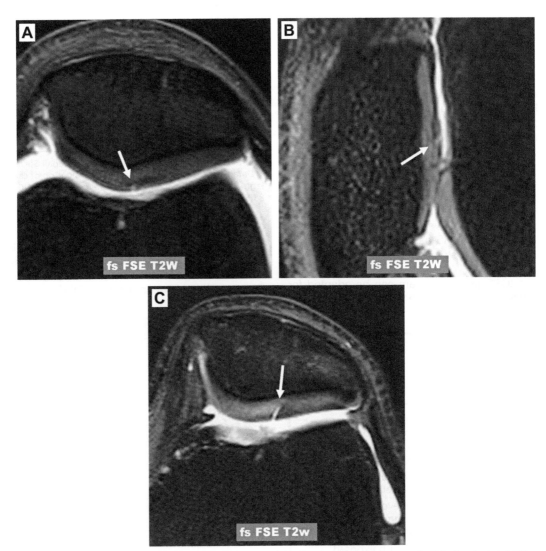

Fig. 11. Partial-thickness cartilage lesions less than 50% in depth (MR imaging grade 2 lesions). Axial (*A*) and sagittal (*B*) images demonstrate a very shallow (less than 50% depth) partial-thickness cartilage fissure in the patella (*arrow*). In a different patient, a deeper (roughly 50% in depth) partial-thickness cartilage fissure is seen within the patella (*C, arrow*).

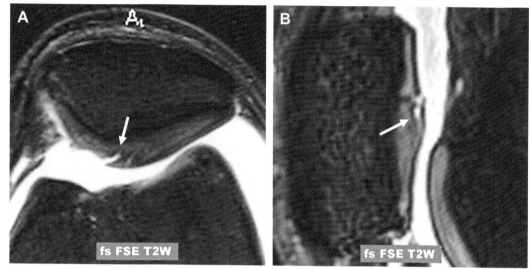

Fig. 12. Partial-thickness cartilage lesion greater than 50% in depth (MR imaging grade 3 lesion) Axial (*A*) and sagittal (*B*) images demonstrate a deep (>50% in depth) cartilage fissure in the patella (*arrow*). Grade 3 cartilage lesions are often treated as full-thickness lesions, as many have a thin component reaching the subchondral bone that may not be obvious on MR imaging.

of osteochondral lesions, for which different grading systems have been developed as outlined in a later section. With the use of the higher resolution imaging afforded by 3-T MR imaging systems, detection of partial-thickness ankle lesions may be more feasible. In the radiology report, it is best to verbally describe the depth of lesion as stratified by the grading system outlined rather than to assign a numeric grade to a lesion, as different referring physicians may use different systems or be unfamiliar with certain grading systems (eg, dictate "partial-thickness defect less than 50% in depth" rather than "grade 2").

Lesion margins

A description of the cartilage lesion margins should include an assessment of both lesion containment and lesion shouldering. Lesion containment refers to the presence or absence native cartilage immediately surrounding the lesion. A lesion is poorly contained if it extends to or beyond the edge of the cartilaginous surface or if the surrounding cartilage is extensively damaged. Such a condition may occur when the lesion is very extensive, or simply because the lesion is positioned at the periphery of the cartilaginous surface. A cartilage lesion centered on a highly curving articular surface, such as the peripheral talar dome, is also effectively poorly contained. Poorly contained cartilage lesions are problematic for two reasons. A poorly contained lesion has a greater tendency to enlarge because it is more vulnerable to extension at points where

it is not contained or protected by surrounding normal cartilage. Also, poorly contained lesions are more difficult to repair because native cartilage is not present on all sides of the lesion to which to anchor and protect repair tissue.

Lesion shouldering refers to the integrity of the edges of the cartilage lesion. If a lesion is "well shouldered," it will demonstrate crisp, vertical edges. A lesion with "poor shoulders" may be effectively larger than one that is well shouldered and may demonstrate margins that are fibrillated or irregular (**Fig. 15**). The extent of these findings should be noted. It is not always possible to determine the status of the margins of the cartilage lesions. Small flaps or regions of associated delamination also contribute to poor shouldering and should be mentioned in the radiology report (**Fig. 16**). Delamination of the cartilage from the subchondral bone can be seen without an overlying cartilage defect or fissure (**Fig. 17**). Such lesions are effectively full-thickness cartilage abnormalities because the delaminated cartilage is unstable.

With any cartilage repair procedure, debridement to clean margins of surrounding normal native cartilage is required before further intervention. Although a lesion may appear to be small, it could become much larger after the necessary debridement of cracked or unstable margins. This action may render the cartilage lesion not amenable to certain treatments. While a description of the lesion containment and shouldering is often helpful preoperatively, MR imaging is not

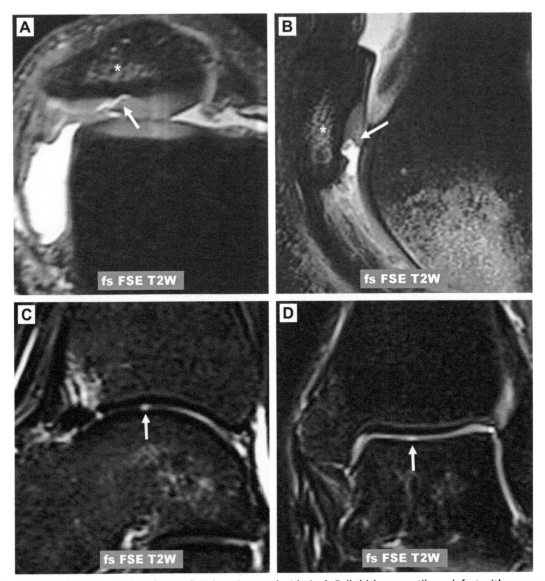

Fig. 13. Full-thickness cartilage lesions (MR imaging grade 4 lesion). Full-thickness cartilage defect with an associated flap is demonstrated in the patella (*A* and *B*, *arrow*). In a different patient, a small, full-thickness cartilage defect is seen as a focus of fluid signal on the central talar dome (*C* and *D*, *arrow*). The finding of focal fluid signal in the expected location of articular cartilage is a particularly helpful sign when cartilage is very thin. As shown, full-thickness cartilage lesions may (*A* and *B*) or may not (*C* and *D*) have subjacent edema-like bone marrow signal (*A* and *B*, *asterisk*).

always accurate in predicting the actual lesion size, and treatment options may change at surgery.

Bone marrow edema and subchondral cysts

Edema-like marrow signal in the subchondral bone is a frequent finding with deep cartilage defects, but can also be observed in the absence of any cartilage abnormality. In some cases, the bone marrow edema can be the only finding that indicates a subtle or occult cartilage injury. When subchondral bone marrow edema is seen, a careful search for associated cartilage lesion should be undertaken (**Fig. 18**). A deep cartilage lesion with associated subchondral bone marrow edema may be evidence that the lesion reaches the subchondral bone plate (see **Fig. 14**). In many cases, the only sign of a cartilage lesion in the ankle may be the presence of subchondral marrow edema.

Bone marrow edema can be graded in terms of both depth and intensity. Superficial bone marrow

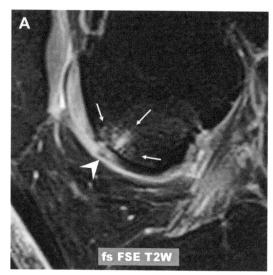
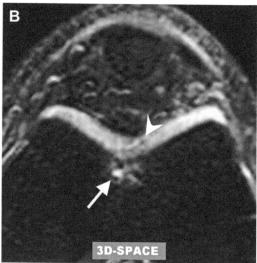

Fig. 14. Full-thickness cartilage lesion (MR imaging grade 4 lesion). Although the cartilage lesion in the trochlea (*A* and *B*, *arrowhead*) has suspected extension to the subchondral bone, the associated bone marrow edema (*A*, *small arrows*) and subchondral cyst (*B*, *large arrow*) raises the confidence that the lesion is truly full-thickness.

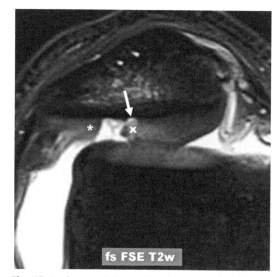

Fig. 15. Lesion containment and margins. It is important to describe the margins of solitary cartilage lesions that may be treated with surgery. This full-thickness cartilage lesion within the lateral patellar facet is "contained" because it has intact cartilage on all sides. When treating this lesion, the surgeon will prepare the defect by debridement of all unstable cartilage at the margins to produce sharp vertical walls. The lateral margin (*asterisk*) of this full thickness has sharp borders while the medial margin (*cross*) has an associated flap (*arrow*) and will require debridement. Noncontained lesions may require a different surgical techniques.

edema is located immediately beneath the subchondral bone plate and extends only a few millimeters in depth. More extensive bone marrow edema can be graded by measuring the depth below the subchondral plate. Some researchers have measured the volume of edema-like marrow signal using image segmentation programs.[34] Generalized edema involving the entire epiphysis, condyle, or talus may occur. The intensity of bone marrow edema can be graded as follows: mild if its signal intensity is less than that of muscle, moderate if the intensity is equal to that of muscle, and intense if the signal intensity is greater than that of muscle.

Subchondral cysts are often evidence that an overlying cartilage lesion reaches subchondral bone. However, subchondral cysts, particularly in the ankle, can also be seen in isolation (ie, without an overlying cartilage lesion) and can cause significant symptoms (**Fig. 19**). If subchondral cysts are identified in the ankle the radiologist should report their size, and also the presence or absence of any overlying cartilage defect. If there is no overlying cartilage defect, the surgeon may opt to take a retrograde approach to repair the subchondral bone, leaving the overlying cartilage untouched and intact. However, if a cartilage lesion is present, the lesion will be treated through an intra-articular approach. At the authors' institution, the ankle surgeons confirm the status of the cartilage overlying the cyst by arthroscopy before performing a drilling procedure. Therefore, they are less concerned about the radiologist's accuracy in

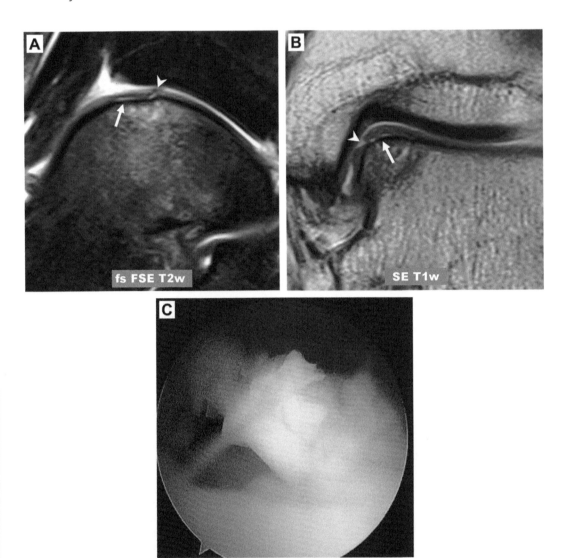

Fig. 16. Traumatic delamination. A young college athlete presented with ankle pain and swelling after a soccer injury. Sagittal (*A*) and coronal (*B*) images show an osteochondral lesion of the medial talar dome with a full-thickness lesion (*arrowhead*) that could be mistakenly called a small fissure. However, closer inspection shows a thin line of fluid signal along the bone-cartilage interface (*arrow*) indicating that a larger cartilage delamination is present. The arthroscopic photo (*C*) shows that the cartilage fragment was easily lifted from the bone. Following debridement and microfracture, the patient returned to the same level of play as before the injury.

determining if there is a cartilage defect than they are about the anterior-posterior location of the lesion that determines the proper arthroscopic portal.

Supporting structures

Damage to the supporting ligamentous structures should be noted in reports of the knee or ankle, as these pathologies may also need to be addressed operatively to ensure optimal joint function and cartilage repair. In knee reports, a specific comment should be made regarding any meniscal damage that is associated with a cartilage lesion. An abnormal meniscus may exacerbate a cartilage

lesion or create a contact surface damaging to cartilage repair tissue (**Fig. 20**). Similarly, for the ankle, the report should state any injury to the medial or lateral ankle ligaments. As discussed earlier, the presence of ankle instability may necessitate a staged procedure if cartilage repair is being contemplated, or the abandonment of a cartilage repair in favor of debridement.

Osteochondral Lesions/Osteochondritis Dissecans

The terms osteochondral lesion and osteochondritis dissecans have been used, at times,

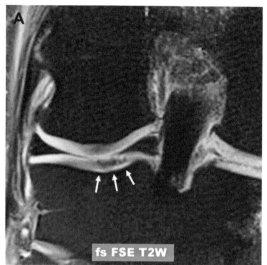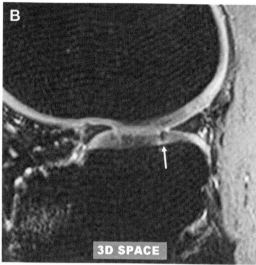

Fig. 17. Delamination in situ. Cartilage on the lateral tibial plateau appears to have an intact surface with a focal low signal region (*A* and *B*). Closer inspection demonstrates a thin high signal line at the interface of the deep cartilage and subchondral bone (*arrows*), which indicates a delamination injury with the separated cartilage remaining within the defect. This easily overlooked finding is particularly important to note in the MR report, as it may not be detectable at the time of arthroscopy without probing because cartilage surface may be intact.

interchangeably to describe articular lesions involving both cartilage and bone. The term osteochondritis dissecans was first used by Konig[35] in 1888, and referred to the development of atraumatic loose joint bodies. This term is now considered a misnomer, however, as no histologic findings of inflammation have been identified to

Fig. 18. Edema-like marrow signal. When bone marrow edema is seen, a careful search for overlying cartilage injury should be made. In this case, focal bone marrow edema in the posterolateral talar dome (*small arrows*) highlights the somewhat subtle overlying chondral injury (*larger arrow*).

warrant the suffix "-itis."[36] Furthermore, although many possible etiological factors for osteochondritis dissecans have been proposed and studied, the exact cause remains elusive and is most likely multifactorial.[36–38] The term osteochondritis dissecans has mostly been used to refer to the development of an apparently atraumatic osteochondral lesion, predominately in the pediatric and young adult population, but the term has also been applied to traumatic lesions. Therefore, to avoid confusion the authors prefer to use the general term osteochondral lesion at their institution.

Osteochondral lesions in the knee
Of all osteochondral lesions, 75% occur in the knee and 4% occur in the ankle.[39] There is a bimodal age distribution of osteochondral lesions in the knee, occurring in patients aged 11 to 13 years and 17 to 35 years. These lesions are classified as juvenile and adult osteochondral forms, respectively, and are distinguished by skeletal maturity.[40,41] A proportion of adult osteochondral lesions represent unrecognized or incompletely healed juvenile osteochondral lesions.[42] Osteochondral lesions of the knee occur slightly more frequently in male patients than in female patients.[43,44] The etiology of osteochondral lesions in the knee continues to be debated but likely relates to a combination of trauma, repetitive microtrauma, and genetics.[36,45,46] A vascular origin has also been proposed, but Chiroff and Cooke found no evidence of avascular necrosis

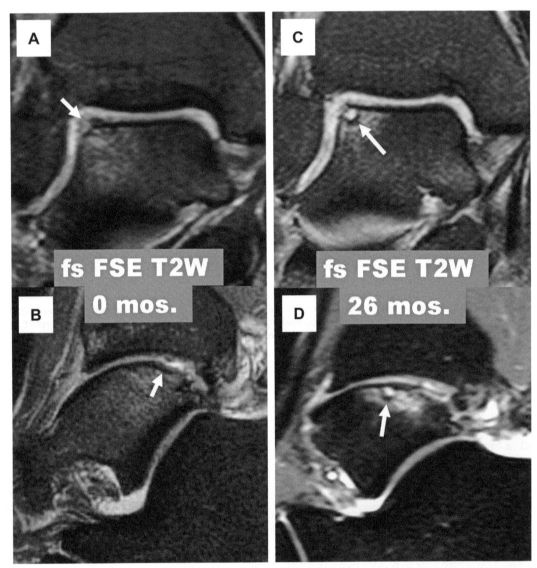

Fig. 19. Development of subchondral cyst of the talus. Cartilage irregularity and slight depression of subchondral bone (*A* and *B*, *small arrows*) are present at the posterior lateral talar dome. Two years later (*C* and *D*), a small subchondral cyst with bone marrow edema has developed (*larger arrows*), likely the cause of the patient's persistent symptoms. It is important to report subchondral cysts and their size as well as the presence or absence of an overlying cartilage defect.

on histologic examinations of osteochondral fragments.[47] More atraumatic lesions occur in the knee than in the ankle.

Patients with osteochondral lesions of the knee often present with vague knee pain, and may report knee clicking or locking.[48,49] On physical examination patients may exhibit focal tenderness, joint effusion, and altered gait (tibial external rotation). Most osteochondral lesions of the knee occur in the medial femoral condyle (80%–90% of cases). The classic lesion is located at the posterolateral aspect of the medial condyle, near

the notch,[34,50] and accounts for 70% of medial femoral condylar lesions.[39] However, osteochondral lesions of the knee also occur in the lateral femoral condyle, trochlea, and patella. The predilection of these lesions for the posterolateral medial femoral condyle may relate to anatomic variation, which allows the medial femoral condyle to abut the tibial spine at its posterolateral aspect, leading to localized chronic trauma.[36] The fact that medial femoral condyle osteochondral lesions of the knee are seen bilaterally in 30% to 40% of patients lends support to the theory that these

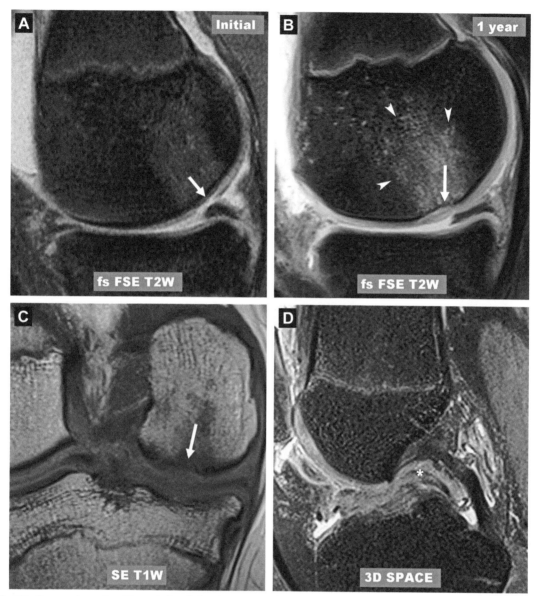

Fig. 20. Progression of cartilage defect following meniscal tear. A small medial meniscus from a tear is seen with a cartilage defect in the medial femoral condyle (A, arrow). One year later (B–D), a bucket handle meniscal tear has developed (D, asterisk), and there is now an osteochondral lesion with a cartilage fragment and subchondral bone depression (B and C, arrow), and increased edema-like marrow signal (B, arrowheads). In the radiology report, it is important to report meniscal pathology in the setting of cartilage disease, as meniscal abnormalities predispose to progression of cartilage damage.

lesions are at least partly related to genetics and/or anatomic variation.

Osteochondral lesions in the ankle

Although the relative percentage of overall osteochondral lesions in the ankle is small compared with the percentage seen in the knee these lesions account for most cases cartilage injury of the ankle. Compared with the bimodal distribution of osteochondral lesions in the knee, there is a single but wider age distribution for patients with osteochondral lesions in the ankle (range, 15–35 years). Similar to the knee, osteochondral lesions in the ankle are slightly more common among men than among women (63% male patients).[28] Most osteochondral lesions in the ankle are believed to have a traumatic origin; however, nontraumatic causes have been noted in up to 24% of cases.[25]

Osteochondral lesions of the lateral ankle more commonly have a traumatic cause than those of the medial ankle (94% of lateral lesions vs 62% of medial lesions).[25] The cartilage surface, subchondral bone plate, and subchondral cancellous bone can be considered as one anatomic unit in the ankle.[51] Lesions of the cartilage, subchondral plate, subchondral bone, or any combination of these regions are frequently grouped together as osteochondral lesions.

Most patients with an osteochondral lesion of the ankle present with nonspecific ankle pain and swelling. Some patients describe joint-catching symptoms and deep ankle pain.[28] In the setting of acute ankle sprain, the incidence of an osteochondral lesion is estimated to be 6.5%.[43] However, the incidence of osteochondral lesions in the ankle is much higher in the setting of persistent ankle pain following a sprain. In a group of patients with 7 months of persistent ankle pain after a sprain, 38% were found to have an osteochondral lesion at arthroscopy.[52] An association between ankle fractures and osteochondral lesions has also been noted. In a study of 86 cases of ankle fracture, 28% of patients with ankle fractures also had a chondral lesion of the talar dome. Distal fibular fractures were found to have the highest association with osteochondral lesions

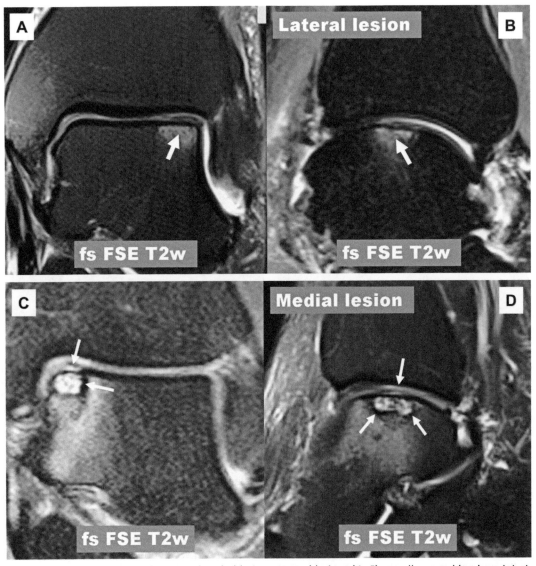

Fig. 21. Medial versus lateral talar osteochondral lesions. Lateral lesions (*A*, *B*), usually caused by shear injuries, are often shallow, disc-shaped lesions (*arrow*), whereas medial lesions (*C*, *D*) are more commonly from impaction, and appear deeper and cylindrical (*arrows*).

Table 3	
Berndt and Harty staging system for osteochondral lesions of the talus as modified by Anderson et al	
Stage	**Description**
I	Focal compression of subchondral bone with intact overlying cartilage
II	Incomplete separation of an osteochondral fragment
IIA	Formation of a subchondral cyst
III	Complete detachment of an osteochondral fragment that remains in place
IV	Complete detachment of an osteochondral fragment that becomes displaced, either at the injury site or remotely within the joint space

Data from Anderson IF, Crichton KJ, Grattan-Smith T, et al. Osteochondral fractures of the dome of the talus. J Bone Joint Surg Am 1989;71:1143–52.

(70%). Osteochondral lesions of the talus were also associated with bimalleolar and trimalleolar fractures, but to a lesser degree than isolated distal fibular fractures.[53] These findings support the theory that most osteochondral lesions of the ankle are traumatic in origin.

Most osteochondral lesions of the ankle are located on the talar dome. Within the talar dome, slightly more lesions are found medially than laterally (56%–62% medial vs 36%–44% lateral).[28] Both medial and lateral osteochondral lesions may be found in the same ankle. Osteochondral lesions of the talus have characteristic shapes depending on their location, due to the differences in

Table 4	
ICRS arthroscopic grading system for osteochondral lesions	
Stage	**Description**
I	Stable lesion with softened but intact overlying cartilage
II	Partial fragment discontinuity, but stable fragment when probed
III	Complete fragment discontinuity, but no fragment dislocation
IV	Complete fragment dislocation, empty defect

From Brittberg M, Peterson L. Introduction of an articular cartilage classification. ICRS Newsletter 1998;1:5–8; with permission.

biomechanics on either side of the ankle joint. Laterally located lesions are typically shallow and may be displaced because of the shearing force that produces them. Medially located lesions, on the other hand, are deeper and cylindrical in shape because of the impaction and torsion forces that create them (**Fig. 21**).[9,44,45,54,55]

Osteochondral lesions of the tibial plafond are unusual, with an incidence ratio of 1:20 with respect to osteochondral lesions of the talar dome.[30] This finding may reflect the more favorable cartilage stiffness parameters of tibial plafond compared with the talus or differences in force distribution related to the contrasting curvatures of the plafond and dome.[56] A study of 38 osteochondral lesions of the distal tibia showed a fairly uniform distribution of lesions across the tibial plafond.[30] This same study showed that kissing lesions of the tibial plafond and talar dome are very rare (1 out of 38 tibial plafond lesions).

Classification of osteochondral lesions

The initial staging system for osteochondral lesions of the talus was established by Berndt and Harty and is composed of 4 stages that correspond with the progression of injury through progressive degrees of trauma (**Table 3**).[54] By MR imaging, it is not clear that osteochondral lesions progress through these stages over time.[57] In 1989, Anderson and colleagues[45] proposed adding a Stage IIa lesion to include the formation of subchondral cysts to the staging system.

Although this staging system has long been established, many studies have shown that it is not accurate in predicting clinical outcomes.[58–60] It has also not been shown to correlate with

Table 5		
Signs of osteochondral lesion instability in adult and juvenile patients		
Adult Patient (Closed Physis)	**Juvenile Patient (Open Physis)**	
High signal line surrounding the fragment	Fluid signal line surrounding the lesion	
Subchondral cyst(s) around the lesion	Multiple breaks in the subchondral bone plate	
Focal chondral or subchondral bone defect	Low signal rim of the osteochondral lesion	
Fluid-filled osteochondral defect	—	

arthroscopic assessment of the cartilage status of the lesion.[27] There is now clinical evidence that osteochondral lesions of both the knee and the ankle should be treated based on the integrity of the overlying cartilage and the stability of the osseous fragment rather than the radiographic stage.[27,56,59,61] The Berndt and Harty staging system has not been shown to correlate with

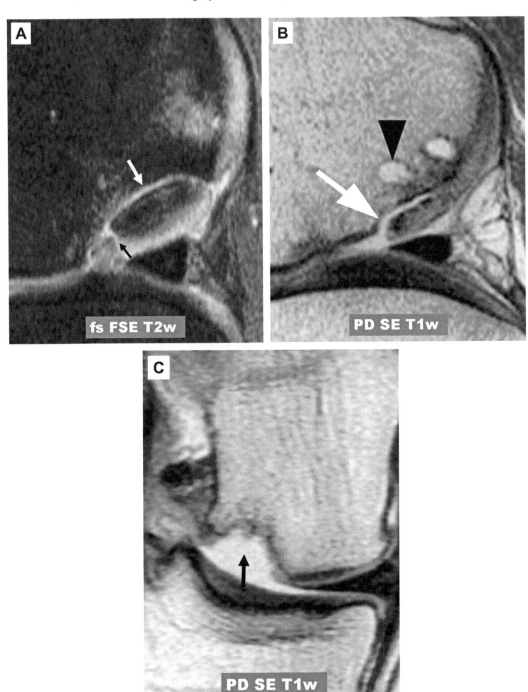

Fig. 22. Signs of osteochondral fragment instability in the adult. Fragment instability may be indicated by a high signal line surrounding the lesion (*A* and *B*, *white arrow*), the presence of subchondral cysts (*B*, *arrowhead*), an empty bone defect filled with fluid (*C*, *arrow*), and/or a high signal line passing into the lesion indicating articular fracture (*A*, *black arrow*). (*From* Winalski CS, Gupta KB. Magnetic resonance imaging of focal articular cartilage lesions. Top Magn Reson Imaging 2003;14:131–44.)

arthroscopic assessment of the cartilage status of the lesion.[27] The ICRS has therefore established an arthroscopic grading system for osteochondral lesions, described initially for the knee, which includes an assessment of the overlying articular cartilage and fragment stability (**Table 4**).

MR imaging for assessment of osteochondral lesions

MR imaging is a valuable tool in the assessment of osteochondral lesions and has proved useful for noninvasive preoperative assessment.[45,62] Studies in the knee have shown the utility of MR imaging to assess osteochondral lesion stability.[40] De Smet and colleagues[63] first showed the ability of MR imaging to evaluate the stability of an osteochondral fragment in the knee and ankle. Four signs of instability were identified (**Table 5**). The first and most common sign is a high signal line surrounding the fragment.[63] The second sign is the presence of cysts surrounding the fragment, which are believed to be related to osseous

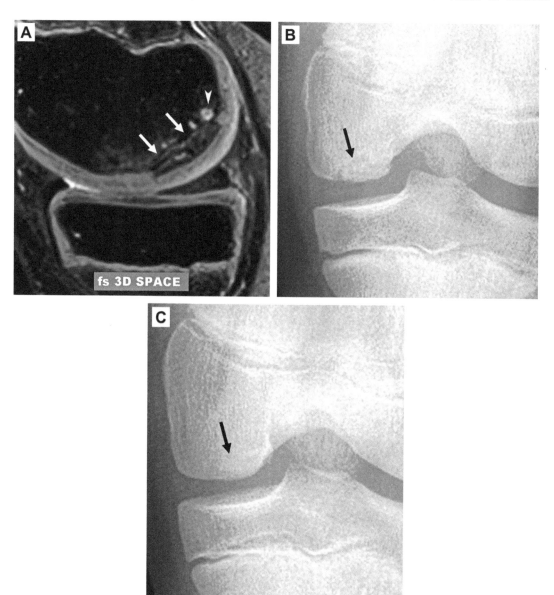

Fig. 23. Stable osteochondral lesion in a juvenile (skeletally immature) patient. Sagittal MR image (*A*) shows an intermediate signal line (*arrows*) beneath the osteochondral lesion of the medial femorally condyle with no fluid-like interface. Radiographs at the time of the MR imaging examination (*B*) and 1 year later (*C*) show progressive healing of the osteochondral lesion (*black arrow*) without surgery. Cysts in association with osteochondral lesions (*A, arrowheads*) do not imply instability in the juvenile as they do in the adult.

resorption due to alteration in biomechanical forces. These cysts are not always related to communication with joint fluid, as they have been seen with intact overlying cartilage at arthroscopy.[64] The third sign is the presence of a focal cartilage and/or subchondral bone plate defect. The fourth sign is the presence of a high signal within the fragment, indicating articular fracture (**Fig. 22**). In the adult (closed physis), any one of these signs has high sensitivity and specificity for detecting an unstable lesion. No relationship between lesion size and stability and lesion location and stability has been identified.[40]

Although these 4 signs also have high sensitivity for detecting unstable osteochondral lesions in the juvenile knee, they have poor specificity. In a study of 36 juvenile osteochondral lesions, the 4 De Smet MR imaging signs of instability had a sensitivity of 100% but a specificity of only 17%.[40] There are multiple reports of children with

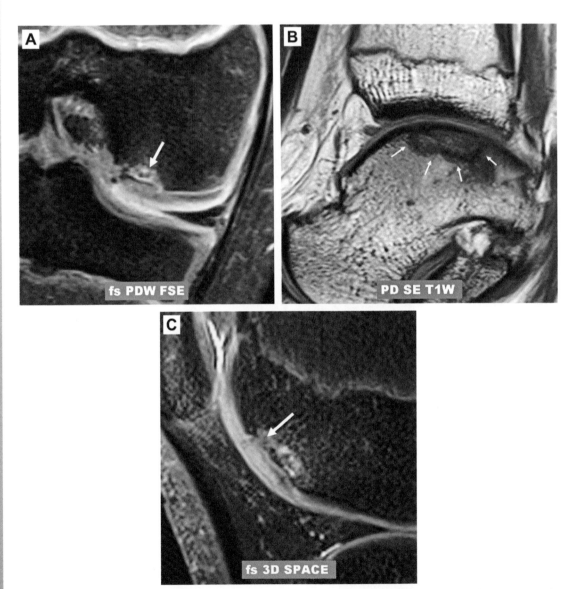

Fig. 24. Three signs of osteochondral lesion instability in the juvenile (skeletally immature) patient. In the juvenile, a high signal line surrounding the osteochondral lesion must be of fluid intensity to imply instability (*A, arrow*). A hypointense rim on T1-weighted images surrounding the osteochondral lesion also implies instability (*B, small arrows*). Multiple breaks in the subchondral bone indicated by intermediate and high signal foci disrupting the subchondral bone adjacent to the osteochondral lesion (*C, arrow*) also indicates instability. In all these osteochondral lesions, the cartilage surface was intact at arthroscopy. Cysts seen in association with osteochondral lesions do not imply instability in the juvenile as they do in the adult.

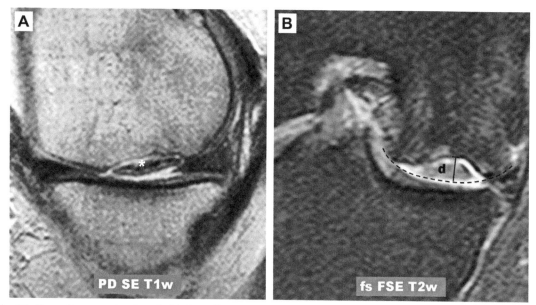

Fig. 25. Reporting an osteochondral lesion. The osseous component (*A, asterisk*), less than 2 mm in depth, is too thin in this case for direct fixation of the fragment. (*B*) The maximum depth (d) of the osteochondral lesion into the subchondral bone is less than 10 mm, suggesting that bone grafting may not be required prior to cartilage repair surgery.

osteochondral lesions with a high signal line or cysts surrounding the lesion that have healed with only conservative management, suggesting that these lesions were not truly unstable. The high signal line and cysts surrounding the lesions are therefore not robust indicators of instability in juvenile cases as they are in adults.[40,65] When 3 different signs are applied, the specificity for instability can be improved significantly, achieving a sensitivity and specificity of 100% (see **Table 5**). The first of these signs is a fluid signal rim surrounding the lesion. Unlike in an adult, the high signal rim surrounding a lesion in a child must have the same signal intensity as joint fluid to imply instability (**Fig. 23**). A second sign is the presence of multiple breaks in the subchondral bone plate, which can be identified by focal regions of high signal within the otherwise low-signal, albeit abnormal contour, subchondral bone. A third sign is a low signal-intensity rim within subchondral bone surrounding the lesion (**Fig. 24**). This low-signal rim, which was only observed in unstable lesions, may represent sclerotic bone formation.[40]

Treatment of osteochondral lesions of the knee is largely dependent on the stability of the lesion. Therefore, when reporting an osteochondral lesion of the knee it is important to provide an age-appropriate assessment of lesion stability based on the criteria shown in **Table 5**. It is also important to note the thickness of the osseous fragment and

the maximum depth of the lesion into subchondral bone, as these features will determine whether direct fixation by screw or pin, or osteochondral plug fixation of the lesion can be attempted. If the osteochondral fragment cannot be directly fixed, bone grafting may be required (**Fig. 25**).

In the ankle the cartilage, subchondral bone plate, and subchondral bone are often grouped as a single anatomic unit. Therefore, isolated cartilage lesions are often classified as osteochondral

Table 6	
Grading system for osteochondral lesions of the ankle	

Grade	Description
0	Normal
1	Hyperintense but morphologically intact cartilage
2	Fibrillation or fissuring of cartilage not extending to bone
3	Chondral flap or exposed bone
4	Loose (unstable) but nondisplaced fragment
5	Displaced fragment

Data from Mintz DN, Tashjian GS, Connell DA, et al. Osteochondral lesions of the talus: a new magnetic resonance grading system with arthroscopic correlation. Arthroscopy 2003;19:353–9.

lesions. An alternative grading system that evaluates the status of the articular cartilage has been devised (Table 6). This system has less stratification of cartilage lesion depth compared with those for the knee, a practical consideration given the thinness of ankle cartilage and associated difficulty in accurately judging lesion depth on MR imaging. The aforementioned age-appropriate criteria for osteochondral lesion instability shown in Table 5 can be applied to assess lesion stability in the ankle as well (ie, in the case of a grade 4 lesion). A study of 40 osteochondral lesions of the ankle found that MR imaging correctly graded 83% of lesions using this grading system, with arthroscopy serving as the gold standard.[66] When the grades were subdivided into disease-positive (grades 2, 3, 4, 5) and disease-negative (grades 0 and 1) groups, MR imaging had a sensitivity of 95% and specificity of 100%[66] for detecting disease. There are numerous treatment options for osteochondral lesions of the ankle, ranging from rest and immobilization to autologous chondrocyte implantation. Use of this grading system can help to stratify patients who would benefit from surgical intervention (grades 2–5) and those who would not (grades 0 and 1).

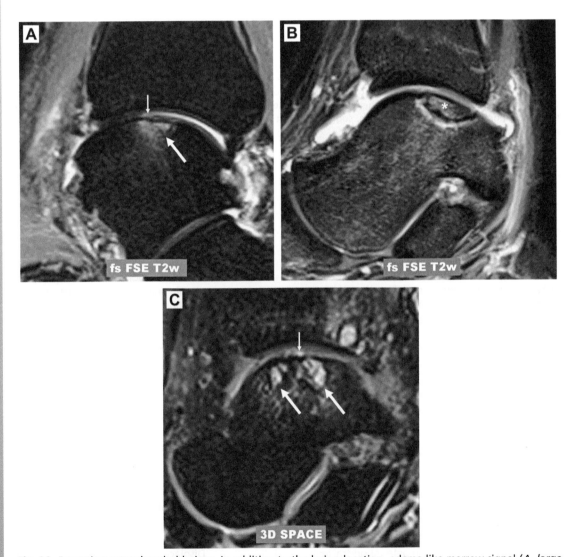

Fig. 26. Reporting osteochondral lesions. In addition to the lesion location, edema-like marrow signal (A, *large arrow*) should be noted, as it can be associated with pain. A measurement of the thickness of the osseous fragment (B, *asterisk*) should be provided. Measurements of subchondral cysts (C, *large arrows*) should be provided, as bone grafting may be necessary. Damage to the overlying cartilage, as present in these examples (A and C, *small arrow*), usually precludes a retrograde repair approach.

Although grading systems provide a basic framework for judging osteochondral lesion severity, radiology reports should be tailored to reflect the treatment practices of the referring surgeons. At the authors' institution, the acuity of the osteochondral ankle lesion, patient age, subchondral bone fragment thickness, and the presence and size of subchondral cysts are most important in guiding therapy. The surgeons consider surgical repair in a young patient if the incident injury has occurred within the past 3 months. If the thickness of the bone fragment is at least 2 mm thick, a direct pin fixation may be attempted as initial therapy. If this initial fixation fails, a more extensive repair such as osteochondral autograft transfer system or autologous chondrocyte implantation would be considered. In older patients and those not requiring optimal joint function, debridement and marrow stimulation, such as microfracture, are usually performed. Painful subchondral cysts are treated with either a debridement and marrow stimulation procedure or bone grafting, depending on size. Therefore, in the radiology report the location of the osteochondral lesion, the thickness of any bone fragment, and the presence and size of any subchondral cysts are emphasized (Fig. 26).

SUMMARY

Cartilage abnormalities in the knee and ankle are a common source of pain, and are often difficult to diagnose clinically and with radiographs. MR imaging is a valuable tool for diagnosing and characterizing cartilage lesions of both the knee and the ankle. In this article the authors describe the normal appearance of articular cartilage and the grading of cartilage lesions in the knee and ankle. Guidelines on how to report cartilage abnormalities are presented and the wide spectrum of image findings illustrated. Knowledge of and familiarity with these aspects will allow the radiologist to provide more accurate and clinically useful reports.

REFERENCES

1. Noyes FR, Bassett RW, Grood ES, et al. Arthroscopy in acute traumatic hemarthrosis of the knee: incidence of anterior cruciate tears and other injuries. J Bone Joint Surg Am 1980;62:687–95.
2. Bedi A, Feeley BT, Williams RJ III. Management of articular cartilage defects of the knee. J Bone Joint Surg Am 2010;92:994–1009.
3. Simon TM, Jackson DW. Articular cartilage: injury pathways and treatment options. Sports Med Arthrosc 2006;14:146–54.
4. Brittberg M, Winalski CS. Evaluation of cartilage injuries and repair. J Bone Joint Surg Am 2003; 85(Suppl 2):58–69.
5. Goddwin DW. MR imaging of the articular cartilage of the knee. Semin Musculoskelet Radiol 2009; 13(4):326–39.
6. Schibany N, Ba-Ssalamah A, Marlovits S, et al. Impact of high Field (3.0T) magnetic resonance imaging on diagnosis of osteochondral defects in the ankle joint. Eur J Radiol 2005;55:283–8.
7. Rush Department of Biochemistry. Available at: http://www.rushu.rush.edu/servlet/Satellite?MetaAttrName= meta_university&ParentId=1225124420159&Parent Type=RushUnivLevel3Page&c=content_block&cid= 1225124420147&level1-p=3&level1-pp=1225124419 893&level1-ppp=1225124419893&pagename= Rush%2Fcontent_block%2FContentBlockDetailWeb. Accessed March 12, 2011.
8. Shepherd DE, Seedhom BB. Thickness of human articular cartilage in joints of the lower limb. Ann Rheum Dis 1999;58:27–34.
9. Raikin SM, Elias I, Zoga AC, et al. Osteochondral lesions of the talus: localization and morphologic data from 424 patients using a novel anatomical grid scheme. Foot Ankle Int 2007;28:154–61.
10. Oakley SP, Portek I, Szomor Z, et al. Poor accuracy and interobserver reliability of knee arthroscopy measurements are improved by the use of variable angle elongated probes. Ann Rheum Dis 2002;61: 540–3.
11. Hardy PA, Nammalwar P, Kuo S. Measuring the thickness of articular cartilage from MR images. J Magn Reson Imaging 2001;13:120–6.
12. van Dijk CN, Reilingh ML, Zengerink M, et al. The natural history of osteochondral lesions in the ankle. Instr Course Lect 2010;59:375–86.
13. Schumacher BL, Su JL, Lindley KM, et al. Horizontally oriented clusters of multiple chondrons in the superficial zone of the ankle, but not knee articular cartilage. Anat Rec 2002;266:241–8.
14. Chubinskaya S, Kuettner KE, Cole AA. Expression of matrix metalloproteinases in normal and damaged articular cartilage from human knee and ankle joints. Lab Invest 1999;79(12):1669–77.
15. Aurich M, Mwale F, Reiner A, et al. Collagen and proteoglycan turnover in focally damaged human ankle cartilage. Arthritis Rheum 2006;54(1):244–52.
16. Shepherd DE, Seedhom BB. The 'instantaneous' compressive modulus of human articular cartilage in joints of the lower limb. Rheumatology 1999;38: 124–32.
17. Treppo S, Koepp H, Quan EC, et al. Comparison of biomechanical and biochemical properties of cartilage from human knee and ankle pairs. J Orthop Res 2000;18:739–48.
18. Huch K. Knee and ankle: human joints with different susceptibility to osteoarthritis reveal different cartilage

cellularity and matrix synthesis in vitro. Arch Orthop Trauma Surg 2001;121:301–6.

19. Fetter NL, Leddy HA, Guilak F, et al. Composition and transport properties of human ankle and knee cartilage. J Orthop Res 2006;24(2):211–9.

20. Orazizadeh M, Cartlidge C, Wright MO, et al. Mechanical responses and integrin associated protein expression by human ankle chondrocytes. Biorheology 2006;43:249–58.

21. Dang Y, Cole AA, Homandberg GA. Comparison of the catabolic effects of fibronectin fragments in human knee and ankle cartilages. Osteoarthritis Cartilage 2003;11(7):538–47.

22. Hendren L, Beeson P. A review of the differences between normal and osteoarthritis articular cartilage in human knee and ankle joints. Foot (Edinb) 2009; 19:171–6.

23. Recht MP, Goodwin DW, Winalski CS, et al. MRI of articular cartilage: revisiting current status and future directions. AJR Am J Roentgenol 2005;185: 899–914.

24. Stephens T, Diduch DR, Balin JI. The cartilage black line sign: an unexpected MRI appearance of deep cartilage fissuring in three patients. Skeletal Radiol 2011;40(1):113–6.

25. Tol JL, Struijs PA, Bossuyt PM, et al. Treatment strategies in osteochondral defects of the talar dome: a systematic review. Foot Ankle Int 2000;21(2):119–26.

26. Kocher MS, Tucker R, Ganley TJ, et al. Management of osteochondritis dissecans of the knee: current concepts review. Am J Sports Med 2006;34: 1181–91.

27. Pritsch M, Horoshovski H, Farine I. Arthroscopic treatment of osteochondral lesions of the talus. J Bone Joint Surg Am 1986;68:862–5.

28. Zengerrink M, Struijs PA, Tol JL, et al. Treatment of osteochondral lesions of the talus: a systematic review. Knee Surg Sports Traumatol Arthrosc 2010; 18:238–46.

29. The ICRS knee cartilage lesion mapping system. ICRS Cartilage Injury Evaluation Package from the International Cartilage Repair Society. Available at: www.cartilage.org. Accessed March 12, 2011.

30. Elias I, Raikin SM, Schweitzer ME, et al. Osteochondral lesions of the distal tibial plafond: localization and morphologic characteristics with an anatomical grid. Foot Ankle Int 2009;30:524–9.

31. Outerbridge RE. The etiology of chondromalacia patellae. J Bone Joint Surg Br 1961;43:752–67.

32. Parisien JS, Vangness T. Operative arthroscopy of the ankle. Three years experience. Clin Orthop Relat Res 1985;199:46–53.

33. Bredella MA, Tirman PF, Peterfy CG, et al. Accuracy of T2-weighted fast spin-echo MR imaging with fat saturation in detecting cartilage defects in the knee: comparison with arthroscopy in 130 patients. AJR Am J Roentgenol 1999;172:1073–80.

34. Mayerhoefer ME, Breitenseher M, Hofmann S, et al. Computer-assisted quantitative analysis of bone marrow edema of the knee: initial experience with a new method. AJR Am J Roentgenol 2004;182: 1399–403.

35. Konig F. Uber freie Korper in der Gelenken. Dtsch Z Klin Chir 1887;27:90–109 [in German].

36. Clanton TO, DeLee JC. Osteochondritis dissecans: history, pathophysiology, and current treatment concepts. Clin Orthop Relat Res 1982;167:50–64.

37. Glancy GL. Juvenile osteochondritis dissecans. Am J Knee Surg 1999;12:120–4.

38. Hefti F, Beguiristain J, Krauspe R, et al. Osteochondritis dissecans: a multicenter study of the European Pediatric Orthopedic Society. J Pediatr Orthop B 1999;8:231–45.

39. Aichroth P. Osteochondritis dissecans of the knee. A clinical survey. J Bone Joint Surg Br 1971;53(3): 440–7.

40. Kijowski R, Blankenbaker DG, Shinki K, et al. Juvenile versus adult osteochondritis dissecans of the knee: appropriate MR imaging criteria for instability. Radiology 2008;248(2):571–8.

41. Cahill BR. Osteochondritis dissecans of the knee: treatment of juvenile and adult forms. J Am Acad Orthop Surg 1995;3:237–47.

42. Garrett JC. Osteochondritis dissecans. Clin Sports Med 1991;10:569–93.

43. Bosien WR, Staples OS, Russell SW. Residual disability following acute ankle sprains. J Bone Joint Surg Am 1955;37(6):1237–43.

44. Canale ST, Belding. RH: Osteochondral lesions of the talus. J Bone Joint Surg Am 1980;62(1):97–102.

45. Anderson IF, Crichton KJ, Grattan-Smith T, et al. Osteochondral fractures of the dome of the talus. J Bone Joint Surg Am 1989;71(8):1143–52.

46. Barrie HJ. Osteochondritis dissecans 1887–1987. A centennial look at König's memorable phrase. J Bone Joint Surg Br 1987;69(5):693–5.

47. Chiroff RT, Cooke CP 3rd. Osteochondritis dissecans: a histologic and microradiographic analysis of surgically excised lesions. J Trauma 1975;15(8): 689–96.

48. Twyman RS, Desai K, Aichroth PM. Osteochondritis dissecans of the knee: a long-term study. J Bone Joint Surg Br 1991;73:461–4.

49. Schenck RC Jr, Goodnight JM. Osteochondritis dissecans. J Bone Joint Surg Am 1996;78:439–56.

50. Loredo R, Sanders TG. Imaging of osteochondral injuries. Clin Sports Med 2001;20:249–78.

51. Bohndorf K. Injuries at the articulating surfaces of bone (chondral, osteochondral, subchondral fractures and osteochondrosis dissecans). Eur J Radiol 1996;22:22–9.

52. Takao M, Uchio Y, Naito K, et al. Arthroscopic assessment for intra-articular disorders in residual ankle disability after sprain. Am J Sports Med

2005;33(5):686–92. Available at: http://dx.doi.org/
10.1177/0363546504270566. Accessed March 12,
2011.

53. Aktas S, Kocaoglu B, Gereli A, et al. Incidence of
chondral lesions of talar dome in ankle fracture
types. Foot Ankle Int 2008;29(3):287–92.

54. Berndt AL, Harty M. Transchondral fractures (osteochondritis dissecans) of the talus. J Bone Joint Surg
Am 1959;41:988–1020.

55. Robinson DE, Winson IG, Harries WJ, et al. Arthroscopic treatment of osteochondral lesions of the
talus. J Bone Joint Surg Br 2003;85(7):989–93.

56. Athanasiou KA, Niederauer GG, Schenck RC Jr.
Biomechanical topography of human ankle cartilage. Ann Biomed Eng 1995;23(5):697–704.

57. Elias I, Jung JW, Raikin SM, et al. Osteochondral
lesions of the talus: change in MRI findings over
time in talar lesions without operative intervention
and implications for staging systems. Foot Ankle
Int 2006;27:157–66.

58. Jurgensen I, Bachmann G, Siaplaouras J, et al.
[Clinical value of conventional radiology and MRI
in assessing osteochondrosis dissecans stability].
Unfallchirurg 1996;99:758–63 [in German].

59. Stone JW. Osteochondral lesions of the talar dome.
J Am Acad Orthop Surg 1996;4:63–73.

60. Bachmann G, Jurgensen I, Siaplaouras J. [The
staging of osteochondritis dissecans in the knee
and ankle joints with MR tomography: a comparison
with conventional radiology and arthroscopy]. For-
tschritte Gebiet Rontgenstrahlen Neuen Bildgeben-
den Verfahren. Rofo 1995;163:38–44 [in German].

61. Bruns J. Osteochondrosis dissecans tali. Results of
surgical therapy. Unfallchirurg 1993;96:75–81.

62. Takao M, Uchio Y, Kakimaru H, et al. Arthroscopic
drilling with debridement of remaining cartilage for
osteochondral lesions of the talar dome in unstable
ankles. Am J Sports Med 2004;32(2):332–6.

63. De Smet AA, Ilahi O, Graf BK. Reassessment of
the MR Criteria for Stability of osteochondritis dissecans in the knee and ankle. Skeletal Radiol 1996;25:
159–63.

64. Yuan HA, Cady RB, DeRosa C. Osteochondritis dissecans of the talus associated with subchondral
cysts. J Bone Joint Surg Am 1979;61:1249–51.

65. Yoshida S, Ikata T, Takai H, et al. Osteochondritis
dissecans of the femoral condyle in the growth
stage. Clin Orthop Relat Res 1998;346:162–70.

66. Mintz DN, Tashjian GS, Connell DA, et al. Osteochondral lesions of the talus: a new magnetic resonance
grading system with arthroscopic correlation.
Arthroscopy 2003;19(4):353–9.

The Current State of Imaging the Articular Cartilage of the Upper Extremity

Humberto G. Rosas, MD[a],*, Michael J. Tuite, MD[b]

KEYWORDS
- Review article • Cartilage • Upper extremity
- Osteochondral injuries

Cartilaginous injuries and degenerative processes involving the joints afflict millions of individuals each year with enormous socioeconomic ramifications.[1–3] Although most imaging studies have centered on the evaluation of the articular cartilage of the knee,[4–9] with the advancement in treatment options, the recent interest in developing disease-modifying drugs, and the necessity to noninvasively monitor the success of treatment, the role of imaging will inevitably continue to expand. Noninvasive methods of acquiring morphologic and physiologic details play an ever-increasing role in the treatment and management of patients with cartilaginous disease. MR imaging, with its excellent tissue contrast, is currently the imaging modality of choice for evaluating articular cartilage. However, imaging of smaller joints, such as those found in the upper extremity, present several challenges secondary to thin overlying cartilage in conjunction with complex surface geometry. Current MR imaging techniques often lack adequate spatial resolution and tissue contrast to appropriately evaluate the articular cartilage of smaller joints. With the introduction of dedicated multichannel extremity coils, higher field strength scanner, and new morphologic and quantitative MR imaging techniques, the future holds promise in overcoming these obstacles.

This article reviews cartilaginous diseases of the upper extremity emphasizing those that can be assessed using current clinical MR imaging protocols and addresses the limitations of current imaging techniques in evaluating the articular cartilage of smaller joints. It also provides a brief overview of novel techniques that may be instituted in the future to improve the diagnostic performance of MR imaging in the evaluation of the articular cartilage of the upper extremity.

SHOULDER

Cartilaginous degeneration within the glenohumeral joint is relatively uncommon, particularly when compared with the weight bearing joints such as the hip or knee. Autopsy studies have shown a relative high frequency of shallow fibrillation involving the glenohumeral joint. However, higher Outerbridge grades II to IV lesions were infrequent in the absence of trauma.[10] The incidence of higher-grade cartilaginous lesions at arthroscopy has been estimated at 5% and supports the autopsy results.[11,12] Therefore, if a past history of trauma or infection is not elicited and imaging demonstrates more diffuse and severe cartilaginous loss, other causes such as crystalline depositions disorders, inflammatory arthritides, metabolic disorders, synovial osteochondromatosis, and neuropathic osteoarthropathy should be considered in addition to primary osteoarthritis (**Figs. 1** and **2**). Rapid chondrolysis

[a] Musculoskeletal Radiology, Department of Radiology, University of Wisconsin School of Medicine and Public Health, University of Wisconsin Hospital and Clinics, F2/422, 600 Highland Avenue, Madison, WI 53792, USA
[b] Musculoskeletal Radiology, Department of Radiology, University of Wisconsin School of Medicine and Public Health, University of Wisconsin Hospital and Clinics, E3/311, 600 Highland Avenue, Madison, WI 53792, USA
* Corresponding author.
E-mail address: hrosas@uwhealth.org

Magn Reson Imaging Clin N Am 19 (2011) 407–423
doi:10.1016/j.mric.2011.02.006
1064-9689/11/$ – see front matter. Published by Elsevier Inc.

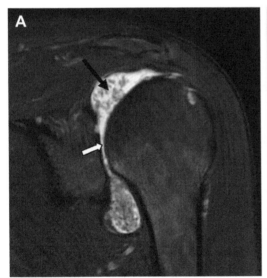
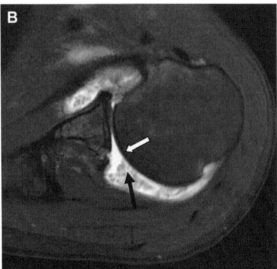

Fig. 1. Rheumatoid arthritis in a 43-year-old woman. Coronal T1-weighted fat-saturated (*A*) and axial proton density (PD)–weighted fat-saturated (*B*) MR arthrographs of the shoulder demonstrate diffuse cartilage loss (*white arrows*) and multiple intra-articular filling defects consistent with rice bodies (*black arrows*).

after arthroscopy has been reported with several plausible causal agents, including the application of thermal or radiofrequency energy typically used for capsulorrhapy,[13–16] intra-articular administration of gentian violet at the time of arthroscopy,[17] and the use of a continuous bupivacaine pump to aid in the management of postoperative pain.[14]

Cartilaginous Abnormalities and Injury Patterns

Several studies have reported an association between cartilaginous lesions and rotator cuff disease, subacromial impingement, and instability. Peterson[18] found that 75% of shoulders demonstrating cartilaginous disease had concomitant

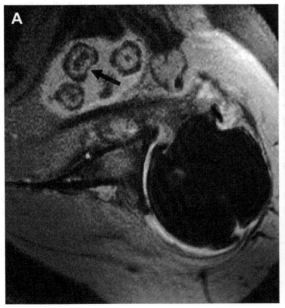
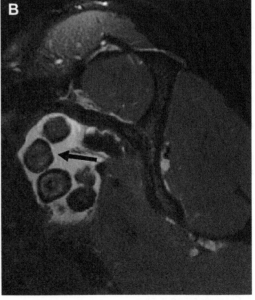

Fig. 2. Synovial osteochondromatosis in a 42-year-old woman. Axial proton density–weighted fat-saturated (*A*) and oblique sagittal T2-weighted fat-saturated (*B*) MR images of the shoulder show multiple ossified bodies (*black arrows*) of approximately equal size distributed throughout the subcoracoid bursa.

findings of attrition or rupture of the rotator cuff. What remains to be determined is if a true relationship exists or if these are 2 independent processes related to aging. Several theories propose a cascade of events tying the processes together. One possibility is that rupture of the rotator cuff leads to leakage of synovial fluid resulting in loss of the intracapsular pressure and decreased perfusion to the articular cartilage. Instability and superior migration of the humeral head predisposes to altered biomechanics and increased wear of articular surfaces. The mechanical forces and relative lack of nutrition ultimately lead to atrophy of the glenohumeral cartilage, osteoporosis of the subchondral bone plate, and collapse of the humeral head, a phenomenon referred to as cuff tear arthropathy.[19] At arthrography, rotator cuff lesions were identified in more than 90% of shoulders with osteoarthritis of the glenohumeral joint.[20] Gartsman and Taverna,[21] however, reported a much lower prevalence of cartilaginous lesions (13%) in a series of 200 patients with reparable full-thickness rotator cuff tears, with only 5% demonstrating lesions defined as major and involving 150 mm^2 or more of exposed areas of bone.

Patients presenting with clinical findings of subacromial impingement reportedly have a higher prevalence of cartilaginous disease. Guntern and colleagues[22] found a prevalence of 29% for humeral cartilaginous lesions and 15% for glenoid cartilaginous lesions in 52 patients with subacromial impingement syndrome undergoing both MR arthrography and arthroscopy. The investigators stressed the importance of interrogating the cartilage on MR imaging and MR arthrography in this subset of patients because early degenerative joint disease can mimic symptoms of shoulder impingement[23] and can alter the treatment plan.

Trauma and instability often coincide with cartilage injury. Acute dislocations can result in cartilage shear injuries[24] (**Fig. 3**) and impaction fractures such as a Hill-Sachs lesion, which when large can involve the articular surface of the humeral head.[25,26] The incidence of cartilage shear injury, osteoarthritis, or Hill-Sachs lesion after an index anterior shoulder dislocation ranges between 24% and 90%.[27–29] Predictors of osteoarthritis in the setting of instability include time to surgery, age of the patient, presence of a Hill-Sachs lesion or glenoid rim impaction fracture, and presence of a rotator cuff tear.[27,30]

More focal cartilage injury patterns have also been described. In a small subset of patients developing acute onset of pain after a single traumatic event, focal cartilaginous lesions were identified along the posterosuperior aspect of the

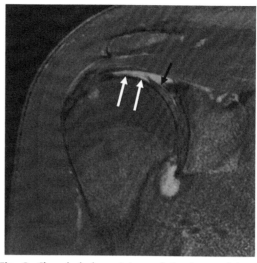

Fig. 3. Chondral shear injury of the humeral head after an acute trauma in a 22-year-old man. Oblique coronal T2-weighted fat-saturated MR image of the shoulder reveals a large focal chondral shear injury overlying the central aspect of the humeral head (*white arrows*). Normal intermediate signal cartilage is present medially (*black arrow*).

humeral head medial to the typical location of a Hill-Sachs lesion.[31] Although all patients had additional pathologic condition involving the shoulder on MR imaging, those undergoing arthroscopy required debridement with good short-term outcomes in individuals with smaller cartilaginous lesions. This cartilaginous injury pattern differs in location and clinical history from the injury pattern near the insertion of the supraspinatus tendon described by Paley and colleagues[32] in 41 symptomatic overhand-throwing professional athletes. The injury pattern occurred in 17% of subjects and typically consisted of Outerbridge grade II or III cartilaginous lesions less than 1 cm in maximal diameter. The cartilaginous lesions were associated with other signs of posterior impingement such as undersurface fraying of the rotator cuff or fraying of the posterosuperior labrum.

Although rare, osteochondral lesions do occur in the glenoid fossa, with the most common imaging features demonstrating either a multiloculated cyst in the subchondral bone plate or a single osteochondral fragment (**Figs. 4** and **5**). Patients typically relay a history of trauma, and a strong association with instability, capsular redundancy, labral injuries, and intra-articular loose bodies have been reported.[33,34] These osteochondral lesions should be differentiated from more common cartilaginous injuries to the glenoid referred to as Bankart lesions. Bankart lesions

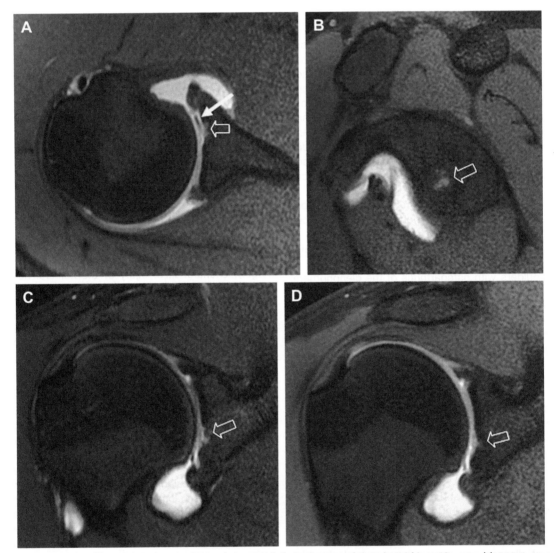

Fig. 4. Focal osteochondral injury involving the anteroinferior aspect of the glenoid in a 19-year-old young man. Axial PD-weighted fat-saturated (*A*), sagittal T2-weighted fat-saturated (*B*), oblique coronal T2-weighted fat-saturated (*C*), and oblique coronal T1-weighted fat-saturated (*D*) MR arthrographs of the shoulder show irregularity of the subchondral bone plate (*block arrows*) with overlying cartilage loss and undermining of the subjacent cartilage (*A, white arrow*) suggesting a cartilage flap.

are the direct result of an anterior dislocation leading to impaction of the humeral head into the anteroinferior glenoid rim. This lesion results in a spectrum of injuries to the glenoid fossa from isolated tears of the anteroinferior labrum to labral injuries with concomitant involvement of the subjacent cartilage or cartilage and bone (osseous Bankart lesion).[35] Trauma secondary to forced adduction of the humeral head against the glenoid cavity with the arm in abduction and external rotation may result in a superficial tear of the anteroinferior labrum with involvement of the subjacent glenoid cartilage (**Fig. 6**), otherwise known as

a glenolabral articular disruption (GLAD).[36,37] In contradistinction to a Bankart or Bankart variant lesion,[35] the GLAD lesion described by Neviaser[36] maintains the integrity of the inferior glenohumeral ligament and is not associated with glenohumeral instability on physical examination or history of dislocation. A less-common injury typically involving the posterior glenoid rim is the glenoid articular rim divot. The cause of this lesion is unknown. However, axial compression has been theorized, with the injury occurring at developmentally weak spots along the fusion sites of the multiple ossification centers of the glenoid.[38,39]

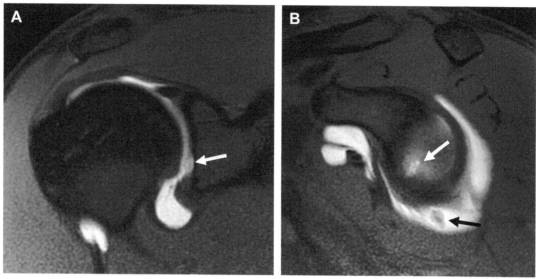

Fig. 5. Isolated chondral injury of the glenoid after a sports injury in a 21-year-old man. Oblique coronal T1-weighted fat-saturated (A) and oblique sagittal T2-weighted fat-saturated (B) MR arthrographs of the shoulder show that contrast extends into the donor site of a full-thickness cartilage shear injury (white arrows) of the glenoid. Associated loose cartilage body similar in size and morphology to the donor site is seen in the axillary recess (B, black arrow).

Imaging

Plain radiographs are typically the initial study performed in conjunction with a directed physical examination in the evaluation of patients with shoulder abnormality, with cross-sectional imaging playing a complementary role. Although the cartilage is not directly visualized, radiographs provide invaluable information regarding alignment, fractures, and soft tissue calcifications essential in the orthopedic management of patients with cartilaginous disease. The most common radiographic examination includes an anteroposterior (AP) view, true AP or Grashey view, scapular Y view, and axillary view.[40] In cases

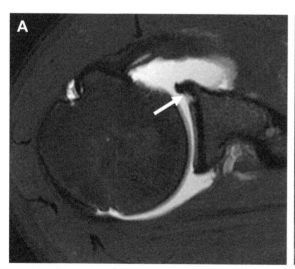
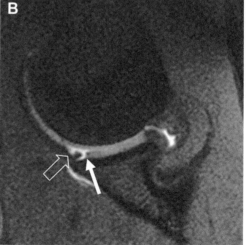

Fig. 6. Glenolabral articular disruption lesion in a 27-year-old man. (A) Axial PD-weighted fat-saturated MR arthrograph of the shoulder demonstrates irregularity of the anteroinferior labrum and adjacent cartilage (arrow). (B) T1-weighted fat-saturated MR arthrograph with the arm positioned in abduction and external rotation better delineates the superficial tearing of the labrum and subjacent full-thickness cartilage injury (white arrow). The inferior glenohumeral ligament (block arrow) remains intact.

of instability, alternative views such as the West Point view,[41] Stryker notch view,[25,42] or Garth view[43] may enhance detection of associated osseous injuries such as the Hill-Sachs or osseous Bankart lesions.

Although MR imaging is currently the modality of choice in the evaluation of the glenohumeral joint with high diagnostic accuracy in evaluating the labroligamentous structures and rotator cuff,[44–47] little has been written regarding its role in detecting cartilaginous lesions. This lack of literature is partly due to the inherent difficulty in evaluating the articular cartilage of smaller joints. Cadaveric studies with MR imaging correlation showed a tendency to overestimate the thickness of the thinner peripheral portion of the humeral articular cartilage and underestimate the thickness of the thicker central portion.[48,49] Interestingly, MR imaging overestimated the thickness of the glenoid cartilage.[49] The same study also noted that the glenoid cartilage was thinnest centrally and significantly thicker inferiorly than superiorly.

Regardless of the sequence used to evaluate the glenohumeral joint, high spatial resolution is required for the adequate detection of cartilaginous lesions. Although optimization of scanning parameters is beyond the scope of this article, spatial resolution is improved by maximizing matrix size while maintaining a small field of view and slice thickness. The trade-off for improved spatial resolution is decreased signal-to-noise ratio (SNR), which can be partly compensated for with the use of dedicated high-performance multi-channel extremity coils.[50]

An additional hurdle in evaluating the articular cartilage of the glenohumeral joint has been the lack of dedicated cartilage-sensitive sequences in shoulder MR imaging protocols. Using conventional MR imaging sequences, Guntern and colleagues[22] reported combined sensitivities and specificities of 76.5% and 69.0%, respectively, for humeral cartilage lesions and 75.0% and 64.5%, respectively, for glenoid cartilage lesions. More recently, the use of a 3-dimensional water-excitation true fast imaging with steady state precession sequence at the time of MR arthrography resulted in improved sensitivities and specificities of 89.5% and 87.0%, respectively, for humeral cartilage lesions and 70.0% and 82.0%, respectively, for glenoid cartilage lesions.[51] This result was especially true for deep cartilage lesions. Causes of diagnostic error included difficulty assessing the thinner peripheral cartilage of the humerus, which would be expected given a mean thickness of 1.24 mm superimposed on the effects of chemical shift.[22,49] Another diagnostic dilemma included evaluation of the interface between the glenoid cartilage and labrum, resulting in the false interpretation of a peripheral cartilage defect.[22]

Given that cartilage imaging is in its infancy, newer cartilage-sensitive sequences for evaluation of the glenohumeral joint have not yet been implemented. However, the recent development of 3-dimensional sequences with higher in-plane spatial resolution, thinner slice thickness, and improved tissue contrast combined with the use of currently available 8-channel shoulder coils and better fat suppression techniques, such as linear combination,[52] water excitation,[53] and iterative decomposition of water and fat with echo asymmetry and least squares estimates (IDEAL),[54] may lead to renewed interest and increased accuracy for evaluating the articular cartilage of the glenohumeral joint. Further research is definitely required.

Despite the anemic state of the literature regarding the articular cartilage of the glenohumeral joint, cartilage assessment requires an understanding of the anatomy and potential pitfalls. Both the humerus and glenoid contain normal bare areas. The bare area of the glenoid represents a small focal area of thinned articular cartilage located centrally overlying a small bony prominence of focal subchondral thickening termed the tubercle of Asskay.[55,56] The location, morphology, and normal underlying bone marrow differentiate this entity from an osteochondral lesion.[57] The larger physiologic bare area of the humeral head should also not be confused for a cartilaginous lesion and is an area devoid of cartilage along the posterolateral aspect of the humeral head extending from the infraspinatus tendon insertion to the articular margin.[58]

ELBOW

The limitations in imaging and evaluating the articular cartilage of the elbow joint are similar to those of the glenohumeral joint. Thin cartilage superimposed on the undulating contours of the articular surfaces of the distal humerus, capitellum, and radial head result in suboptimal visualization of the articular cartilage. This suboptimal visualization is predominantly because of lack of adequate in-plane resolution of the currently available MR imaging techniques.[59–62] However, MR imaging has played an important role in diagnosing and characterizing more focal processes involving the articular cartilage and the underlying subchondral bone of the elbow joint such as osteochondritis dissecans (OCD), impaction injuries, and intra-articular loose bodies.

Cartilaginous Abnormalities and Injury Patterns

OCD most commonly involves the anterolateral aspect of the capitellum; however, it has also been described in the radial head, ulna, and trochlea (**Fig. 7**).[63,64] Repetitive valgus stress and a precarious vascular supply have been theorized to predispose to the development of capitellar OCD lesions.[65–68] Adolescent athletes aged between 12 and 16 years make up the majority of individuals with this condition, with the highest incidence reported in pitchers and gymnasts.[66,67,69,70] Despite aggressive therapy, the prognosis can be poor, with long-term follow-up demonstrating the presence of degenerative joint disease and persistent pain in approximately 50% of patients.[71,72]

Treatment of patients with OCD of the elbow depends primarily on the stability of the OCD lesion. Stable lesions are generally treated conservatively with activity modification, muscle conditioning, and, occasionally, splinting and have a high likelihood of spontaneously healing. Unstable lesions or stable lesions refractory to conservative measures require surgical interventions such as abrasion chondroplasty or microfracture. Internal fixation, excision, or bone grafting is reserved for larger, typically acutely dislodged OCD lesions.[73–76]

Although elbow radiographs serve as the initial screening examination in patients with suspected OCD of the elbow, Kijowski and colleagues[77] showed radiographs to be fairly insensitive, with only a 47% detection rate at the time of initial interpretation. MR imaging has the ability to detect radiographically occult OCD lesions in the early stages of the disease process as well as to provide relevant anatomic detail influencing treatment options, such as lesion size, location, and stability. Both stable and unstable lesions demonstrate a hypointense rim on T1-weighted images with variable signal intensity centrally. Although studies have advocated the use of MR arthrography or intravenous contrast enhancement to stage OCD lesions,[78,79] Kijowski and colleagues showed that

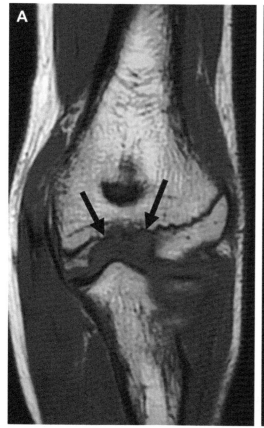
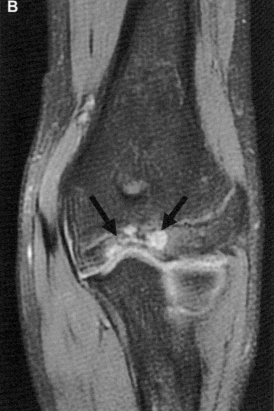

Fig. 7. Lateral trochlear OCD lesion in a 15-year-old boy. Coronal T1-weighted (*A*) and coronal PD-weighted fat-saturated (*B*) MR images of the elbow show a well-circumscribed lateral trochlear OCD lesion (*arrows*). Although a rare lesion, lateral trochlear OCD lesions tend to be much larger than medial trochlear OCD lesions.

noncontrast MR imaging can determine the stability of the osteochondral fragment (Fig. 8).[80–82] All arthroscopically proven unstable OCD lesions demonstrated either a rim of high signal intensity or marginal cysts on fluid-sensitive sequences. If contrast-enhanced MR imaging is performed, enhancement of the OCD lesion after the administration of intravenous contrast suggests an intact blood supply and viability of the fragment. A peripheral ring of enhancement at the interface between the fragment and adjacent subchondral bone is thought to represent enhancing granulation tissue and suggests instability of the lesion.[78] Imbibition of

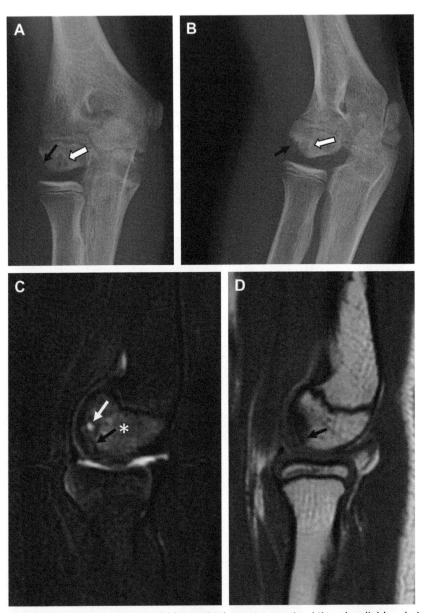

Fig. 8. Unstable capitellar OCD in a16-year-old boy. Initial anteroposterior (A) and radial head view (B) radiographs of the elbow demonstrate a subchondral lucency with central ossifications involving the capitellum (*black arrows*) and suggestion of cysts along the margin of the lesion (*white arrows*). Subsequent sagittal T2-weighted fat-saturated (C) and sagittal T1-weighted (D) MR images of the elbow demonstrate a low signal intensity rim (*black arrows*), intermediate signal centrally, adjacent bone marrow edema (C, *asterisk*), and a marginal cyst (C, *white arrow*). The family refused treatment, and follow-up sagittal T2-weighted fat-saturated (E) and sagittal T1-weighted (F) MR images demonstrate interval dislodgment of an osteochondral fragment (*white arrows*).

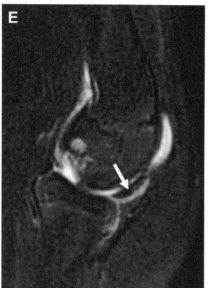

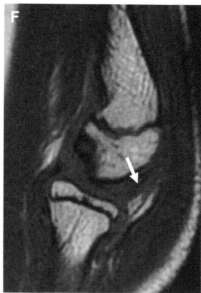

Fig. 8. (*continued*)

intra-articular contrast between the OCD fragment and the native bone at the time of MR arthrography is a result of disruption of the articular surface and is highly suggestive of an unstable lesion.[79]

An OCD lesion should be differentiated from normal cartilage pseudodefects, which occur in both the capitellum and ulna. The articular surface of the trochlear notch has a characteristic bare area at the junction of the anterior one-third and posterior two-thirds and divides the sigmoid notch into the coronoid process anteriorly and the olecranon posteriorly.[83,84] The pseudodefect of the capitellum (**Fig. 9**) represents the normal abrupt transition between the articular surface of the posteroinferior capitellum and subjacent nonarticular portion of the lateral epicondyle.[85] On sagittal images with the elbow in extension, this pseudodefect becomes readily apparent with the normal loss of contact between the articular surface of the posterolateral radius and the adjacent capitellar pseudodefect. There is no misinterpretation because OCD lesions are located more anteriorly within the capitellum and typically have signal abnormalities involving either the subjacent bone plate or the marrow. Caution should be taken in relying solely on the location because posterior capitellar impaction injuries have recently been described in the literature.[86,87] Most articles noted an association with acute trauma, typically either posterior elbow dislocation or posterolateral rotatory elbow instability. Given the clinical history and associated imaging findings, including a high prevalence of lateral collateral ligament injuries

and fractures of the radial head and coronoid processes,[88] the mechanism proposed for this type of injury is impaction of a posteriorly dislocated radial head into the capitellum. Rosenberg and colleagues[88] described several MR imaging findings that help to differentiate an impaction injury from a pseudodefect of the capitellum, including bone marrow edema, subchondral hyperintense T2 signal in an arclike configuration, subarticular cyst, and subcortical linear signal abnormality as well as the aforementioned associated ligamentous and osseous injuries.

Finally, osteochondrosis can affect the elbow, which typically occurs in a younger patient population when compared with OCD and impaction type injuries. Osteochondrosis is a self-limiting disease of children aged between 5 and 12 years and occurs during periods of active ossification of the epiphyseal centers of the elbow. The condition can involve the capitellum (Panner disease) or trochlea (Hegemann disease).[89–91] Although some investigators postulate that osteochondrosis and OCD represent different stages of the same pathologic process,[92] these 2 conditions should be considered as 2 distinct clinical entities because they affect different patient populations and have extremely different prognoses and long-term outcomes. Unlike in patients with OCD, residual deformity or development of intra-articular loose bodies is rare in patients with osteochondrosis. Given the relatively benign course of Panner and Hegemann diseases, MR imaging is infrequently used for further characterization.

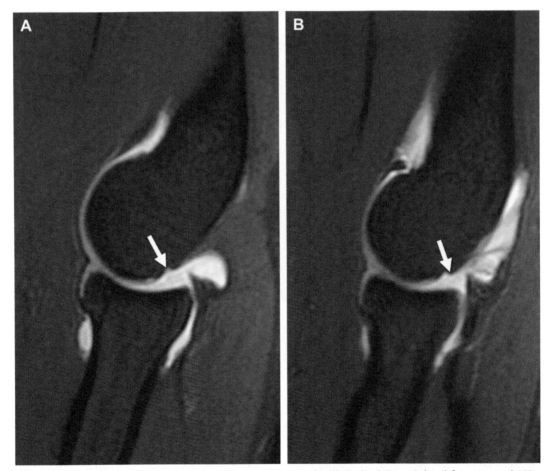

Fig. 9. Capitellar pseudodefect (*arrows*) in a 21-year-old man. (*A, B*) Sagittal T1-weighted fat-saturated MR arthrographs of the elbow show a normal groove at the junction of the posterolateral aspect of the capitellum and lateral epicondyle.

Typical imaging features, however, include fragmentation of the ossifying epiphysis with diffuse hypointense T1 signal and hyperintense T2 signal when compared with a more focal process often involving the articular surface in patients with OCD and impaction injuries.

Imaging

Radiographs remain the primary imaging modality in evaluating patients with elbow pain, providing indispensable details regarding alignment, fractures, loose bodies, and soft tissue calcifications. Secondary signs of cartilaginous disease such as joint space narrowing, malalignment, or frank osseous changes, however, occur late in the disease process. This is problematic because long-term follow-up studies have reported that chondral and osteochondral lesions of the elbow result in osteoarthritis in more than 50% of cases.[71,72] As cartilage repair techniques continue to advance[93–96] and with the recent interest in developing disease-modifying osteoarthritis drugs,[97,98] it will become imperative to diagnose early cartilaginous disease with a high degree of accuracy using noninvasive methods. The same obstacles encountered when imaging the articular cartilage of the glenohumeral joint are also found within the elbow joint: thin overlying cartilage compounded by curved articular surfaces.

Adequate morphologic detail on imaging requires thin sections of the order of 1 mm and in-plane resolution approaching 0.15 mm as well as techniques to eliminate chemical shift artifacts at the bone-cartilage interface.[62,99,100] In addition, fat suppression, which decreases chemical shift, and increases the dynamic range and overall contrast between cartilage and the surrounding tissue,[101] can fail because the elbow cannot always be positioned at the isocenter of the scanner. The required spatial resolution is beyond the capabilities of most currently available MR imaging techniques, likely accounting for the relatively sparse literature on the subject matter and reported low sensitivities and specificities for detecting cartilaginous lesions within the elbow joint. A cadaveric study evaluating computed tomographic (CT) arthrography versus MR arthrography in detecting cartilaginous lesions of the elbow joint reported overall sensitivities of 80% and 93% and overall specificities of 78% and 95% for CT and MR arthrographies, respectively.[102] Most cartilaginous lesions were in the radiohumeral compartment, with sensitivities highest for lesions involving the radial head and capitellum and lowest for lesions involving the ulna.

The challenges faced in imaging smaller joints with complex surface anatomy and thin overlying cartilage are currently being solved by implementing new MR imaging techniques to allow for higher diagnostic performance when evaluating articular cartilage. Although a detailed description of newer cartilage-sensitive sequences is beyond the scope of this article, advancements include 3-dimensional spoiled gradient-echo and balanced steady-state free precession techniques. Both techniques have been shown to increase the detection of cartilaginous lesions in the knee joint[103–105] and have certain advantages and disadvantages. As alluded to earlier in the shoulder section, new fat suppression techniques such as linear combination,[52] water excitation,[53] and IDEAL[54] should, in theory, correct for field inhomogeneity, particularly when imaging off center, and allow for better cartilage assessment within the elbow joint.

WRIST

MR imaging has increasingly played a role in the evaluation of chronic wrist pain, with reported high diagnostic accuracy for detecting injuries involving the tendons, scapholunate ligament, lunotriquetral ligament, and central portion of the triangular fibrocartilage.[106–110] Although cartilage loss may be a potential cause for wrist pain and its presence can alter both medical and surgical treatments, the current literature is fairly deficient with most studies performed before the development of multichannel extremity coils, cartilage-sensitive sequences, and high field strengths scanners. The difficulties in visualizing the articular cartilage of the wrist joint are no different from those in visualizing the remainder of the upper extremity or any small joint for that matter: complex articular surfaces with thin overlying cartilage.

Cartilaginous Abnormalities and Injury Patterns

Several conditions would benefit in improved cartilage imaging of the wrist joint. The extent of cartilage loss is one of the main determinants in choosing between performing a partial wrist fusion and total wrist arthrodesis.[111] A partial wrist fusion may preserve up to 52% of motion, a significant difference in functionality for a patient.[112] In the treatment of patients with Keinbock disease or scapholunate advanced collapse, the state of the overlying articular cartilage may mean the difference between performing a proximal row carpectomy and a 4-corner fusion.[113,114] A proximal row carpectomy relies on intact cartilage overlying the lunate fossa and capitate head, allowing for a direct painless articulation between the 2 structures. A noninvasive imaging technique that could accurately characterize the extent of cartilage loss within the wrist joint for preoperative planning would limit the need for arthroscopy, currently the gold standard. Wrist arthroscopy although safe, has an overall complication rate of 5.2%.[115] Mutimer and colleagues[116] showed only fair correlation with a κ value of 0.38 between arthroscopy and MR imaging in evaluating the cartilage of the wrist joint and concluded that the diagnostic accuracy of MR imaging in its current state was insufficient to replace arthroscopy in assessing the painful degenerative wrist. The study, however, failed to state the imaging parameters used during the MR imaging examination and likely did not incorporate newer cartilage-sensitive sequences in the imaging protocol.

With the development of effective disease-modifying antirheumatic drugs and the trend toward aggressive early treatment in an attempt to minimize progression of disease and improve functional outcomes,[117–119] the effect and role of wrist imaging in patients with rheumatoid arthritis has greatly expanded recently. Optimally, treatment should be instituted before the development of irreversible structural damage, typically during the early inflammatory stages of rheumatoid arthritis. Imaging should provide not only a static picture of the disease but also prognostic data to tailor treatment regiments. Benton and colleagues[120] studied and scored several MR imaging features in patients with early rheumatoid arthritis including bone marrow edema, synovitis, erosions, and tendonitis over a 6-year span with imaging at baseline, 1 year, and 6 years and compared the results with inflammatory and clinical markers as well as functional outcomes. The investigators concluded that the early features of rheumatoid arthritis on MR imaging, particularly the presence of bone marrow edema, could predict 6-year functional outcomes. Longitudinal studies on the value of imaging inflammatory arthritides to accurately predict prognosis and evaluate response to therapy rely on reproducible scoring schemes such as the Rheumatoid Arthritis Magnetic Resonance Imaging Score (RAMRIS)[121,122] and the Simplified Rheumatoid Arthritis Magnetic Resonance Imaging Score (SAMIS).[123] The current scoring methods do not directly evaluate cartilage loss but instead evaluate the extent of erosions, bone marrow edema, and synovitis. As MR imaging techniques improve and higher accuracy in detecting superficial cartilage loss is obtained, analysis of disease state and progression will likely include the documentation of cartilage volume and the presence or absence of early cartilaginous degeneration.

Imaging

Studies with surgical or gross pathologic correlation have evaluated the diagnostic performance of MR imaging for detecting cartilaginous lesions of the wrist joint.[116,124,125] Haims and colleagues[124] reported only fair interobserver agreement (κ value, 0.279–0.360) with low sensitivities in the distal radius (27%), the scaphoid (31%), the lunate (41%), and the triquetrum (18%) when compared with arthroscopy. Specificities for the same regions ranged from 75% to 93%. The investigators found no statistical difference in accuracy when evaluating high-grade versus low-grade cartilaginous lesions, indirect

MR arthrogram versus unenhanced MR imaging studies, location of cartilaginous lesions, sex, age, or presence of disease at multiple sites. Saupe and colleagues[125] compared 1.5-T with 3.0-T scanners for detecting cartilaginous lesions in cadaveric wrist specimens using the same imaging parameters and found slightly increased sensitivities and specificities ranging from 43% to 52% and 82% to 89%, respectively, for 1.5-T scanners and 48% to 52% and 82%, respectively, for 3.0-T scanners. Sensitivities were highest in evaluation of the proximal carpal row (67%–71%) and lowest in the evaluation of the distal carpal row (14%–24%). No statistically significant difference in diagnostic performance was seen at different field strengths, but interobserver agreement increased at 3.0 T (κ value = 0.634) when compared with 1.5 T (κ value = 0.267). However, it must be considered that neither of the above-mentioned studies used dedicated multichannel wrist coils or intra-articular contrast. More SNR-efficient 8-channel wrist coils enable higher-resolution imaging,[50] and previous studies evaluating cartilaginous lesions of the knee have demonstrated improved diagnostic performance with MR arthrography compared with MR imaging.[126,127] In addition, these previous studies did not include newly developed cartilage-sensitive sequences, which provide higher in-plane resolution, thinner slices, greater tissue contrast, and more robust fat suppression. Additional studies are warranted to determine which sequence is best suited for evaluating the articular cartilage of smaller joints such as the

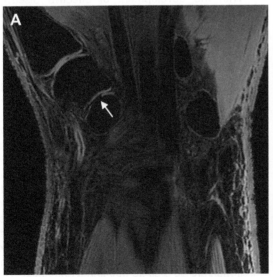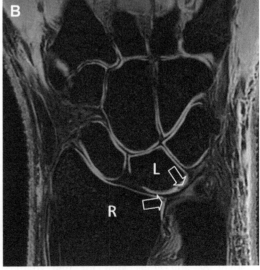

Fig. 10. (A, B) Coronal multiple echo recombined gradient echo MR images of the wrist demonstrate a full-thickness cartilage defect overlying the distal pole of the scaphoid (A, white arrow) as well as subtle partial-thickness cartilage fissures (B, block arrows) of the lunate (L) and distal radius (R).

wrist. Newly developed 3-dimensional techniques such as multiple echo recombined gradient echo (**Fig. 10**) and fast spin echo-Cube (GE Healthcare, Milwaukee, WI, USA) may provide the necessary anatomic detail.

SUMMARY

Imaging the articular cartilage of the upper extremity poses several challenges related to the thin overlying cartilage and complex surface geometry, which is compounded by the inadequate spatial resolution of currently available MR imaging techniques. Additional factors include suboptimal tissue contrast and failure of fat suppression secondary to off-isocenter imaging. Recent advancements such as the development of dedicated multichannel extremity coils, more SNR-efficient 3-dimensional MR imaging techniques, and more robust methods of fat suppression should lead to improved diagnostic performance for evaluating the articular cartilage of the small joints of the upper extremity.

REFERENCES

1. Brandt KD. Osteoarthritis. Clin Geriatr Med 1988; 4(2):279–93.
2. Peyron JG. Epidemiological aspects of osteoarthritis. Scand J Rheumatol Suppl 1988;77:29–33.
3. From the Centers for Disease Control and Prevention. Arthritis prevalence and activity limitations–United States, 1990. JAMA 1994;272(5):346–7.
4. Kijowski R, Blankenbaker DG, Davis KW, et al. Comparison of 1.5- and 3.0-T MR imaging for evaluating the articular cartilage of the knee joint. Radiology 2009;250(3):839–48.
5. Kijowski R, Blankenbaker DG, Woods MA, et al. 3.0-T evaluation of knee cartilage by using three-dimensional IDEAL GRASS imaging: comparison with fast spin-echo imaging. Radiology 2010; 255(1):117–27.
6. Kijowski R, Blankenbaker DG, Klaers JL, et al. Vastly undersampled isotropic projection steady-state free precession imaging of the knee: diagnostic performance compared with conventional MR. Radiology 2009;251(1):185–94.
7. Wong S, Steinbach L, Zhao J, et al. Comparative study of imaging at 3.0 T versus 1.5 T of the knee. Skeletal Radiol 2009;38(8):761–9.
8. Mohr A. The value of water-excitation 3D FLASH and fat-saturated PDw TSE MR imaging for detecting and grading articular cartilage lesions of the knee. Skeletal Radiol 2003;32(7):396–402.
9. Disler DG, McCauley TR, Kelman CG, et al. Fat-suppressed three-dimensional spoiled gradient-echo MR imaging of hyaline cartilage defects in

10. Meachim G, Emery IH. Cartilage fibrillation in shoulder and hip joints in Liverpool necropsies. J Anat 1973;116(Pt 2):161–79.
11. Outerbridge RE, Dunlop JA. The problem of chondromalacia patellae. Clin Orthop Relat Res 1975;(110):177–96.
12. Iannotti JP, Naranja RJJ, Warner JJ. Surgical management of shoulder arthritis in the young and active patient. In: Complex and revision problems in shoulder surgery. Philadelphia: Lippincott-Raven; 1997. p. 289–302.
13. Caffey S, McPherson E, Moore B, et al. Effects of radiofrequency energy on human articular cartilage: an analysis of 5 systems. Am J Sports Med 2005;33(7):1035–9.
14. Petty DH, Jazrawi LM, Estrada LS, et al. Glenohumeral chondrolysis after shoulder arthroscopy: case reports and review of the literature. Am J Sports Med 2004;32(2):509–15.
15. Levine WN, Clark AM Jr, D'Alessandro DF, et al. Chondrolysis following arthroscopic thermal capsulorrhaphy to treat shoulder instability. A report of two cases. J Bone Joint Surg Am 2005;87(3): 616–21.
16. Sanders TG, Zlatkin MB, Paruchuri NB, et al. Chondrolysis of the glenohumeral joint after arthroscopy: findings on radiography and low-field-strength MRI. AJR Am J Roentgenol 2007;188(4):1094–8.
17. Tamai K, Higashi A, Cho S, et al. Chondrolysis of the shoulder following a "color test"-assisted rotator cuff repair–a report of 2 cases. Acta Orthop Scand 1997;68(4):401–2.
18. Petersson CJ. Degeneration of the gleno-humeral joint. An anatomical study. Acta Orthop Scand 1983;54(2):277–83.
19. Neer CS 2nd, Craig EV, Fukuda H. Cuff-tear arthropathy. J Bone Joint Surg Am 1983;65(9): 1232–44.
20. Kernwein GA. Roentgenographic diagnosis of shoulder dysfunction. JAMA 1965;194(10):1081–5.
21. Gartsman GM, Taverna E. The incidence of glenohumeral joint abnormalities associated with full-thickness, reparable rotator cuff tears. Arthroscopy 1997;13(4):450–5.
22. Guntern DV, Pfirrmann CW, Schmid MR, et al. Articular cartilage lesions of the glenohumeral joint: diagnostic effectiveness of MR arthrography and prevalence in patients with subacromial impingement syndrome. Radiology 2003;226(1):165–70.
23. Ellman H, Harris E, Kay SP. Early degenerative joint disease simulating impingement syndrome: arthroscopic findings. Arthroscopy 1992;8(4):482–7.
24. Choi YS, Potter HG, Scher DM. A shearing osteochondral fracture of the humeral head following

an anterior shoulder dislocation in a child. HSS J 2005;1(1):100–2.

25. Hill HA, Sachs MD. The grooved defect of the humeral head. A frequently unrecognized complication of disclocations of the shoulder joint. Radiology 1940;25:306–11.

26. Richards RD, Sartoris DJ, Pathria MN, et al. Hill-Sachs lesion and normal humeral groove: MR imaging features allowing their differentiation. Radiology 1994;190(3):665–8.

27. Cameron ML, Kocher MS, Briggs KK, et al. The prevalence of glenohumeral osteoarthrosis in unstable shoulders. Am J Sports Med 2003;31(1):53–5.

28. Calandra JJ, Baker CL, Uribe J. The incidence of Hill-Sachs lesions in initial anterior shoulder dislocations. Arthroscopy 1989;5(4):254–7.

29. Hintermann B, Gachter A. Arthroscopic findings after shoulder dislocation. Am J Sports Med 1995;23(5):545–51.

30. Buscayret F, Edwards TB, Szabo I, et al. Glenohumeral arthrosis in anterior instability before and after surgical treatment: incidence and contributing factors. Am J Sports Med 2004;32(5):1165–72.

31. Carroll KW, Helms CA, Speer KP. Focal articular cartilage lesions of the superior humeral head: MR imaging findings in seven patients. AJR Am J Roentgenol 2001;176(2):393–7.

32. Paley KJ, Jobe FW, Pink MM, et al. Arthroscopic findings in the overhand throwing athlete: evidence for posterior internal impingement of the rotator cuff. Arthroscopy 2000;16(1):35–40.

33. Yu JS, Greenway G, Resnick D. Osteochondral defect of the glenoid fossa: cross-sectional imaging features. Radiology 1998;206(1):35–40.

34. Shanley DJ, Mulligan ME. Osteochondrosis dissecans of the glenoid. Skeletal Radiol 1990;19(6):419–21.

35. Bankart AS, Cantab MC. Recurrent or habitual dislocation of the shoulder-joint. Br Med J 1923;2(3285):1132–3.

36. Neviaser TJ. The GLAD lesion: another cause of anterior shoulder pain. Arthroscopy 1993;9(1):22–3.

37. Sanders TG, Tirman PF, Linares R, et al. The glenolabral articular disruption lesion: MR arthrography with arthroscopic correlation. AJR Am J Roentgenol 1999;172(1):171–5.

38. Snyder SJ, Banas MP, Belzer JP. Arthroscopic evaluation and treatment of injuries to the superior glenoid labrum. Instr Course Lect 1996;45:65–70.

39. Snyder SJ, Banas MP, Karzel RP. An analysis of 140 injuries to the superior glenoid labrum. J Shoulder Elbow Surg 1995;4(4):243–8.

40. Merrill V. Shoulder Girdle. In: PW B, editor. Merrill's atlas of radiographic positions and radiologic procedures. 8th edition. St Louis: Mosby; 1995. p. 126–47.

41. Rokous JR, Feagin JA, Abbott HG. Modified axillary roentgenogram. A useful adjunct in the diagnosis of recurrent instability of the shoulder. Clin Orthop Relat Res 1972;82:84–6.

42. Hall RH, Isaac F, Booth CR. Dislocations of the shoulder with special reference to accompanying small fractures. J Bone Joint Surg Am 1959;41(3):489–94.

43. Garth WP Jr, Slappey CE, Ochs CW. Roentgenographic demonstration of instability of the shoulder: the apical oblique projection. A technical note. J Bone Joint Surg Am 1984;66(9):1450–3.

44. Hodler J, Kursunoglu-Brahme S, Snyder SJ, et al. Rotator cuff disease: assessment with MR arthrography versus standard MR imaging in 36 patients with arthroscopic confirmation. Radiology 1992;182(2):431–6.

45. Gusmer PB, Potter HG, Schatz JA, et al. Labral injuries: accuracy of detection with unenhanced MR imaging of the shoulder. Radiology 1996;200(2):519–24.

46. Palmer WE, Brown JH, Rosenthal DI. Labral-ligamentous complex of the shoulder: evaluation with MR arthrography. Radiology 1994;190(3):645–51.

47. Bencardino JT, Beltran J, Rosenberg ZS, et al. Superior labrum anterior-posterior lesions: diagnosis with MR arthrography of the shoulder. Radiology 2000;214(1):267–71.

48. Hodler J, Loredo RA, Longo C, et al. Assessment of articular cartilage thickness of the humeral head: MR-anatomic correlation in cadavers. AJR Am J Roentgenol 1995;165(3):615–20.

49. Yeh LR, Kwak S, Kim YS, et al. Evaluation of articular cartilage thickness of the humeral head and the glenoid fossa by MR arthrography: anatomic correlation in cadavers. Skeletal Radiol 1998;27(9):500–4.

50. Kneeland JB, Hyde JS. High-resolution MR imaging with local coils. Radiology 1989;171(1):1–7.

51. Dietrich TJ, Zanetti M, Saupe N, et al. Articular cartilage and labral lesions of the glenohumeral joint: diagnostic performance of 3D water-excitation true FISP MR arthrography. Skeletal Radiol 2010;39(5):473–80.

52. Vasanawala SS, Pauly JM, Nishimura DG. Linear combination steady-state free precession MRI. Magn Reson Med 2000;43(1):82–90.

53. Kornaat PR, Ceulemans RY, Kroon HM, et al. MRI assessment of knee osteoarthritis: Knee Osteoarthritis Scoring System (KOSS)–inter-observer and intra-observer reproducibility of a compartment-based scoring system. Skeletal Radiol 2005;34(2):95–102.

54. Gold GE, Reeder SB, Yu H, et al. Articular cartilage of the knee: rapid three-dimensional MR imaging at 3.0 T with IDEAL balanced steady-state free

precession–initial experience. Radiology 2006; 240(2):546–51.

55. Warner JJ, Bowen MK, Deng XH, et al. Articular contact patterns of the normal glenohumeral joint. J Shoulder Elbow Surg 1998;7(4):381–8.

56. Paturet G, editor. Textbook of human anatomy. Paris: Masson et Cie Libraries de L'Academie de Medecine; 1951. p. 119.

57. Ly JQ, Bui-Mansfield LT, Kline MJ, et al. Bare area of the glenoid: magnetic resonance appearance with arthroscopic correlation. J Comput Assist Tomogr 2004;28(2):229–32.

58. Rudez J, Zanetti M. Normal anatomy, variants and pitfalls on shoulder MRI. Eur J Radiol 2008;68(1): 25–35.

59. Waldschmidt JG, Rilling RJ, Kajdacsy-Balla AA, et al. In vitro and in vivo MR imaging of hyaline cartilage: zonal anatomy, imaging pitfalls, and pathologic conditions. Radiographics 1997;17(6):1387–402.

60. Disler DG, Recht MP, McCauley TR. MR imaging of articular cartilage. Skeletal Radiol 2000;29(7): 367–77.

61. Trattnig S, Mlynarik V, Huber M, et al. Magnetic resonance imaging of articular cartilage and evaluation of cartilage disease. Invest Radiol 2000; 35(10):595–601.

62. Rubenstein JD, Li JG, Majumdar S, et al. Image resolution and signal-to-noise ratio requirements for MR imaging of degenerative cartilage. AJR Am J Roentgenol 1997;169(4):1089–96.

63. Patel N, Weiner SD. Osteochondritis dissecans involving the trochlea: report of two patients (three elbows) and review of the literature. J Pediatr Orthop 2002;22(1):48–51.

64. Vanthournout I, Rudelli A, Valenti P, et al. Osteochondritis dissecans of the trochlea of the humerus. Pediatr Radiol 1991;21(8):600–1.

65. Haraldsson S. On osteochondrosis deformas juvenilis capituli humeri including investigation of intraosseous vasculature in distal humerus. Acta Orthop Scand Suppl 1959;38:1–232.

66. Brown R, Blazina ME, Kerlan RK, et al. Osteochondritis of the capitellum. J Sports Med 1974;2(1): 27–46.

67. Mitsunaga MM, Adishian DA, Bianco AJ Jr. Osteochondritis dissecans of the capitellum. J Trauma 1982;22(1):53–5.

68. Woodward AH, Bianco AJ Jr. Osteochondritis dissecans of the elbow. Clin Orthop Relat Res 1975;(110):35–41.

69. Takahara M, Shundo M, Kondo M, et al. Early detection of osteochondritis dissecans of the capitellum in young baseball players. Report of three cases. J Bone Joint Surg Am 1998;80(6):892–7.

70. Casey M, Vade A, Lomasney L, et al. Radiologic case study. Osteochondritis dissecans of the capitellum. Orthopedics 2002;25(8):802, 878–80.

71. Bauer M, Jonsson K, Josefsson PO, et al. Osteochondritis dissecans of the elbow. A long-term follow-up study. Clin Orthop Relat Res 1992;(284): 156–60.

72. Takahara M, Ogino T, Sasaki I, et al. Long term outcome of osteochondritis dissecans of the humeral capitellum. Clin Orthop Relat Res 1999;(363):108–15.

73. Bradley JP, Petrie RS. Osteochondritis dissecans of the humeral capitellum. Diagnosis and treatment. Clin Sports Med 2001;20(3):565–90.

74. Schenck RC Jr, Goodnight JM. Osteochondritis dissecans. J Bone Joint Surg Am 1996;78(3): 439–56.

75. McManama GB Jr, Micheli LJ, Berry MV, et al. The surgical treatment of osteochondritis of the capitellum. Am J Sports Med 1985;13(1):11–21.

76. Brownlow HC, O'Connor-Read LM, Perko M. Arthroscopic treatment of osteochondritis dissecans of the capitellum. Knee Surg Sports Traumatol Arthrosc 2006;14(2):198–202.

77. Kijowski R, De Smet AA. Radiography of the elbow for evaluation of patients with osteochondritis dissecans of the capitellum. Skeletal Radiol 2005; 34(5):266–71.

78. Peiss J, Adam G, Casser R, et al. Gadopentetate-dimeglumine-enhanced MR imaging of osteonecrosis and osteochondritis dissecans of the elbow: initial experience. Skeletal Radiol 1995;24(1): 17–20.

79. Kramer J, Stiglbauer R, Engel A, et al. MR contrast arthrography (MRA) in osteochondrosis dissecans. J Comput Assist Tomogr 1992;16(2):254–60.

80. Steinbach LS, Schwartz M. Elbow arthrography. Radiol Clin North Am 1998;36(4):635–49.

81. Carrino JA, Smith DK, Schweitzer ME. MR arthrography of the elbow and wrist. Semin Musculoskelet Radiol 1998;2(4):397–414.

82. Kijowski R, De Smet AA. MRI findings of osteochondritis dissecans of the capitellum with surgical correlation. AJR Am J Roentgenol 2005;185(6): 1453–9.

83. Rosas H, Lee K. Imaging acute trauma of the elbow. Semin Musculoskelet Radiol 2010;14(4): 394–411.

84. Wang AA, Mara M, Hutchinson DT. The proximal ulna: an anatomic study with relevance to olecranon osteotomy and fracture fixation. J Shoulder Elbow Surg 2003;12(3):293–6.

85. Rosenberg ZS, Beltran J, Cheung YY. Pseudodefect of the capitellum: potential MR imaging pitfall. Radiology 1994;191(3):821–3.

86. Feldman DR, Schabel SI, Friedman RJ, et al. Translational injuries in posterior elbow dislocation. Skeletal Radiol 1997;26(2):134–6.

87. Faber KJ, King GJ. Posterior capitellum impression fracture: a case report associated with

posterolateral rotatory instability of the elbow. J Shoulder Elbow Surg 1998;7(2):157–9.

88. Rosenberg ZS, Blutreich SI, Schweitzer ME, et al. MRI features of posterior capitellar impaction injuries. AJR Am J Roentgenol 2008;190(2):435–41.

89. Panner H. A peculiar affection of the capitellum humeri, resembling Calve-Perthes' disease of the hip. Acta Radiol 1927;8:617–8.

90. Kobayashi K, Burton KJ, Rodner C, et al. Lateral compression injuries in the pediatric elbow: Panner's disease and osteochondritis dissecans of the capitellum. J Am Acad Orthop Surg 2004;12(4):246–54.

91. Beyer WF, Heppt P, Gluckert K, et al. Aseptic osteonecrosis of the humeral trochlea (Hegemann's disease). Arch Orthop Trauma Surg 1990;110(1):45–8.

92. Singer KM, Roy SP. Osteochondrosis of the humeral capitellum. Am J Sports Med 1984;12(5):351–60.

93. Sato M, Ochi M, Uchio Y, et al. Transplantation of tissue-engineered cartilage for excessive osteochondritis dissecans of the elbow. J Shoulder Elbow Surg 2004;13(2):221–5.

94. Nakagawa Y, Matsusue Y, Ikeda N, et al. Osteochondral grafting and arthroplasty for end-stage osteochondritis dissecans of the capitellum. A case report and review of the literature. Am J Sports Med 2001;29(5):650–5.

95. Jackson DW, Scheer MJ, Simon TM. Cartilage substitutes: overview of basic science and treatment options. J Am Acad Orthop Surg 2001;9(1):37–52.

96. Nehrer S, Minas T. Treatment of articular cartilage defects. Invest Radiol 2000;35(10):639–46.

97. Qvist P, Bay-Jensen AC, Christiansen C, et al. The disease modifying osteoarthritis drug (DMOAD): is it in the horizon? Pharmacol Res 2008;58(1):1–7.

98. Hunter D, Hellio Le Graverand-Gastineau M. How close are we to having structure-modifying drugs available? Med Clin North Am 2009;93(1):223–34.

99. Schenck RC Jr, Athanasiou KA, Constantinides G, et al. A biomechanical analysis of articular cartilage of the human elbow and a potential relationship to osteochondritis dissecans. Clin Orthop Relat Res 1994;(299):305–12.

100. Milz S, Eckstein F, Putz R. Thickness distribution of the subchondral mineralization zone of the trochlear notch and its correlation with the cartilage thickness: an expression of functional adaptation to mechanical stress acting on the humeroulnar joint? Anat Rec 1997;248(2):189–97.

101. van Leersum M, Schweitzer ME, Gannon F, et al. Chondromalacia patellae: an in vitro study. Comparison of MR criteria with histologic and macroscopic findings. Skeletal Radiol 1996;25(8):727–32.

102. Waldt S, Bruegel M, Ganter K, et al. Comparison of multislice CT arthrography and MR arthrography for the detection of articular cartilage lesions of the elbow. Eur Radiol 2005;15(4):784–91.

103. Disler DG. Fat-suppressed three-dimensional spoiled gradient-recalled MR imaging: assessment of articular and physeal hyaline cartilage. AJR Am J Roentgenol 1997;169(4):1117–23.

104. Recht MP, Piraino DW, Paletta GA, et al. Accuracy of fat-suppressed three-dimensional spoiled gradient-echo FLASH MR imaging in the detection of patellofemoral articular cartilage abnormalities. Radiology 1996;198(1):209–12.

105. Hargreaves BA, Gold GE, Beaulieu CF, et al. Comparison of new sequences for high-resolution cartilage imaging. Magn Reson Med 2003;49(4):700–9.

106. Golimbu CN, Firooznia H, Melone CP Jr, et al. Tears of the triangular fibrocartilage of the wrist: MR imaging. Radiology 1989;173(3):731–3.

107. Schweitzer ME, Brahme SK, Hodler J, et al. Chronic wrist pain: spin-echo and short tau inversion recovery MR imaging and conventional and MR arthrography. Radiology 1992;182(1):205–11.

108. Zlatkin MB, Chao PC, Osterman AL, et al. Chronic wrist pain: evaluation with high-resolution MR imaging. Radiology 1989;173(3):723–9.

109. Schweitzer ME, Natale P, Winalski CS, et al. Indirect wrist MR arthrography: the effects of passive motion versus active exercise. Skeletal Radiol 2000;29(1):10–4.

110. Bencardino JT. MR imaging of tendon lesions of the hand and wrist. Magn Reson Imaging Clin N Am 2004;12(2):333–47, vii.

111. Nagy L. Salvage of post-traumatic arthritis following distal radius fracture. Hand Clin 2005;21(3):489–98.

112. Meier R, van Griensven M, Krimmer H. Scaphotrapeziotrapezoid (STT)-arthrodesis in Kienbock's disease. J Hand Surg Br 2004;29(6):580–4.

113. Tomaino MM, Miller RJ, Cole I, et al. Scapholunate advanced collapse wrist: proximal row carpectomy or limited wrist arthrodesis with scaphoid excision? J Hand Surg Am 1994;19(1):134–42.

114. Cohen MS, Kozin SH. Degenerative arthritis of the wrist: proximal row carpectomy versus scaphoid excision and four-corner arthrodesis. J Hand Surg Am 2001;26(1):94–104.

115. Beredjiklian PK, Bozentka DJ, Leung YL, et al. Complications of wrist arthroscopy. J Hand Surg Am 2004;29(3):406–11.

116. Mutimer J, Green J, Field J. Comparison of MRI and wrist arthroscopy for assessment of wrist cartilage. J Hand Surg Eur Vol 2008;33(3):380–2.

117. Bukhari MA, Wiles NJ, Lunt M, et al. Influence of disease-modifying therapy on radiographic outcome in inflammatory polyarthritis at five years: results from a large observational inception study. Arthritis Rheum 2003;48(1):46–53.

118. Emery P. Evidence supporting the benefit of early intervention in rheumatoid arthritis. J Rheumatol Suppl 2002;66:3–8.

119. Emery P, Breedveld FC, Dougados M, et al. Early referral recommendation for newly diagnosed rheumatoid arthritis: evidence based development of a clinical guide. Ann Rheum Dis 2002;61(4):290–7.

120. Benton N, Stewart N, Crabbe J, et al. MRI of the wrist in early rheumatoid arthritis can be used to predict functional outcome at 6 years. Ann Rheum Dis 2004;63(5):555–61.

121. Ostergaard M, Peterfy C, Conaghan P, et al. OMERACT Rheumatoid Arthritis Magnetic Resonance Imaging Studies. Core set of MRI acquisitions, joint pathology definitions, and the OMERACT RA-MRI scoring system. J Rheumatol 2003;30(6):1385–6.

122. Lassere M, McQueen F, Ostergaard M, et al. OMERACT Rheumatoid Arthritis Magnetic Resonance Imaging Studies. Exercise 3: an international multicenter reliability study using the RA-MRI Score. J Rheumatol 2003;30(6): 1366–75.

123. Cyteval C, Miquel A, Hoa D, et al. Rheumatoid arthritis of the hand: monitoring with a simplified MR imaging scoring method–preliminary assessment. Radiology 2010;256(3):863–9.

124. Haims AH, Moore AE, Schweitzer ME, et al. MRI in the diagnosis of cartilage injury in the wrist. AJR Am J Roentgenol 2004;182(5):1267–70.

125. Saupe N, Prussmann KP, Luechinger R, et al. MR imaging of the wrist: comparison between 1.5- and 3-T MR imaging–preliminary experience. Radiology 2005;234(1):256–64.

126. Gagliardi JA, Chung EM, Chandnani VP, et al. Detection and staging of chondromalacia patellae: relative efficacies of conventional MR imaging, MR arthrography, and CT arthrography. AJR Am J Roentgenol 1994;163(3):629–36.

127. Mathieu L, Bouchard A, Marchaland JP, et al. Knee MR-arthrography in assessment of meniscal and chondral lesions. Orthop Traumatol Surg Res 2009;95(1):40–7.

Index

Note: Page numbers of article titles are in **boldface** type.

A

Aggrecans, 251
Ankle, and knee, articular cartilage of, how to report
  lesions of, 382–403
      MR imaging of, **379–405**
  articular cartilage of, normal MR appearance of,
    380–382
    versus knee cartilage, 379–380
  normal, articular cartilage of, 381–382, 383
  osteochondral lesions in, 395–397, 401
Arthritides, inflammatory, 339–354
    clinical signs of, 340
    crystalline-induced, and infectious, MR
      imaging assessment of, **339–363**
    MR imaging definitions in, 343
    MR imaging technique in, 340–341,
      342, 343, 344
    treatment of, 340
Arthritis. See also *Arthritides.*
  infectious, 358–360
  juvenile idiopathic, 347–351, 352
  psoriatic, 352–353, 354
  rheumatoid. See *Rheumatoid arthritis.*
Arthropathy(ies), crystalline-induced, 354–358
  neuropathic, 359
Arthroplasty, total hip, femoroacetabular
  impingement after, 369
Articular cartilage, abnormalities of, and injury
  patterns, 408–410
  as acellular and avascular, 250–251
  as joint-specific, 216
  biochemical properties of, 250–251
  biochemistry and physiology of, MR imaging
    of, 253–254
  biomechanical studies of, 215–216
  clinical imaging of, 218–226
  compositional imaging of, in osteoarthritis
    knee, 311
  degenerative and posttraumatic lesions of,
    appearance of, 230–233
  fast spin-echo image of, 219, 222
  functional anatomy and physiology of,
    250–253
  histology of, 215
  imaging sequences of, technique and
    performance of, 366, 367, 369
  lesions of, classification of, 387

    detection in MR imaging, factors influencing,
      365–366
    grading system for, 387
    of knee and ankle, how to report, 382–403
    solitary, of knee and ankle, how to report,
      385–392
  morphologic assessment of, importance of,
    229–230
  morphologic imaging of, **229–248**
    sequences of, 233–236
  MR imaging appearance of, **215–227**
  MR imaging methods for evaluating, pros and
    cons of, 250
  MR imaging of, 216–218, 229
    overview of, 323–324
  multicompartmental disease of, 383, 384
  of ankle, normal, 381–382, 383
    versus knee cartilage, 379–380
  of elbow, 412–417
  of glenohumeral joint, imaging of, 412
  of hip joint, conventional MR imaging and MR
    arthrography of, 369–373
    MR physiologic imaging of, 373–375
  of knee, normal, 381, 382
    versus ankle cartilage, 379–380
  of knee and ankle, lesions of, 379
    MR imaging of, **379–405**
    normal, MR imaging appearance of, 380–382
  of upper extremity, current state of imaging of,
    407–423
  of wrist, abnormalities and injury patterns of,
    417–419
  partial thickness, 389
  physiology of, MR imaging of, **249–282**
  repair of, autologous chondrocyte implantation in,
    331–334
    matrix-assisted autologous chondrocyte
      implantation in, 331–334
    microfracture in, 324–325, 326
    osteochondral allograft in, 327–329, 330
    osteochondral autograft transfer in, 325–327,
      328, 329
    synthetic resorbable scaffolds in, 330–331, 332
  repair procedures, MR imaging assessment of,
    323–337
    parameters in, 324
    types of, MR imaging assessment of, 324–334
  split-line studies of, 216, 217

Magn Reson Imaging Clin N Am 19 (2011) 425–428
doi:10.1016/S1064-9689(11)00021-3
1064-9689/11/$ – see front matter © 2011 Elsevier Inc. All rights reserved.

mri.theclinics.com

Articular (*continued*)
    structure of, and signal intensity, 217, 220
    swelling pressure of, 251, 252
    three dimensional virtual models of, 375
    type II collagen fibrils in, 252
    unicompartmental disease of, 384
    zones of, 289

B

Bone attrition, subchondral, MR imaging of, 304
Bone erosions, in rheumatoid arthritis, 344–346, 347, 348
Bone marrow edema, grading of, 390–391
    in rheumatoid arthritis, 344, 345, 346, 349
Bone marrow lesions, and radiographic progression of osteoarthritis, 285–286
    subchondral, MR imaging of, 300–303, 304
Boston-Leeds osteoarthritis knee score, 296, 297–299
Bursae, in osteoarthritis of knee, 310

C

Capitellum, osteochondritis dissecans of, 414–415
    pseudodefect of, 415, 416
Cartilage, articular. See *Articular catilage.*
Cartilage imaging, high field strength, in articular cartilage imaging, 242–243
Cartilage imaging sequences, limitations of, 240–242
    morphologic, diagnostic performance of, 236–240
Chondral injury, hypothetical model of, 289
Chondrocalcinosis, 357, 358
Chondrocyte implantation, autologous, in articular cartilage repair, 331–334
Contrast-enhanced imaging, 258–262
Cruciate ligament, anterior, tears of, in osteoarthritis, 309, 310
    posterior, tears of, in osteoarthritis, 309
Cystlike lesions, subchondral, MR imaging of, 303–304
Cysts, periarticular, around knee, in osteoarthritis, 309–311
    subcondral, 391, 394

D

Dactylitis, 353, 354
Delayed gadolinium-enhanced MR imaging of cartilage, 258–261, 313–314, 374
Diffusion-weighted imaging, of articular cartilage, 271–272, 315
Driven equilibrium Fourier transform, three-dimensional, to assess articular cartilage, 234–235, 249
Dual echo steady-state sequence, 249
    three-dimensional, to assess articular cartilage, 234
    to assess articular cartilage, 233

E

Elbow, articular cartilage of, 412–417
    osteochondritis dissecans of, 413–414

F

Fast spin-echo image, of articular cartilage, 219, 222
Femoral condyle(s), articular cartilage of, 216, 217
    with normal cartilage, 219
Femoral head, cartilage lesion on, imaging of, 239–240
Femoroacetabular impingement, after total hip arthroplasty, 369
    cam-type, 367
    pincer-type, 367
Fluctuating equilibrium MR imaging, 249

G

Glenohumeral joint, articular cartilage of, imaging of, 412
Glenoid, chondral injury of, 409–410, 411
Glenolabral articular disruption lesion, 410, 411
Gout, acute, 355, 356
    tophaceous, 356
Gradient-echo sequences, three-dimensional, for cartilage imaging, 234

H

Hip, as common site of osteoarthritis, 365
    early degeneration of, MR imaging of, *365–378*
    osteoarthritis of, early, causes of, 366–369
    pain in, MR imaging in, 365
    total arthroplasty of, femoroacetabular impingement after, 369
Humeral head, chondral shear injury of, 409

J

Joint effusion, in osteoarthritis of knee, 308–309
    in rheumatoid arthritis, 342
Joint space, narrowing of, in rheumatoid arthritis, 346, 347, 349, 350, 351
Juvenile idiopathic arthritis, 347–351, 352

K

Knee, abnormalities of, T2-weighted fast spin-echo image of, 230, 231
    and ankle, articular cartilage of, MR imaging of, **379–405**
        lesions of articular cartilage of, how to report, 382–403
    articular cartilage of, normal MR appearance of, 380–382

versus ankle cartilage, 379–380

malalignment of, causes of, 284
  in osteoarthritis, rapid structural damage
    in, 285
  techniques for estimating, 285
  without osteoarthritis, 285
normal, articular cartilage of, 381, 382
osteoarthritis of, joint effusion in, 308–309
  MR imaging in research of, **295–321**
    techniques available for, 295–296
  radiographic, knee pain in, 285
osteochondral lesions in, 393–395
osteoporosis of, structural abnormalities in, MR
  imaging-detected, to predict pain and
  progression, 300–315
pain in, in cartilage lesions, T2-weighted fast
  spin-echo imaging in, 241, 242
periarticular cysts around, in osteoarthritis,
  309–311
semiquantitative scoring MR imaging-based
  systems for assessment of, 296–300
Knee osteoporosis scoring system, for assessment
  of knee, 296, 297–299, 302

L

Loose bodies, in osteoarthritis of knee, 311

M

Magnetization transfer MR imaging, 269–271
Meniscal disease, tibiofemoral cartilage loss in,
  305, 306
Meniscal dysfunction, in osteoarthritis, 286–287
Meniscal extrusion, in tibiofemoral cartilage loss,
  305–307
Meniscal tears, surgery in, 287
Meniscectomy, total, osteoarthritis after, 287–288
Microfracture, in articular cartilage repair,
  324–325, 326
MR arthrography, and conventional MR imaging,
  of articular cartilage of hip joint, 369–373
  indirect, in evaluation of hip, 373
MR imaging, and effect of filtering on spatial
  resolution, 220, 223
  bandwidth of, effect on signal density and spatial
    resolution, 219, 222
  effect of partial volume averaging on, 221, 223

N

Neuropathic arthropathy, 359

O

Osteoarthritis, after total meniscectomy, 287–288
  definition of, 283
  hip as common site of, 365

meniscal dysfynction in, 286–287
of hip, early, causes of, 366–369
of knee, joint effusion in, 308–309
  MR imaging in research of, **295–321**
    techniques available for, 295–296
prevalence of, 229, 249
rapidly progressive, biomechanical
  considerations in, **283–294**
tears of anterior cruciate ligament in, 309, 310
tears of posterior cruciate ligament in, 309
Osteochondral allograft, in articular cartilage repair,
  330, 337–329
Osteochondral autograft transfer, in articular cartilage
  repair, 325–327, 328, 329
Osteochondral junction, 289, 290
  delamination injury of, 289, 291
Osteochondral lesions, 392–403
  in ankle, 395–397
    grading system for, 401
  in knee, 393–395
  MR imaging for, 399–403
Osteochondral unit, cartilage and subchondral bone
  as, 288
  injuries of, 288–291
Osteochondritis dissecans, 392–403
  of capitellum, 414–415
  of elbow, 413–414
  of trochlea, 413
Osteochondromatosis, synovial, 408
Osteomyelitis, with nonviable tissue, 358
Osteoporosis, of knee, structural abnormalities in,
  MR imaging-detected, to predict pain and
  progression, 300–315

P

Patella, acute osteochondral fracture of, 216, 218
  articular cartilage of, 216, 217
  cartilage of, T2-weighted fast spin-echo image of,
    225, 226
Patellar facet, lateral, chondral delaminaion of, 291
  medial, full-thickness vertical fissure of, 289, 290
Psoriatic arthritis, 352–353, 354

R

Rheumatoid arthritis, joint effusion in, 342
  MR imaging in, 342–347
  of shoulder, 408
  prevalence of, 341–342

S

Sacroiliitis, 354, 355
Scaffolds, synthetic resorbable, in articular cartilage
  repair, 330–331, 332
Semiquantitative scoring systems, MR imaging-
  based, for assessment of whole knee joint,
  296–300

Shoulder, articular cartilage loss in, T2-weighted fast
    spin-echo image of, 225
    cartilaginous degeneration of, 407–412
    rheumatoid arthritis of, 408
Sodium MR imaging, 254–255, 256, 257
Spin-echo image, fast, sequences of, two- and
    three-dimensional, 233–234
    T2-weighted fast, of articular cartilage loss in
        shoulder, 225
        of cartilage of patella, 225, 226
        of tibial plateau, signal intensity on, 218, 221
Spondyloarthropathies, seronegative, 351–354
Steady-state free precession imaging, balanced,
    249–250
        three-dimensional, to assess articular
            cartilage, 235–236, 249
Synovitis, active, 343
    and tenosynovitis, 342
    whole-knee, in osteoarthritis, 307–308

T

T2 mapping, functional cartilage, 266, 267
    in show matrix changes, 264
T2 maps, heat scale and color scale, 265
T2 relaxation time mapping, 262–266
Tendinitis, calcific, 357, 358

Tenosynovitis, 349
    synovitis and, 342
Tesla(3-) scanner, improved spatial resolution with,
    222, 224
Tibial plateau, articular cartilage of, 216, 217
        structure of, 216, 217
    T2-weighted spin-echo image of, signal intensity
        on, 218, 221
T1p imaging, 255–257, 258, 314–315
Trochlea, osteochondritis dissecans of, 413

U

Upper extremity, articular cartilage of, current state of
    imaging of, 407–423
UTE MR imaging, 266–269, 270

W

Whole-Organ Magnetic Resonance Imaging Score,
    283
Whole-organ MR imaging scoring system, for
    assessment of knee, 296, 297–299, 302
Wrist, articular cartilage of, abnormalities and injury
    patterns of, 417–419

Moving?

Make sure your subscription moves with you!

To notify us of your new address, find your **Clinics Account Number** (located on your mailing label above your name), and contact customer service at:

Email: journalscustomerservice-usa@elsevier.com

800-654-2452 (subscribers in the U.S. & Canada)
314-447-8871 (subscribers outside of the U.S. & Canada)

Fax number: 314-447-8029

Elsevier Health Sciences Division
Subscription Customer Service
3251 Riverport Lane
Maryland Heights, MO 63043

*To ensure uninterrupted delivery of your subscription, please notify us at least 4 weeks in advance of move.

ELSEVIER

Printed and bound by CPI Group (UK) Ltd, Croydon, CR0 4YY

03/10/2024

01040357-0011